AN ILLUSTRATED COLOUR TEXT

PSYCHOLOGY AND SOCIOLOGY APPLIED TO MEDICINE

AN ILLUSTRATED COLOUR TEXT

PSYCHOLOGY AND SOCIOLOGY APPLIED TO MEDICINE

Edited by

MIKE PORTER BA MPhil
Senior Lecturer,
Department of General Practice,
University of Edinburgh, UK

BETH ALDER PhD C.Psychol
Senior Lecturer,
Department of Epidemiology and Public Health,
University of Dundee, UK

CHARLES ABRAHAM BA DPhil
Reader in Health and Social Psychology,
School of Social Sciences,
University of Sussex, UK

Foreword by KEITH MILLAR

Illustrated by ROBERT BRITTON

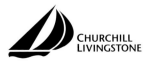
CHURCHILL
LIVINGSTONE

EDINBURGH LONDON NEW YORK OXFORD PHILADELPHIA ST LOUIS SYDNEY TORONTO 1999

CHURCHILL LIVINGSTONE
An imprint of Elsevier Science Limited

© Churchill Livingstone, a division of Harcourt Brace and Company
Limited 1999
© Harcourt Publishers Limited 2000
© Elsevier Science Limited 2002. All rights reserved.

First Edition 1999
   Reprinted 2000, 2001, 2002

ISBN 0 4430 4971 8

British Library Cataloguing in Publication Data
A catalogue record for this book is available from the British Library

Library of Congress Cataloging in Publication Data
A catalog record for this book is available from the Library of Congress

Note
Medical knowledge is constantly changing. As new information becomes
available, changes in treatment, procedures, equipment and the use of drugs
become necessary. The authors and publishers have, as far as it is possible,
taken care to ensure that the information given in this text is accurate and up to
date. However, readers are strongly advised to confirm that the information,
especially with regard to drug usage, complies with current legislation and
standards of practice.

 your source for books,
journals and multimedia
in the health sciences
www.elsevierhealth.com

For Churchill Livingstone

Publisher: Timothy Horne
Project manager: Ninette Premdas
Project editor: Jim Killgore
Design: Sarah Cape
Page make-up: Kate Walshaw
Project controller: Nancy Arnott

The
publisher's
policy is to use
paper manufactured
from sustainable forests

Printed in China by RDC Group Limited
C/04

CONTRIBUTORS

Charles Abraham BA DPhil
Reader in Health and Social Psychology, School of Social Sciences, University of Sussex, UK

Beth Alder PhD C.Psychol
Senior Lecturer, Department of Epidemiology and Public Health, University of Dundee, UK

Jacqueline M. Atkinson BA PhD C.Psychol Hon. MFPHM
Senior Lecturer, Departments of Public Health and Psychological Medicine, University of Glasgow, UK

Pamela J. Baldwin BA MPhil PhD C.Psychol
Clinical Psychologist, Working Minds Research, Blackford Pavilion, Astley Ainslie Hospital, Edinburgh, UK

Kenneth Boyd MA BD PhD FRCP(Edin)
Senior Lecturer in Medical Ethics, Department of Geriatric Medicine, University of Edinburgh, UK

Lloyd Carson MA PhD
Lecturer in Psychology, School of Psychology, University of St Andrews, UK

Sarah Cunningham-Burley BSocSc PhD
Senior Lecturer in Medical Sociology, Department of Public Health Sciences, University of Edinburgh, UK

George Deans BSc MSc PhD C.Psychol
Consultant Clinical Psychologist and Honorary Clinical Senior Lecturer, Department of General Practice and Primary Care, University of Aberdeen Medical School, UK

Morag L. Donaldson MA PhD
Senior Lecturer, Department of Psychology, University of Edinburgh, UK

Mary Gilhooly BS MEd MPhil PhD C.Psychol
Professor of Health Studies and Director of the Centre of Gerontology and Health Studies, University of Paisley, UK

Cynthia A. Graham BA MAppSc PhD
Assistant Professor of Clinical Psychology, Department of Psychiatry, Adjunct Assistant Professor of Psychology, Department of Psychology, Indiana University, USA

Richard Hammersley MA PhD
Director, Social Sciences Research Training Unit, Department of Sociological Studies, University of Sheffield, UK

Jane Hopton MA
Research Psychologist, Department of General Practice, University of Edinburgh, UK

Gail Johnston BSocSc PhD RGN Dipl. District Nursing
Research Fellow, Department of Epidemiology and Public Health, University of Dundee, UK

Marie Johnston BSc PhD C.Psychol FBPsS FRSE
Professor, School of Psychology, University of St Andrews, UK

Michael P. Kelly BA(Hons) MPhil PhD Hon.MFPHM
Head of School and Professor, School of Social Sciences, University of Greenwich, UK

Pauline Lightbody BA PhD C.Psychol
Research Fellow, Centre of Gerontology and Health Studies, University of Paisley, UK

Susan Llewelyn BA MSc PhD FBPsS
Course Director, Oxford Regional Training Course in Clinical Psychology, Warneford Hospital, Oxford, UK

Hannah M. McGee PhD Reg.Psychol FPsSI C.Psychol AFBPsS
Professor, Health Services Research Centre, Department of Psychology, Royal College of Surgeons in Ireland, Dublin

Pauline McGoldrick BSSc MSc D Clin Psychol
Clinical Lecturer in Health Psychology/Clinical Psychologist, Unit of Dental and Oral Health, Dundee Dental Hospital and School, University of Dundee, UK

Kenneth Mullen MA MLitt PhD
Lecturer, Division of Behavioural Science, Department of Psychological Medicine, University of Glasgow, UK

Sheina Orbell BSc PhD
Senior Lecturer, Department of Psychology, University of Sheffield, UK

Mike Porter BA MPhil
Senior Lecturer, Department of General Practice, University of Edinburgh, UK

Edwin R. van Teijlingen MA PhD
Lecturer in Public Health, Department of Public Health, University of Aberdeen, UK

Peter Wright MA DPhil
Senior Lecturer in Psychology, University of Edinburgh, UK

Sally Wyke BSc PhD
Senior Research Fellow, Department of General Practice, University of Edinburgh, UK

Editorial Panel
Mike Porter
Beth Alder
Charles Abraham
Richard Hammersley
Sarah Cunningham-Burley
Marie Johnston

FOREWORD

There was a time, not so long ago, when 'behavioural science' was seen by many in medical education as an irrelevant part of the curriculum that used up time that might otherwise be devoted to subjects that 'really mattered'. Even worse, it was taught by social scientists, those most troublesome of creatures who, if not outright seditious in questioning the conventional practice of medicine, were certainly taking a liberty in suggesting that doctors should know more about their patients' psychological processes and social circumstances if they were to make a decent job of serving their health needs.

But times change and a significant catalyst for change has been the UK General Medical Council. The GMC has always been a powerful advocate of the behavioural sciences in its various recommendations on the structure of the UK medical curriculum, but none more so than in its innovative document Tomorrow's Doctors. Gone is the requirement for students to spend a mind-numbing nine-to-five existence in lectures and laboratories as the passive, force-fed recipients of information that few would ever need even in a lifetime spent in medical practice. Now the focus is upon 'student-centred learning'— an active process of seeking out information, evaluating it and making decisions about what to do with it. And a significant part of that focus is upon understanding patients as individuals who live in society and whose character, experiences and circumstances will affect their interaction both with medical practitioners and the whole bureaucracy of the health-care system.

This book embodies absolutely the ethos of the GMC's 'new look' for medical education with a style that encourages enquiry and evaluation. The 'spreads' on each topic provide synopses of key issues and questions, and it is then up to the student to pursue further detail through the references provided or by a literature search. An active learning process is encouraged which is both effective and interesting for the reader. The use of illustrative 'case studies' helps bring home to the student the real-life relevance of psychological and social issues across a range of medical conditions and health care in general.

The editors have drawn together a team of writers whose experience in teaching and research in behavioural science gives excellent coverage and authority to the topics addressed. The result is that the book provides the foundation to serve the GMC's recommendation that behavioural science be integrated with teaching in other disciplines throughout the five years of the new medical curriculum. Hitherto, many textbooks in behavioural science have been aimed at the medical student in the old 'pre-clinical curriculum' where, in the first two years of the course, learning of 'basic science' was the order of the day, and teaching in behavioural science often followed suit by covering rather basic processes or concepts in psychology and sociology. The broad coverage of the present book provides the potential to serve students throughout their medical training, even in the later years of the curriculum where the focus inevitably is upon advanced clinical issues. As an aside, the fact that the book demonstrates that behavioural science can be integrated with other disciplines throughout the curriculum is confirmation of the extent to which research in health psychology and medical sociology now informs and contributes to understanding in clinical medicine (the past decade's profusion of new journals of health psychology is testament in itself).

The final section of the book asks the reader to consider 'How do you fit in to all of this?' and presents some of the realities of working in medicine. Most students realise quite early in their course that a career in medicine will not have the glamour and excitement portrayed in television's medical 'soap' dramas. Those who are approaching the end of their undergraduate training will find useful advice to cope with what lies ahead, and perhaps explicit articulation of their anxieties and concerns about how they will meet the demands of their career. Society's attitude to medicine has changed radically over the past quarter century and we, as patients, have become 'consumers' who expect more and, indeed, may demand more of health services. We are more likely to expect to be equal partners in decisions made about our health and to have little hesitation about complaining when we are dissatisfied or when things go wrong. These realities are addressed in this book and it can only be of benefit to student readers. Those who read and internalise this book's behavioural and social perspective of medical practice can look forward to a clearer understanding of patients' needs and to justifying patients' confidence in them.

1998

Keith Millar
PhD C.Psychol FBPsS
Professor of Behavioural Science
Department of Psychological Medicine
University of Glasgow

PREFACE

This textbook aims to provide medical students with a broad and stimulating introduction to psychological and sociological concepts, theories and research as they apply to medicine. If medicine is to be effective in maintaining people's health and well-being, it must be sensitive to the ways in which health and illness make sense within people's lives and how people understand their relationships with doctors and other health care professionals. These, and other issues, are addressed by researchers working in health psychology and medical sociology. For these reasons both psychology and sociology are seen as essential to the medical curriculum (General Medical Council, 1994).

The book has been designed and written primarily to take account of the needs of students who are embarking on the new integrated, systems-based and problem-based, medical courses which have been introduced in the UK and elsewhere.

The material is presented in accessible, two-page 'spreads'. Each spread addresses a discrete topic with its own case study, questions for further thought and key points. However, the spreads are cross-referenced so that the book also forms an integrated whole.

Of course, none of these topics can be adequately covered in two pages. Yet all can be introduced in this way. Each spread includes key references which may be followed up by the student, but individual course organisers and tutors will undoubtedly want to recommend further reading which links the material to their particular courses or modules.

The teaching and learning of psychology and sociology in relation to health, illness and medicine is often hampered by two important factors. First, psychology and sociology (unlike biomedical sciences) deal with aspects of our everyday experience. It is all too easy to believe that we already know what there is to be known about such familiar things, as for example 'Why people don't take their doctor's advice'. One of the key tasks of psychologists and sociologists is, as Fritz Heider put it, to cut through this 'veil of obviousness'. Secondly, the very fact that people do attempt to understand and make sense of their personal and social worlds makes it difficult to conduct behavioural and social research without, in some way, influencing what they tell us and their behaviour.

Thus, for example, asking patients whether they took their medication or not may, if not carefully asked, elicit responses which patients think researchers want to hear rather than their real reasons. Asking doctors why patients don't take their medicines may start the doctor thinking about their own part in the process and change their behaviour. Such opportunities for bias and influence make it particularly important for students to think critically and to check the assumptions, methods and findings of different research studies.

The references have, therefore, been included not just to encourage students to read more deeply into a topic, but also to think critically about the reasoning and the evidence presented. Both psychology and sociology are enlivened by debate and discussion. Details of research studies are often given in boxes and students are encouraged to be critical. Evidence-based medicine is a concept that is as applicable to behavioural science as it is to clinical practice.

The book is divided into nine sections beginning with a description of normal human development and common health problems associated with the life span. The second section seeks to address the question 'How does the person develop?' and focuses on the development of some key psychological processes, for example the development of language, personality and sexuality. The third section seeks to address the question 'In what ways are our behaviour and health constrained by the social contexts within which we live?' and also includes spreads on the concepts and measurement of health, illness and disease. Section 4 presents a more specific discussion of how social and personal factors interact to influence our risk of ill health. The topic of risk-taking behaviour is developed further in Section 5 where issues of illness prevention and health promotion are discussed in terms of both the behaviour of individuals and the behaviour of governments and large organisations.

Sections 6 and 7 shift the perspective from health promotion to illness behaviour. Section 6 focuses on what people do when they feel ill or anxious about their health and on their experience of consultations and of hospitals. Doctors' communication skills are also reviewed. Section 7 selects a number of specific disorders and examines how people experience and respond to them. A range of ways of helping people to cope with illness and disability are also described.

Section 8 examines some of the problems and issues associated with different ways of organising health services, and Section 9 reviews the experience of being a medical student and a junior doctor, concluding with a discussion of basic professional and ethical issues.

It is doubtful if any introductory textbook could be comprehensive and we are aware of some important topics which have not been covered, and others which have received more of a psychological than a sociological approach, and vice-versa. We hope, however, that the breadth of coverage and the style of presentation will be attractive to students, stimulate their interest in the psychosocial aspects of health, illness and medical practice, and encourage them to pursue their interests in greater depth.

Some editorial control has been exercised by both the editorial panel and the principal editors, but final responsibility for each spread has been left to individual authors. Our thanks to the editorial panel and to our authors for responding so willingly to our comments and suggestions, and for writing to such a tight word limit.

M.P.
B.A.
C.A.

CONTENTS

HOW DO HEALTH SERVICES WORK? 140

HOW DO YOU FIT INTO ALL OF THIS? 148

PREGNANCY AND CHILDBIRTH

This textbook appropriately starts at the beginning of life, at birth. It is also appropriate to use one of the most 'natural' life events as an introduction to the behavioural sciences. The birth of humans differs from births in other mammals in our social construction of the event. Our social behaviour is guided by institutions and customs, not merely by instinctual needs; and perhaps nothing illustrates this basic sociological principle better than the sheer diversity of human practices at the time of childbirth, and their responsiveness to historically changing influences. In other words, where and how and in whose presence a woman gives birth differs from one social setting to another. Human societies everywhere prescribe certain rituals and restrictions to pregnant and labouring women. For example, the place of delivery is often prescribed, be it a special village hut or a special obstetric hospital.

Pregnancy and childbirth are important life events which are often influenced by doctors. Obstetrics is an important part of medical training. Every medical student is required to attend a certain number of deliveries. Doctors may be directly involved, in providing ante-natal or post-natal care or attending the birth, or more indirectly through the provision of infertility treatment, through the provision of birth control methods, or as back-up for midwives in case something unexpected happens during a normal delivery.

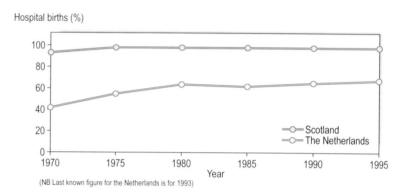

Hospital births (%)

Fig. 1 **Percentage of births in hospital in Scotland and the Netherlands.** Sources: Common Services Agency (Scotland); Central Bureau voor de Statistiek (The Netherlands).

THE NATURE OF PREGNANCY AND CHILDBIRTH

There are two major contrasting views on the nature of pregnancy and childbirth (see Table 1). One argues that pregnancy and childbirth are normal events in most women's life cycle. This is often referred to as the psychosocial model. It is estimated that some 85% of all babies will be born without any problems and without the presence of a special birth attendant. Many of the risks in childbirth can be predicted, and consequently pregnant women most at risk can be selected for a hospital delivery in a specialist obstetric hospital. The remainder of pregnant women can opt for a less specialist setting such as a delivery in a community hospital or a home delivery. A proponent of this view is Tew (1990), who discovered to her own surprise whilst preparing epidemiological exercises for medical students in Nottingham that routine statistics did not support the widely-accepted view that increased hospitalisation of birth had caused the decline in mortality of mothers and their new-born babies.

Secondly, the view most commonly held in nearly all Western societies is that pregnancy and particularly labour are risky events, where many things could go wrong. This is referred to as the biomedical model. Childbirth is, therefore, potentially pathological. Since we do not know what will happen to an individual pregnant woman, each woman is best advised to deliver her baby in the safest possible environment. The specialist obstetric hospital with its high-technology screening equipment supervised by obstetricians is regarded as the safest place to give birth. In short, this view states that pregnancy and childbirth are only safe in retrospect.

Consequently, the majority of deliveries occur in hospital. Figure 1 contrasts the percentage of hospital births in the Netherlands with Scotland, where Scotland is representative of the trend in most industrialised countries.

 STOP THINK　Pregnancy can be regarded as a 'normal state of health' in that it occurs without serious problems to most women in their lifetime. Pregnancy can also be seen as an 'illness' in that many women, for example, have morning sickness, experience a slowing down in physical functioning, seek medical care and/or deliver in hospital. How do you regard pregnancy and childbirth, and why?

CHANGING MATERNITY CARE

The place of delivery

Maternity services in the 1990s in Britain are moving through a period of significant change in which the need of the woman to be centrally involved in her care is given greater emphasis. This represents a change from the previous 50–60 years when the trend was towards more hospital deliveries. For example, in Britain, an official report published in 1959 recommended that 70% of all births should take place in hospital, while a similar report in 1970 recommended 100% hospital deliveries on the grounds of safety. Political opinion changed in the late 1980s towards more choice for women, and consequently more

Table 1 **Models of childbirth**

Model	Psychosocial 'Childbirth normal/ natural until pathology occurs'	Biomedical 'Childbirth only normal in retrospect'
Emphasis	Normality Social support Woman = active Health Individual	Risk Risk reduction Woman = passive Illness Statistical

deliveries outside obstetric units. The Winterton Report (1992) proposed a move away from total hospitalisation: 'The policy of encouraging all women to give birth in hospital cannot be justified on grounds of safety.'

The birth attendant

The two views of childbirth also differ regarding who is the desired attendant at birth. If one holds the view that pregnancy and childbirth are only safe in retrospect then the only acceptable birth attendant is a consultant obstetrician, a specialist present just in case something goes wrong. If one holds the view that childbirth is a normal part in the life cycle of most women then the most desirable birth attendant is the expert in normal deliveries, the midwife or the GP. Throughout history, midwives have been and continue to be the major health care attendants at the birthing process. Over the past three centuries in most industrialised countries female midwives have slowly lost control over childbirth to male doctors.

What does 'pregnancy' mean for:

- a midwife?
- an obstetrician?
- a pregnant woman?

Case study
The Dutch example

The Netherlands is the only industrialised country where the proportion of all deliveries taking place outwith specialist hospitals is substantial. Every year approximately one third of all deliveries take place in Dutch homes. Britain and the Netherlands are neighbouring countries with fairly similar levels of health care provision and a similar quality of specialist obstetric care; perinatal mortality rates do not differ substantially between the two countries. (Perinatal mortality rate refers to the number of stillbirths (after 28 weeks' gestation) plus the number of deaths occurring in the first 7 days after the delivery, divided by all live births and stillbirths.) Other outcome indicators suggest that the Dutch programme is superior.

A number of factors have been suggested for this difference in the organisation of maternity care:

- Pregnant women in the Netherlands are not regarded as patients, unless something goes wrong or the delivery is expected to be difficult for previously assessed reasons.
- Practical help is provided in the form of maternity home-care assistants, who look after the mother and new-born baby at home for up to 8 days following the birth. They wash the baby, give advice on breast or bottle feeding, look after other children in the household, walk the dog, etc.
- In case of low-risk pregnancies, the fee for a GP will be reimbursed only if there is no practising midwife in the area, and only in instances of high-risk pregnancies will the fee of an obstetrician be reimbursed.
- Midwives are trained to be independent and autonomous practitioners. They are not trained as nurses first, but attend a separate three-year midwifery course. The importance of independent training is first that nurses are trained to deal with illness and disease, whilst midwives are trained to deal with normal childbirth; and secondly that the hierarchical relationship between nurses and doctors tends to play a part in the medical decision-making process.
- Most midwives are practising as independent practitioners in the community, similar to most dentists in Britain. As private entrepreneurs they have to be more consumer-friendly to attract customers.
- All major political parties agree that the midwife is the obvious person to provide maternity care and that deliveries should preferably take place at home.

One could, of course, argue that Britain and the Netherlands are different countries and therefore not comparable. However, the populations in these two neighbouring countries are not too different in terms of national income, the physiology of the average woman, life expectancy and many other socio-economic indicators. Although the funding of health care is different, the organisation of service provision and the quality of medical care is fairly similar. For example, the majority of all deliveries in Britain and the Netherlands are attended by midwives. In fact one can turn the question of comparability round and ask, for example: Why is the proportion of home births equally low in Britain, Germany and the USA, while their organisation of health care in general, and of maternity care in particular, is so different?

Pregnancy is often a time of great expectations and excitement relating to the birth and parenthood. Women in modern Western society have, on average, only two babies in their lifetime. At the same time, as obstetricians and/or midwives might attend deliveries many times a week or even a day, their expectations are considerably different from those of the expecting mother, and not only because the baby is not their own. Their priorities can be guided by medical requirements, hospital policies, or availability of resources. Such differences can easily lead to misunderstanding and dissatisfaction by the new parents (especially if the parties have not been able to get to know each other). Considering the role and status of health professionals (see pp. 152–153) it is more likely that the mother is disappointed than the birth attendant.

Pregnancy
and childbirth

- Biological events are never purely biological but always partly socially constructed.
- Where, how and in whose presence a woman gives birth differs from one culture to another.
- There are two different ways of looking at pregnancy and childbirth: (a) pregnancy is a normal event in most women's lives and (b) childbirth is a risky event and only normal in retrospect.
- Pregnant women and health professionals are likely to see the birth differently.
- Different ways of organising health care can have profound effects on professionals and health service users.

REPRODUCTIVE ISSUES

The practice of medicine is closely involved with reproductive issues, and pregnancy and childbirth may be the most important point of contact with the medical profession. Reproductive issues are relevant to all of us throughout our lives and for many reasons, but they have particular relevance to health. Both psychological and physical health are influenced by sexuality and fertility. A disease syndrome or health problem which is apparently unrelated to reproduction may have been affected by a previous pregnancy, infertility problem or miscarriage. The stage of the reproductive career will affect decisions about managing a problem. Reproductive changes over the life span particularly affect women, and from puberty onwards biological changes, social changes, and psychological changes have powerful effects.

THE MENSTRUAL CYCLE

The biological basis of the menstrual cycle is the changing hormone production related to the ovary. It is important to be aware of the underlying biological changes even when considering people's social behaviour. Follicular stimulating hormone (FSH) and luteinising hormone (LH) are released from the pituitary, and stimulate the growth of ovarian follicles (the follicular phase). These secrete oestradiol and as the level rises the FSH levels fall because of negative feedback. An LH surge is triggered and this provokes ovulation from the now mature ovarian follicle. The remaining follicle becomes the corpus luteum and secretes progesterone as well as oestradiol. These changes are shown in Figure 1. After ovulation, oestradiol and progesterone levels fall (the luteal phase) and the endometrial lining is shed during menstruation.

Menstrual pain is experienced by many women and may be helped by relaxation techniques as well as drugs. Menstruation may be perceived negatively, and there are religious and social taboos surrounding behaviour during menstruation. Sexual intercourse may be avoided and myths such as not washing hair during menstruation may be pervasive. 'Feminine hygiene' (sanitary towels and tampons) has only recently been advertised on television in the UK, and even so, fluid being absorbed had to be blue rather than red. Many women notice changes during different phases of the menstrual cycle. In Premenstrual Syndrome (PMS) symptoms such as breast tenderness, irritability or depression increase in the pre-menstrual week and improve in the post-menstrual week. The association of phases of the menstrual cycle and psychological changes is weak (Slade 1984), although the media, many women and their partners may believe that mood is related to the phase of the menstrual cycle. This may be because of:

- negative connotations of menstruation in society
- attribution of negative moods to a salient event such as menstruation
- selective recall or attention
- external attribution of negative events as being outside control.

PREGNANCY

During pregnancy and childbirth:

- Women and their partners come into contact with the medical profession and health professionals, perhaps for the first time as adults.
- Admission to maternity hospital may be the first admission to hospital.
- They are experiencing a role transition.

A woman who is pregnant experiences both physical and psychological changes. These begin in pregnancy when there are physical changes in muscle tone, size and shape of the body, stress incontinence and frequency, and fatigue. She may give up work, change her role in her family, and feel that her body image has changed. There may be changes in her self concept and feelings of self-efficacy. She may worry about being a good parent.

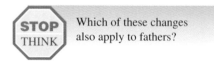

Which of these changes also apply to fathers?

CHILDBIRTH

The context of childbirth is changing (see pp. 2–3) but wherever it takes place it is likely to involve the experience and management of pain (see pp. 132–133). Pain control may be managed differently in hospital and relaxation may be learned in ante-natal classes but most women request some kind of pain relief. Parous women report higher pain thresholds than non-parous women of the same age.

Many women attend ante-natal classes to prepare for the birth and it is now accepted that fathers may be present at the birth. The delivery of a baby is a moving and emotional event and is rated as one of the most significant events in people's lives.

Changes in mood

The transition to parenthood can be seen as a developmental crisis and there are emotional and social changes during pregnancy and in the first post-natal year.

In the first post-natal year the mother:

- adjusts to the demands of a young baby
- may give up work and change her perceived status
- may have a different relationship with her partner
- may have a different relationship with her mother.

She may also miss her former social contacts, the structure and routine of

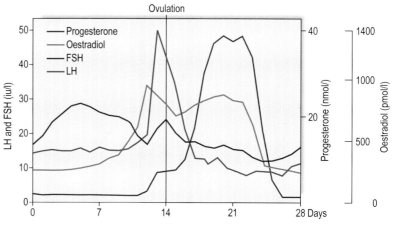

Fig. 1 **Plasma hormone concentrations during the menstrual cycle.**

work, and may feel isolated from former colleagues. About 10% of women experience post-natal depression, and a further 10–15% experience emotional distress in the first post-natal year (Cox 1986) (Fig. 2).

Of course there are positive aspects too:

- Both partners may feel reassured about their gender role; they may feel more 'feminine' or more 'masculine'.
- There is a high status attached to becoming a parent and they may feel more mature and confident.
- Parenting is rated as a very positive experience by most parents.

Not all pregnancies end in the birth of a healthy baby. About 20% end in miscarriage before 20 weeks. If the couple has not told their family and friends that they are expecting a baby, the loss from early miscarriage may not be recognised. About half of mothers experiencing miscarriage suffer from clinical depression. Their grief remains hidden and unspoken and it may be similar to that experienced by a woman who has been diagnosed as infertile. She may feel a loss of the image of herself as a pregnant woman and as a parent. She may believe that she may never be able to bear children, and feel guilt and anger (Hunter 1993).

THE MENOPAUSE

The menopause means literally the last period, but the term climacteric or perimenopause is used to describe the years either side of the menopause. Many women have several years of irregular periods and the climacteric can take place at any time between 40 and 60.

Loss of production of oestrogen, as ovulation declines, results in recognised physical changes such as vasomotor symptoms of hot flushes, night sweats and vaginal dryness; psychological symptoms such as increased depression, irritability, or low libido are often reported.

There is little association between menopausal status and psychological symptoms and probably only vasomotor symptoms are associated with the time of the menopause.

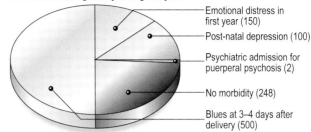

Fig. 2 **Incidence of post-natal morbidity for every 1000 women having a baby during one year.**

Women may encounter more stressful events during the climacteric, and family and sociocultural factors may be more important than changes in hormones. Physical changes may cause depression in post-menopausal women, and certain health problems may begin in middle age such as diabetes mellitus, weight gain and urinary incontinence.

Different perspectives have been presented in order to account for changes during the menopause.

Biomedical model
The menopause is seen as a hormone deficiency disease. Vasomotor symptoms occur because of a decline in the levels of oestrogen produced by the ovary. These symptoms respond well to oestrogen therapy and a number of well-controlled studies have shown the benefits of this therapy. However, although all women suffer declining levels of oestrogen, not all report either vasomotor symptoms or psychological changes.

Cultural model
Society may take a negative view of the menopause. In some societies in which ageing is associated with increased status and wisdom the menopause is seen positively. Mayan Indians in rural Mexico experience loss of oestrogen production in the same way as Western women, although it occurs at a relatively early age

(usually between 41 and 54). In a study of 54 women it was found that they did not report hot flushes or night sweats, nor did they suffer from osteoporosis (Martin et al 1993). The interviewer was a Mayan nurse's aide and fluent in Spanish and Mayan. From their hormone levels about 80% would be expected to have hot flushes but not one of the 54 women reported them. This suggests a strong cultural component. Women may see the menopause negatively, as a loss of femininity, or positively as an end to the demands of childbearing. Health professionals may be able to promote a more positive view.

Psycho-social model
Symptoms may be associated with stressful life events. If menopausal symptoms are assessed using standardised scales it is found that life stress contributes far more than menopausal status to menopausal symptoms, and worries about work and adolescent children are major factors influencing depression. Children leaving home may be a cause of grief, but there may be just as many problems if they do not leave home and remain dependent.

Case study
Mrs Jones is 52, widowed and works part time as an office assistant, She lives with her two daughters. Anne is 25 and has a steady relationship with her boyfriend. She has a 4-week-old baby. Jane is 17 and is still at school, but has little chance of leaving with any paper qualifications. Mrs Jones is often irritable and has dropped out of her usual social activities. Anne has bouts of weepiness and lacks confidence in her abilities as a mother. Jane is disillusioned with study and stays out late in pubs. She has episodes of erratic behaviour.

How would you explain the behaviour in Mrs Jones and her two daughters, assuming either a biological model or a socio-cultural explanation?

Reproductive issues
- Biological, psychological and social changes related to reproduction have powerful effects on women's lives.
- There are physical changes during the menstrual cycle and they may be related to negative psychological changes.
- Pregnancy and childbirth affect mood and relationships in both men and women.
- The menopause is an endocrinological event but it is associated with negative changes which may have psychosocial origins.

DEVELOPMENT IN EARLY INFANCY

The twentieth century has seen dramatic shifts in how we view infancy. The importance of both good medical care and the right psychological environment are now widely accepted. Psychologists have demonstrated that even new-born infants have impressive cognitive and perceptual abilities and learning capacity. A mother goes through an intensive period of getting to know and understand her infant in the first weeks after birth, and she gains a unique insight into interpreting the baby's needs. This makes her observations of great importance should medical complications arise. It is important that doctors treating babies understand more about the baby's competence and listen to what the mother has to say. This spread will discuss changing ideas on what is meant by 'bonding', give examples of the communicative abilities of infants, and show how recognising differences in behaviour of infants may contribute towards improving breast-feeding success.

ASSESSMENT SHORTLY AFTER BIRTH

Infants who fuss and cry a great deal, or who are apathetic and unresponsive to social stimuli, can be at risk of neglect by their mothers. Tests designed to evaluate the neonate's neurological well-being can also be used to encourage mothers to become more sensitive and responsive care-givers. The Brazleton Neonatal Assessment Scale (NBAS) evaluates the neonate's neurological status and respon-siveness to environmental stimuli. It is designed to be administered within a few days of birth and assesses not only the quality of some 20 inborn reflexes, but also the infant's state and reactions to stimuli such as ringing a bell or watching a moving light. If the baby is extremely unresponsive, the low NBAS score would suggest possible neurological dysfunction. If the baby is simply slow, especially when responding to social stimulation, this may be a warning sign for later emo-tional problems.

Because the NBAS is designed to elicit the baby's more engaging characteristics such as cooing, gazing and smiling, it has potential as a teaching aid. Myers (1982) taught parents of healthy, full-term babies how to conduct the NBAS with their own infants and found that after 4 weeks, by comparison with an untrained control group, such parents were both more con-fident in their role and more satisfied

with their babies. Mothers of premature and other high-risk infants similarly become more responsive in interacting with their babies. If you are sceptical about the expressive abilities of neonates see Figure 1.

BONDING AND ATTACHMENT

In the early 1970s a very influential view developed from the work of two paediatricians, Klaus and Kennell. They suggested that for new mothers to fall in love with their babies, referred to as maternal bonding, it was essential that only minimal separation of the infant from its mother should occur after birth. Technically maternal bonding has come to mean a rapid and irreversible change said to take place in the mother within a period immediately following birth and which lasts no more than a few hours or days at the most and during which prolonged contact between mother and baby must occur if maternal feelings are to be properly mobilised. This 'super-glue' theory of maternal love proved very influential, and failure to bond properly was frequently cited as the reason for all kinds of problems ranging from failure to thrive in infancy to cases of child abuse and adolescent delinquency. In one New York hospital this belief reached such heights of absurdity that mothers who had not held their babies after birth were given polaroid photographs to look at so they could bond adequately!

The origins of bonding theory lay in work with animals where there is good evidence for such a critical period in the formation of maternal attachment to

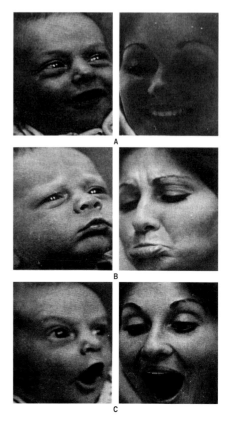

Fig. 1 **A model's happy, sad and surprised expressions, and an infant's corresponding expressions.** (Reprinted with permission from Field T M, Wodson, Greenberg R, Cohen D 1982 Discrimination and imitation of facial expression in neonates. Science 218: 179–181 Copyright 1982 American Association for the Advancement of Science)

the new-born, but many careful studies in the past two decades have shown that there is no evidence of any long-term effects of enforced separation in the period

---

Case study

Mothers often remark that their baby looks happy, sad, or is smiling and this may be put down to harmless self-deception, but experiments (see Field et al 1982) with babies as young as 36 hours show that they are indeed able to imitate facial expressions (Fig. 1). A series of three expressions (happy, sad, surprised) were posed by an adult and observed by 74 neonates, and both baby's and model's faces were videotaped simultaneously using a split-screen technique. Observers subsequently coded the facial expressions of the infants and looked for matches to the model. The chance probability of guessing the facial expression correctly would be 33%, but surprised was correctly guessed on 76% of trials, happy on 58%, and sad on 59%. Videotapes of the model's faces eliminated shaping or reinforcing the neonate's responses as a possible explanation for the result. The authors con-cluded that there is an innate ability to compare the sensory information from facial expressions with the proprioceptive feedback of the movements involved in matching that expression.

immediately after birth. Hence a generation of doctors and nurses can be relieved of guilty feelings with the necessary forced separation following caesarean section or illness at birth. It is interesting that these ideas, although without scientific foundation, revolutionised practice in post-natal wards, allowing babies to sleep in cots at the side of their mothers. (For a good account of this controversy, see Schaffer 1990.)

PROMOTION OF BREASTFEEDING

It is widely accepted that breastfeeding conveys a number of health advantages to the baby, such as providing increased protection against gastrointestinal upset through the presence of antibodies, and longer term influences in the form of decreased susceptibility to eczema. In a developing world context, breastfeeding is an important contraceptive agent because the increased levels of prolactin in the mother delay the return of ovulation and therefore increase birth spacing. It is possible that other advantages of breastfeeding stem more from the act itself rather than any biochemical differences between breast milk and formula. Milk feeds are not a continuous sequence of sucking but are interrupted by removal of the bottle or breast for a variety of reasons such as choking, winding, posseting of milk, changing to another breast, etc. When filmed, feeds are analysed to see if it is the baby or the mother who initiates the break in feeding. For bottle-fed babies the interruptions are found to be almost entirely under the control of the mother, but for breastfed infants there is a predominantly baby-determined pattern. Observations such as this, and other instances of what is known as 'turn-taking' suggest that reciprocity in the context of feeding is more evident in breastfeeding. Many psychologists have become interested in feeding because they see this kind of interaction as the source of subsequent social communication.

Despite all the obvious health advantages to the baby, regular surveys of infant feeding practice mounted by the Office of Population Censuses and Surveys indicate that there are persisting regional and social class variations in the extent of breastfeeding (Fig. 2). Whereas 75% of mothers in the South of England will attempt to breastfeed at birth, in Scotland only 50% will try. By six weeks of age, one third of these mothers will have given up. Even greater discrepancies are evident from breakdown by social class with almost 90% of social classes I and II attempting breastfeeding compared with 60% for social classes IV and V. There are also important differences in the behaviour of the babies, and how mothers interpret these seems to depend on the method of feeding. For example, bottle-fed infants begin to sleep through the night at a significantly earlier age than do breastfed babies; they are also offered solid foods at an earlier age. Breastfeeding mothers regard changes in the frequency of feeding as the most important sign of hunger in their babies, whereas bottle-feeding mothers mention changes in the avidity with which the infants suck from the bottle as most important.

Providing premature babies with human breast milk delivered through a nasogastric tube improves their cognitive development as measured by increases in IQ at a later age. This suggests that some component of breast milk, perhaps long-chain fatty acids, is particularly important for the optimal development of the immature brain. When intelligence (pp. 30–31) was measured at school age, in children delivered at full-term, breast-fed infants were at an advantage and remained so even when the associated educational and socio-economic differences were discounted. These long-term influences on development are especially interesting examples of how early experience can exert an enduring influence in unexpected ways.

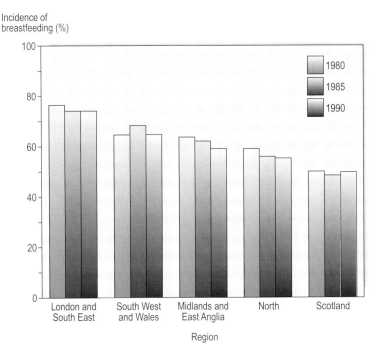

Incidence of breastfeeding (%)

Fig. 2 **Incidence of breastfeeding by region** (1980, 1985 and 1990, Great Britain). (Source: White A, Freeth S, O'Brien M 1992 Infant Feeding 1990. OPCS, Social Survey Division. HMSO, London)

STOP THINK
- How often have you seen a mother breastfeeding her baby ? What are the barriers which make women disinclined to breastfeed publicly?
- Find a mother with a baby under the age of one year and watch her 'talking' to the baby. Do you see any evidence of turn-taking?
- What makes a baby smile? Draw two large dots on a piece of paper and hold this about twelve inches in front of the baby. Add more dots where the nose and mouth should be. Compare the response of babies at about three months and eight months.

Development in early infancy
- Babies in the first week of life can distinguish facial expressions.
- Prolonged contact between mother and infant in the first week of life is not essential for successful mothering to occur.
- Breastfeeding has both immediate and long-term health benefits for the baby.

CHILDHOOD AND CHILD HEALTH

Childhood is a process of transition from high dependency towards autonomy. The risk of serious ill-health interfering in this process has been significantly reduced in most industrialised countries, but there is still a disproportionate excess of deaths and of morbidity amongst children of poorer families. This spread will show that the experience of childhood health and illness is strongly socially-patterned, and that such experience is likely to have long-term consequences.

CHILDREN'S HEALTH

Minor ill-health is relatively common in children, and can, therefore, be seen as relatively 'normal'. Serious disorders of growth and development are relatively rare and will not be discussed here (see pp. 118–119). It should be noted, however, that the decline in serious infectious diseases in children in industrialised countries has meant that congenital disorders have become relatively more predominant.

Very few children in industrialised countries die between the ages of 1 and 14 (Fig. 1). The improvements in children's mortality have occurred steadily over the last 150 years (Fig. 2), largely as a result of improvements in living conditions, sanitation and nutrition which have resulted in a decline in mortality from infectious disease. Alongside these trends, fertility control, advances in immunisation and medical treatment, and greater access to health services have contributed to improvements in children's health. However, deaths from accidents remain a major cause for concern.

By contrast, there appears to have been an increase in self-reported chronic illness among children since this data has been collected in Britain from the early 1970's (Fig. 3), with respiratory illness being the main concern.

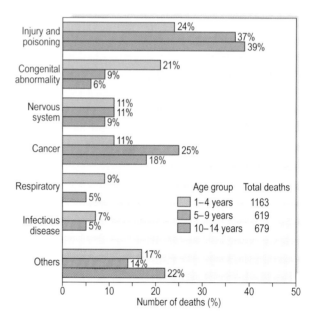

Fig. 1 **Causes of death in childhood (UK, 1990).** (After Woodroffe et al 1993)

PSYCHOLOGICAL HEALTH AND WELL-BEING

There is evidence that adverse family factors, such as a marriage with low mutual support or maternal depression, are related to behaviour problems in children aged 3, and to the onset of behaviour problems when older. However, the patterns of problem behaviour, such as sleep disturbance, challenging behaviour and temper tantrums, do not always disappear if the adverse stress factors are reduced. Counselling and psychotherapy approaches to behaviour problems would suggest that learned patterns of behaviour are often deeply internalised in the subconscious and may be difficult to change (see pp. 126–127).

Research into depression amongst working-class mothers suggests that childhood experience of loss of mother before the age of 11, neglect, and physical and sexual abuse before age 17 are strongly associated with depression (see pp. 114–115). Depression in young men is similarly associated with neglect and abuse as children.

ACCIDENTS

Although the childhood death rate from accidents in the UK has been falling, accidents are the major cause of death in children

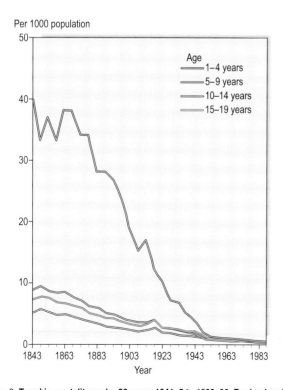

Fig. 2 **Trend in mortality under 20 years 1841–5 to 1986–90, England and Wales.** (From Woodroffe et al 1993)

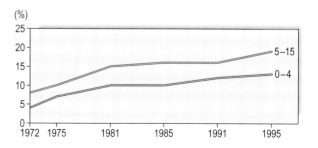

Fig. 3 **The percentage of children age 0–4 and 5–15 reporting longstanding illness, disability or infirmity.** (From: Living in Britain 1995 Office of National Statistics, Crown copyright 1997)

and, like most other causes of death in children, are strongly associated with social class.

Most childhood accidental deaths occur on the roads, though the number of road traffic accidents has fallen slightly despite an increase in the volume of traffic. Even so, children from social class V are more than four times likely to die as pedestrians than children in social class I. Although mortality from injury and poisoning has also declined in all social classes, the differential in mortality for children aged 0–15 in social classes IV and V has increased compared with children in classes I and II.

Studies of children's ability to comprehend danger suggest that children younger than age 7 can be taught that something specific is dangerous but that they are unable to generalise from it. For example, being told not to touch a specific fire will not be related to other fires. Furthermore, younger children do not have the ability to interpret traffic speed.

Although accidents are the major cause of childhood death, they are fortunately relatively rare. However, accidents which result in injury are relatively common and also class related. Injuries to children in social class IV and V are also likely to be more severe. Factors which help to explain this association are: overcrowding leading to higher risk of falls or burns/scalds; relative deprivation leading to older and less safe cooking equipment, fires, wiring, furniture and safety equipment; unprotected roads, particularly fast arterial roads; inadequate play facilities and difficulty supervising children in high-rise blocks.

Risk of specific cause of accidental death and injury varies by sex and changes considerably as children get older. At all ages, boys are more likely than girls to die from an accident or to have an accidental injury, with road-traffic accidents accounting for an increasing proportion of accidents involving boys as they get older. Three types of explanation have been made:

- boys are subjected to more 'rough and tumble' play and to risk-taking than girls
- parents are more likely to supervise girls than boys
- boys are more 'accident prone' because they are encouraged to be more active.

STOP THINK It has been suggested that attempts to educate parents about the risks of accidents and to encourage them to take more responsibility for supervision leads to victim blaming, and to feelings of guilt and defensive anger. What do you think about this and can you think of a more appropriate childhood accident prevention policy?

Accidents to children occur more frequently in households where the mother is depressed. Brown and Davison (1978) suggest that the explanation lies in the following process. As the mother becomes depressed she provides less attention and takes less interest in her children. In order to attract her attention, the children behave more aggressively or problematically, but she withdraws further, which elicits even more extreme behaviour, leading to the increased risk of an accident arising from their behaviour and her lack of supervision.

RESPIRATORY ILLNESS

On average, a child (aged < 5) will have 6–8 respiratory illnesses per year. These illnesses account for about 80% of consultations by this age group with general practitioners,

Case study

In a study of a Glasgow housing estate, Helen Roberts et al (1993) found that mothers saw accidents as just one element of their generally risky insecure lives. They pointed to defects in the design and upkeep of their environment which contributed to the high accident rate: balconies with gaps that small children could fall through, poor kitchen design, inappropriate electrical wiring and switching, inadequate thermostatic control of immersion heaters, dangerous window design and inadequate locks, inadequate play facilities, inadequately protected roads and repair work, broken glass left by glaziers, inadequate rubbish stores and refuse collection.

They considered that only a tiny minority of parents were irresponsible and that professionals and contractors were often responsible for not admitting the design faults and putting them right.

Now repeat the Stop and Think exercise.

which is about five times the frequency of consultation for other common conditions. About 30% of all consultations for children aged < 11 years are for respiratory disease.

As with accidents, there is a strong relationship between social class and respiratory illness. Dampness in the house appears to be a significant factor in increasing the incidence and severity of respiratory illness in children, even when allowing for cigarette smoking in the household (see pp. 56–57). In contrast, whilst the incidence and prevalence of asthma has been increasing in the UK in recent years making it the most common chronic disease in children, there is no clear relationship with social class.

POVERTY, ILLNESS AND CHILD DEVELOPMENT

Children in households with low incomes are more likely to experience ill-health, and are more likely to spend more time absent from school. This in turn can affect their chances of performing well at school and consequently lead to reduced employment opportunities when they leave school. The combined effect of the threefold increase in the numbers of children living in poverty in the UK since 1979 (Dennehy et al 1997), and the ill-health effects of poor working conditions and unemployment (see pp. 58–61) are strong predictors of poorer health in later life for many of these youngsters.

Childhood and child health
- The health of children in industrialised countries has improved considerably over the last 100 years.
- These improvements have largely arisen from improvements in sanitation and standards of living.
- Accidents, and particularly pedestrian accidents, are the major cause of death in children.
- Respiratory illness is the major cause of morbidity in children
- Both accidents and respiratory illness are strongly related to social class and poverty.

ADOLESCENCE

Adolescence describes a period of transition between childhood and the adoption of full adult roles. This transition used to be rapid or immediate after puberty and sometimes involved a formal initiation rite, but these days many people in their mid-twenties have still not taken on all adult responsibilities. The ages at which different adult activities are permitted vary. Thus adolescents are expected to behave in some ways like adults, in others like children. Parents and children often disagree about which roles are appropriate at a given age. Since the 1950s there has also been increasing identification of 'youth' as having a separate identity and market, which helps to make adolescence seem separate. This is largely a cultural rather than a biological phenomenon.

SOURCES OF STRAIN

The physical changes of puberty are important for adolescents, but the psychological changes attributed to adolescence are caused by the difficulties of adolescent roles as much as by physiological changes. Adolescents have near-adult intellectual abilities (although not necessarily adult knowledge or experience) and soon acquire adult physical abilities. More important developmental issues are emotional, sexual and moral ones (Table 1). The influential theorist Eric Erikson (1968) described adolescence as a time of forming adult identity.

Two sources of strain are:

- *Having to choose and adjust to adult roles*. Many adolescents experiment with a variety of roles and behaviours before settling down with what suits them. This experimentation often includes activities which seem extreme to adults; for example, young fashions often offend older sensibilities.

- *Disputes over rights and responsibilities*. Adolescents often complain that adults expect them to have adult responsibilities without adult freedoms: to be responsible enough to baby-sit, but not responsible enough to choose when to have sex. Adults often feel the opposite, that adolescents expect adult freedoms without adult responsibilities: to be free to choose what time to come in, but not to be willing to help with housework.

Despite these strains, most adolescents have a fairly untroubled time and get on relatively well with their parents (Table 2). Most adolescents' interests and aspirations are similar to adults'. For example, one recent survey found that the most popular leisure activities for 18-year-olds were watching TV, listening to music and reading, hardly rebellious activities! Furthermore 78% of them had always been in work or education.

STOP THINK Are you an adolescent? Your first response may be no, yet as a student you probably experience role conflict, when you are told to take responsibility for your own learning while having the curriculum imposed on you. You probably have also experienced the strain and uncertainty of having to cope with practical and emotional matters on your own.

Are there activities which are still not appropriate for people of your age? Consider or discuss with classmates at what age the following activities become acceptable or normal:

- going steady
- sexual intercourse
- marriage
- drinking alcohol
- moving out of one's parents' house
- going to university to study mathematics
- going to university to study medicine.

Table 1 **Key differences between the adult and the child**

Children	Adults
Legally dependent	Legally responsible
Financially dependent	Financially independent
Not sexually active	Sexually active
Barred from many vices	Permitted vices: drinking, smoking, gambling
May not marry	May marry
May not vote or be elected to government	May vote and stand for election
Must be educated	May reject further education

Table 2 **Effects of combined parenting styles on adolescent development**

Two dimensions of parenting style	Hostile Cold, neglects or ignores child's needs, uses punishment to control behaviour	Loving Warm, accepts child's needs, attends to child, uses praise to control behaviour
Authoritarian Makes strict, rigid, unrealistic demands on child's behaviour	*Parent is consistently strict and punishing.* Some parents may be physically or sexually abusive. Adolescent develops internalised anger: neuroses, depression or anxiety, suicide attempts.	*This extreme combination of styles is unlikely* because rigid demands require ignoring child's needs. In less extreme form, the child may become an 'over-achiever' in an unsuccessful effort to please the parent.
Authoritative Has clear expectations for behaviour but these are flexible, realistic and negotiable	*This combination of styles is unlikely* because hostility precludes clear flexible expectations.	*Parent provides good guidance.* **The ideal combination** likely to lead to well-adjusted adult.
Permissive Makes few demands on behaviour and provides few guidelines for child	*Parent largely ignores child's behaviour and punishes inconsistently.* Some parents may be physically or sexually abusive. Adolescent develops externalised anger: acting out behaviour, delinquency, drug abuse.	*Parent treats child too much as an equal: child is 'spoiled'.* Major role conflicts, less extreme acting out behaviour. Child forced to 'be the parent'.

TROUBLED ADOLESCENTS

However, about 20% of adolescents will experience more problems. Many troubled adolescents abuse drugs or alcohol, engage in some criminal activities, may do poorly or drop out of school and are likely also to be depressed or unhappy. They are also likely to engage in behaviour inappropriate for their age, although not considered a problem for older people. Both sexual intercourse and drinking alcohol are considered age-inappropriate for people under 14 (note this is not just a legal definition, but a social norm). For most, this is a temporary phase lasting a few years, but some troubled adolescents become adults with problems. Early

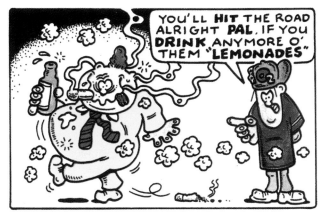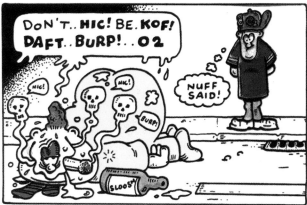

Fig. 1 **Health education information designed for young people is now widely available.** This cartoon dealing with the effects of 'alcopops' is reproduced with permission from the Health Education Board for Scotland, from O_2, Issue 3, 1994.

intervention can help some adolescents, but there is also a risk of labelling someone as mentally ill, drug-addicted or delinquent, actually making problems worse (see pp. 120–121).

The two most common social psychological explanations of risk-taking in adolescents are that they have a sense of invulnerability and are unable or unwilling to think in abstract ways about the future consequences of their own actions. More sociological explanations have suggested that risk-taking behaviour is a part of a youth sub-culture which provides identity and meaning within a larger or dominant adult culture which is seen as irrelevant, unrewarding (or even punitive) and meaningless to their experience and life chances.

Youth is perceived as a time of resilience when a young body can cope with overindulgence: young people will take exercise more because of concerns about attractiveness than health. Even a simple review of the health statistics tends to support this. With the exception of accidents for boys, young people are generally much healthier than older people, and recent evidence has shown that there is no class gradient in health at age 15 (West et al 1990).

HEALTH CARE NEEDS OF ADOLESCENTS

Compared to children and older people, adolescents rarely use health services and their morbidity and mortality rates are low. They are, however, a special target for prevention and health promotion programmes against substance abuse, risky sexual behaviour and suicide (Fig. 1). Drug abuse, alcohol abuse (including accidents while intoxicated) and suicide are among the leading causes of death of adolescents. A difficulty for prevention is that adolescents rarely envisage their own mortality. Adolescents may also have special health concerns related to their rapid physical development, including concerns about their sexual development, acne, allergies, fatigue, headaches, and concerns about body size, diet and exercise.

The provision of health care to adolescents can be problematic. In hospital, because they use few beds, they are often put in children's wards, which they may find patronising, or in adult wards which they may find threatening and lonely. They also tend to be sensitive to condescending attitudes by staff and may rebel or be uncooperative with their health care. Finally, many adolescents are somewhat uncomfortable about their bodies and they may find aspects of health care exceptionally embarrassing.

Case study

Jane is 16. When they discovered that she was dating a boy of another religion, her devout parents threw her out of the house and she got a place in a hostel for homeless women. Shortly afterwards she registered with a new GP and presented, afraid she was pregnant because her period was late. The pregnancy test was negative and on discussion the GP found that Jane was ignorant of the basic facts about sexual function. She had literally slept with her boyfriend while homeless, without intercourse, but believed that this would cause pregnancy. Additionally, she was unaware that an irregular menstrual cycle was normal for young women.

The GP provided some basic sex education and gave Jane a leaflet. The GP also discovered that Jane believed that she had to leave school because she had left home, although she was planning to go to university. The GP thought this was false and told Jane to check with hostel staff, then as she seemed hesitant, and with her consent, phoned the hostel to check this. Being only 16, Jane was entitled to a grant to continue her education. She had also been in care at age 12–13 because physical abuse had been suspected. This meant that she was also entitled to other benefits. Thanks in part to this help the GP formed a relationship of trust with Jane and when she was feeling suicidal a few months later, she rapidly sought the GP's help. At that time, rather than prescribe medication which might be abused, the GP arranged that she attended once a week for 6 weeks to discuss her problems. After a couple of weeks her mood was much improved and she never actually attempted suicide.

Adolescence

- Adolescence is a period of transition between child and adult roles.
- Strain in adolescence can occur when there is conflict over appropriate roles and behaviours.
- Most adolescents have a fairly untroubled time.
- About 20% go through a period of delinquency or problem behaviour, but most get over it.
- Adolescent morbidity and mortality rates are low, and they make little use of health care.
- Special health problems are substance abuse, risky sexual behaviour, depression and suicide.

ADULTHOOD AND MID AGE

This section considers the psychosocial changes that occur in adulthood and their relation to health and illness.

Most children long to be grown up, and grown-ups are seen as having rights and privileges that are strongly desired by children (see pp. 10–11). However, they do not always recognise the accompanying responsibilities of adulthood. Young adults grapple with problems of budgeting, relationships, demands of work and study. On the other hand, health is probably better in early adulthood than at any other time of life. As people get older they may begin to worry about the negative consequences of ageing. This realisation may not be inevitable and may occur at different ages for different people, or indeed, for men and women. At some point the anticipation of the next birthday may be tinged with apprehension about the ageing process.

The ages between seventeen and forty are often described as early adulthood and, until relatively recently, would be regarded as the prime of life. Individuals and society emphasise growth and development on each birthday. In the UK, the eighteenth birthday is seen as being culturally important. Other important milestones may be the legal age of consent to sexual intercourse, drinking alcohol in pubs, or voting. It is also a healthy time of life and young adults are the age group that are least likely to consult doctors apart from health related to reproduction (see pp. 4–5).

MARRIAGE

During adulthood most people will form a relationship with the opposite sex, and most formalise the relationship by getting married. Marriage is still popular even though the divorce rate is rising. The number of single parents is increasing (Fig. 1) and the age at marriage is getting later (Fig. 2). Homosexual partnerships may serve the same function as heterosexual marriage and are becoming increasingly accepted in our society.

There is considerable evidence that men benefit from marriage in terms of physical and mental health, but for women being married can have disadvantages. Being single, widowed or divorced is associated with lower rates of depression in women than it is in men. Blaxter et al (1987) found that men living with a spouse had lower illness scores than men living alone, but for women there was no difference. The protective effect of marriage for men could be linked to social support.

Although marriage appears to be good for men's health, men suffer more severely from loss of their wives by bereavement or breakdown of marriage, and they are more likely to suffer from a range of health problems.

Patients who consult with physical symptoms may be having marital problems, and sometimes these can disrupt their medical treatment. These may involve depression associated with childbirth or sexual problems, or major health and social problems if the wife has been physically abused. A marital separation may be followed by depression and would certainly impede recovery from illness or surgery. Knowledge of the psychology of relationships can help us understand the context of change in health and illness.

Many people live in single households. In the UK in 1991, 26% of all households consisted of one single person. Forty-five percent of adults over twenty years of age were married, fourteen percent were single, the remainder being widowed or divorced. In women in the age group over 74, only twenty-eight percent were married and fourteen percent were single with the remainder being widowed or divorced.

Single women tend to be viewed negatively by society. Women may lack confidence in their ability to survive by themselves. The maintenance of our identity comes from others and our feelings of self worth may be closely linked to the emotional support received in a relationship. However, being single and independent may be advantageous to some women compared with being a traditional wife, and it may be easier for them to avoid emotional and sexual complications.

If a single or widowed woman is ill there may be practical problems. Women often earn less than men and they may not have had employment that has generous sick pay arrangements. The absence of a partner at home may make convalescence difficult.

TRANSITIONS

One perspective on ageing has been given by Erikson. His theory suggests that mid age is a time of conflict between generativity (guiding the next generation) and stagnation (concern with own

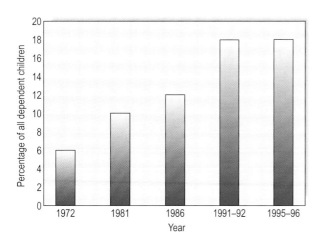

Fig. 1 **Percentage of dependent children with lone mothers.** (Social Trends 27, 1997 edition. HMSO, London)

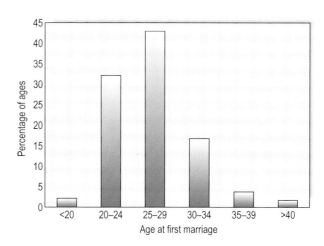

Fig. 2 **Age at first marriage (1993).** (Social Trends 26, 1996 edition. HMSO, London)

needs). Mid age will be associated with different patterns of health and illness, and assessment of a middle-aged patient may have to include their relationship with their own increasingly ageing parents as well as their dependent teenage children

Bond and Coleman (1990) suggest that there has recently been a social reconstruction of middle age. This attempts to establish an ever increasing distance between the middle years (mid 30's to late 60's) and 'geriatric' old age (see pp. 14–15).

Men are sometimes said to go through a 'mid-life crisis'. Half of the men in a study of forty men aged between 37 and 41 identified a period of uncertainty, anxiety and change (Levinson 1978). They saw mid-life as a last chance to achieve goals but others saw mid-life as a dead end, and life as pointless. Men at this stage also become aware of changing physical strength and vigour. Yet the years between maturity and the beginning of old age may be regarded as the prime of life, and a time when many men are at the peak of their careers and are still in good physical health. For these people illness is unexpected and may be perceived as being 'unfair'. It may also be seen as being a failure of medical care or as a result of an unhealthy lifestyle.

- Do you see mid age as the prime of life? What age do you think your health will start to deteriorate?

PREVENTIVE HEALTH IN ADULTHOOD

The time perspective of the young adult may be limited to the demands of their jobs, marriage and bringing up families, but in mid age people may make positive plans for retirement. As people enter mid age they may increasingly focus on preventive health measures and may begin to prepare for retirement. At this time there may be an intense interest in health shown by joining clubs or fitness programmes and attending for screening. Stressful events may occur with relative frequency in mid adulthood and there has been much interest in the link between coping with stress and heart disease in mid age (see p. 104). If elderly parents die or suffer chronic illness when their offspring are mid aged this may focus attention on illness (and health).

Youth and beauty are culturally associated and the association is perpetuated by media images. A youthful physical appearance is a source of power for woman, although men's power depends on wealth and occupation. This has been described as the double standard of ageing. The Association of Graceful Ageing, Health and Moral Attractiveness developed in the 1920's illustrates the anxieties that are reflected in the belief that a healthy mid age will somehow postpone the ageing

process. Physical attractiveness bears little relationship to health in reality. Those who are physically attractive may be assumed to be healthy even though they are not.

There are noticeable changes in physical appearance with increasing age, such as greying hair and loss of skin elasticity. In an ageist society these become negative attributes and generate a vast cosmetic industry. However, greying hair and cragginess of features in men may denote increasing maturity and competence.

Child rearing may dominate the ages between 20 and 45 and much of the contact between adults and the medical profession may be about the health of the children. The mother may consult her general practitioner frequently, and this will allow a relationship to develop which may be valuable when she becomes older and more likely to be ill herself.

- At what age do you think adults consider concealing their age?
- Why should there be a double standard for ageing for men and women? Is it changing?

HEALTH CHANGES AND AGE

The menopause has been held to be responsible for the increase in women's psychological problems in mid age but the evidence for a causal relationship is weak (see p. 5).

The menopause is part of normal development and is defined in medical terms as having occurred when twelve months have elapsed since the last menstrual period.

Sensory abilities progressively decline in adulthood. People's sight deteriorates and a sure sign of reaching mid age is when newspapers are read at arm's length. Sometimes patients at outpatient clinics or admitted to hospital may not carry reading glasses with them, and may not be able to read simple instructions or consent forms.

Hearing also declines slowly but there is little loss of psychomotor skills during mid age.

On the plus side knowledge, confidence and maturity increase with age and as yet are still valued by society. As medical technology increases we are likely to live longer so that the mid age adult should have many healthy and productive years before an extended third age in retirement.

Case study

Forty-year-old Mr Harris and his wife (who works part time as a care assistant) have three children at school, four parents living and an elderly grandmother of 90. Mr Harris lost his job as a printer when his firm was modernised. How would you expect him to view middle age? His wife is concerned about the health of her father, who is a heavy smoker. She is grieving for the loss of her younger sister who died of breast cancer. How would you expect her to view mid age?

Adulthood and mid age

- The age of entry to adulthood is usually considered as being about eighteen but there are differences in social, cultural and psychological milestones.
- Marriage is more beneficial for health in men than in women. Marital problems may affect health.
- In mid age, adults become increasing interested in preventive health.
- Adults spend much time in parenting in mid age and their main contact with the medical profession may be through their children, or their elderly parents
- Physical events such as the menopause and changes in sensory abilities signal the ageing process, but are not directly related to loss of function in mid age.

AGEING

HEALTH IN OLD AGE

It is widely believed by many health care professionals that most old people are physically frail and suffer from multiple disorders. While it is true that the prevalence of disease increases with age, most old people live independent and mobile lives, free from major incapacitating disease (Sidell 1995). Problems with hearing and vision increase with age, and taste and smell sensitivity decrease with age. However, only about 4% of the over-65s reside in long-stay care, and most of those are over 75 years old. Perhaps one of the reasons health care professionals think that all old people are infirm and ill is that this is the group they encounter most frequently in their daily lives.

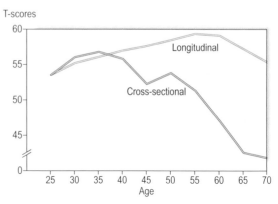

Fig. 1 **Graph showing findings from cross-sectional and longitudinal studies of intelligence and age.**

Examples of ageism are not difficult to find. In 1962, a British physician wrote in The Lancet that it is 'normal' for people over the age of 75 to be:

'frail and unsteady, dozing by day and wakeful by night, confused about people and places, forgetful and untidy, repetitive and boring, selfish and petty perhaps and consumed by a fear of death'.

STOP THINK Which of the following statements do you think are true and which are false?

• Most old people are frail and infirm and a high proportion reside in institutions.
• Old people have no interest in or capacity for sexual relations.
• Intelligence declines with age.
• Old people are incapable of learning new things.
• Depression is a major problem in the elderly.
• Most old people are poor.

If you think that all of these statements are true then you appear to accept the 'myths' of ageing. Myths are stereotypes that predispose us to think about and act towards people in particular ways.

THE AGEING MIND

It is commonly believed that all old people are senile, incapable of learning new things and depressed, and that intelligence declines with age. It is, of course, true that all old people are 'senile' – the word means 'old'. But, to what extent do our intellectual capacities decline with age?

At one time there appeared to be a substantial body of evidence showing that intelligence declines with age (p. 31). The evidence was drawn from cross-sectional studies of performance on intelligence tests. These studies fairly consistently showed that older cohorts, compared with younger cohorts, performed less well on the intelligence tests.

However, as the findings from longitudinal studies emerged, the picture changed quite dramatically (K W Schaie 1996). As can be seen in Figure 1, when the same individuals are tested over time, there is very little change in test performance, i.e. intelligence does *not* decline with age.

Does the ability to learn decline with age? Although it is widely believed that 'you can't teach an old dog new tricks', there is almost no information about learning in old dogs. However, there is now much research on human learning and problem solving which compares the performance of different age groups.

Learning requires two things: the research subject has to get the information 'in' and then, when tested, he or she must get the learned material 'out'. If the performance of old people is worse than that of younger subjects one must devise an experiment to find out which aspect of learning accounts for the differences in test performance. Most studies of what is called 'pacing' have shown that old people need longer to get the learned material 'out'. In pacing studies the experimenter varies the amount of time that subjects have to produce the answer. Results show that, if no time limit is set, performance on learning tasks of older and younger subjects is similar. However, reducing the amount of time to recall the answer leads to decrements of performance for older people (Bromley 1990). Thus, it appears that it takes longer for older people to search their memory stores to retrieve information. Doctors and nurses should, therefore, allow more time for older patients to 'find' the answers to questions. Repeatedly filling the silence with another question will lead to a breakdown in communication (see pp. 92–93).

Another interesting area where older and younger subjects differ is in the ability to filter-out irrelevant information. This is sometimes referred to as the 'cocktail party' effect. When young people go to a party they have little difficulty filtering out the irrelevant conversations taking place around them. Older people find this difficult. Studies of this phenomenon involve asking subjects to listen to headphones in which one message is played to the left ear and a different message to the right ear. The subject is asked to follow only one message (these experiments are called 'dichotic listening experiments'). As people age, test performance indicates that more and more information from the 'wrong' ear appears in the test (Stuart-Hamilton 1994).

These findings are relevant to the practice of medicine in two ways:

• When taking a case history or explaining something to an older patient one should ensure that there are as few distracting and 'irrelevant' noises about as possible; patients find it stressful to have to struggle to listen to and concentrate on one particular conversation (see pp. 92–93).
• It is not uncommon for middle aged patients to visit their GPs asking to have their hearing tested or for wax to be removed from their ears. Testing often reveals no wax and little decrement in the acuity of the patient's hearing. The patient goes away puzzled and frustrated and still convinced that he or she is going deaf. Explanation of this 'central processing' phenomenon usually provides reassurance.

Will all old people eventually develop dementia and suffer from depression? Only a minority will develop dementia. One often sees figures like 1 in 10 over

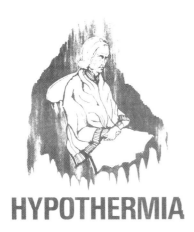

HYPOTHERMIA

Fig. 2 **Image of ageing presented in a health promotion leaflet.**

65 and 1 in 4 over 75 years develop dementia. It is unclear where these figures have come from – certainly not from epidemiological studies. Epidemiological studies indicate that roughly 1% of the 65–75-year-olds and 10% of those over 75 will develop dementia (Ineichen 1987). Depression is also not as common amongst the elderly as some writers have made out. A recent review of the literature has noted that old people are not more prone to depression than younger people. Yet one continues to see books stating that depression in the elderly is a major health hazard.

SEXUALITY

Another common belief is that old people are not interested in, and have no capacity for, sexual relations (see pp. 28–29). Although there have been few studies on sexuality in the elderly, those that exist have found that older people are interested in sex. However, opportunities for sexual relations are often limited, especially for women. Widowed and divorced men often marry younger women and this greatly reduces the numbers of sexual partners available for older women. Although there is much talk of 'toy boys', the reality for older women is that sexual relations with younger men are still frowned upon in society (Blytheway 1995).

Health care professionals often feel uncomfortable thinking or talking about sexual matters with older people. This may have to do with powerful incest taboos that exist which make it hard for us to think about our parents as sexual beings. We may generalize these feelings about our parents to all older people.

Uneasiness about sexuality in elderly people may also be the reason why health care professionals fail to provide opportunities for sexual relations for old people who live in residential care.

POVERTY AND OLD AGE

What is your image of old people? Is it like the one in Figure 2 which appeared in a health promotion leaflet? This is certainly a prevalent media view of old people.

Poverty is a relative concept, and research does show that, as a group, elderly people are financially worse off than younger people. This is particularly true of Britain in comparison with some other European countries. In Britain, nearly three out of five older people live in or on the margins of poverty compared with less than one-quarter of those under pension age (Walker 1993). Furthermore, many elderly people do not claim state benefits to which they are entitled because they resent the intrusion of means testing into their private lives.

While one would not wish to belittle the problems faced by those elderly people who have minimal financial resources (and hypothermia can indeed be a severe risk for them), the danger is that old people themselves will be 'blamed' for their poverty. Rather than ask questions about the way society is structured, for example with people forced to retire at 65, we may lapse into the view that old people are poor because they did not save for their old age.

WORKING WITH OLD PEOPLE

How many health care professionals choose to specialize in areas related to old people? Unfortunately, most studies indicate that health care professionals would rather work with young patients. A review of twelve studies on attitudes to the elderly amongst doctors and medical students revealed that most doctors and medical students preferred to work with younger people (Palmore 1977). When asked, few medical students say they want to specialize in geriatric medicine. This is interesting given that, except for those specializing in pediatrics and obstetrics, most specialties involve care of the elderly. Most people with cancer are old, as are most people with cardiovascular disease.

BELIEFS AND BEHAVIOUR

False beliefs about ageing may have very negative effects on old people. They may also lead to unrealistic fears for the future in adult children. Society as a whole may come to view the elderly as a burden, rather than a resource. More importantly, the behaviour of doctors may be influenced by negative stereotypes of the elderly.

Case study

Two persons in similar physical condition may be differentially designated dead or not. For example, a young child was brought into the emergency room with no registering heartbeat, respiration, or pulse — the standard 'signs of death' — and was, through a rather dramatic stimulation procedure involving the co-ordinated work of a large team of doctors and nurses, revived for a period of eleven hours. On the same evening, shortly after the child's arrival, an elderly person who presented the same physical signs, with — as one physician later stated in conversation — no discernible differences from the child in skin color, warmth, etc, arrived in the emergency room and was almost immediately pronounced dead, with no attempts at stimulation instituted. A nurse remarked, later in the evening, 'They (the doctors) would never have done that to the old lady (attempt heart stimulation) even though I've seen it work on them too'. During the period when emergency resuscitation equipment was being readied for the child, an intern instituted mouth-to-mouth resuscitation. This same intern was shortly relieved by oxygen machinery, and when the woman arrived, he was the one who pronounced her dead. He reported shortly afterwards that he could never bring himself to put his mouth to 'an old lady like that'. (Sudnow 1967).

Ageing

- Most elderly people can, and often do, live independent and mobile lives.
- Myths or stereotypes held by health care professionals can limit the self-esteem and independence of older people.
- There is no evidence that intelligence declines with age, but recall may take longer.
- Opportunities for sexual relations are often limited, particularly for older women.
- Older people are more likely to be poor than younger adults, but are often too 'proud/independent' to claim state benefits to which they are entitled.

DEATH AND BEREAVEMENT

In the course of their career, doctors will often have to care for people who are coming to terms with the loss of someone through death. The terms bereavement, grief and mourning are often used interchangeably to describe a person's reaction to loss. The process after the death, during which individuals learn to adjust to the loss, is known as bereavement; grief can be described as the emotional response to that loss; while mourning refers to the expression of grief (Stroebe and Stroebe 1987). Most people who experience the loss of someone close recover gradually using their own coping resources with the support of family and friends. In some situations where there is a difficulty in coping there may be a need for special help from health professionals. For example, sometimes the death of a spouse can result in the deterioration of the elderly partner or an increase in their dependence on other members of the family. The bereavement period can provide the opportunity for doctors to assess the needs of the surviving spouse or family and to intervene where appropriate with relevant back-up and services (Cartwright 1982).

DETERMINANTS OF GRIEF

Many factors can affect the way in which someone reacts to being bereaved. These may have happened before the bereavement, for example a childhood experience, a previous life crisis like divorce or mental illness, or the type of relationship the bereaved person had with the deceased. The reaction may also be influenced by the bereaved person's present circumstances, for example their age, sex, religion, type of personality or even cultural background. It may also be determined by the circumstances of the bereaved after the death, for example the amount of support they have, and other stresses in their life, such as young children. These have been referred to as the antecedent, concurrent and subsequent determinants of grief (Parkes 1975).

Cultural and religious beliefs of individuals will affect how they display grief and how they should behave in the bereavement period. Strict rules govern the preparation of the body after death and the rituals associated with burial and mourning among different ethnic groups (Firth 1993). For example, in Western society, the preparation of the body for burial has largely been taken over by health professionals or funeral directors, while among Asian communities, these rituals remain an important part of family duty.

THE MOURNING PROCESS

In the same way that the dying process has been described as a series of stages (Kubler-Ross 1970), the process of mourning has similarly been defined as a series of phases which must be passed through by the bereaved before grief can be resolved (see pp. 108–109). Parkes (1975) describes these phases as numbness, yearning, disorganisation and despair and reorganisation. Worden (1991) prefers to describe the process as a series of tasks which must be worked through. He describes these as accepting the reality of the loss, working through the pain, adjusting to an environment in which the deceased is missing and moving on with life. Although these theories can be a useful way of beginning to understand the complexity of the grief process, individual reactions will vary and may not conform to a specific pattern.

NORMAL GRIEF

Normal grief reactions can include a huge range of different types of feelings, moods, symptoms and behaviours. Worden (1991) has classified examples of these under four headings. These are illustrated in Figure 1.

RISK FACTORS

Faulkner (1995) suggests that the reaction to loss may not be normal if:

- a difficult relationship with the deceased has existed before the death; for example, the bereaved person may have been over-dependent on the dead person or disliked them
- the death has been violent (e.g. murder) or sudden or unexplained (e.g. suicide)
- the nature of the bereaved's involvement in the death has been unsatisfactory; for example, the bereaved person may not have had time to say goodbye, may not have visited the person before the death or may not have been present at the death
- the bereaved person has previously experienced difficult losses; for example, divorce or mutilating surgery (Faulkner 1995).

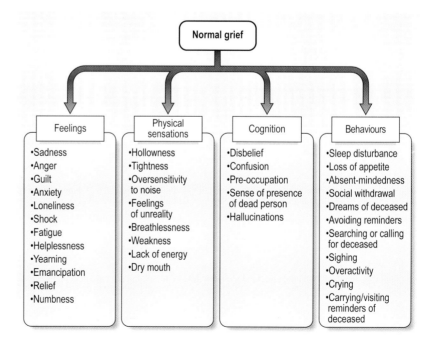

Fig. 1 **A typology of normal grief.** (Worden 1991)

Case study

Ethel was a 61-year-old woman whose husband Jack had died 6 months earlier after a sudden heart attack. At around the same time her youngest daughter, Ruth, had left home to start a university course in a city about 30 miles away from where they lived. Her two elder children were both married and living abroad. Previously a lively woman, with many and varied interests, Ethel had shared most of these with her husband as they both enjoyed early retirement. Lately, however, Ethel had become withdrawn and morose and seemed to have lost all interest in anything. She had stopped going to the clubs of which she was a member and preferred instead to spend her days looking at old family photos or going through her husband's belongings which she refused to part with. She constantly phoned her daughter in tears and said she did not want to carry on living without her husband. As a result Ruth felt guilty at having left her mother to cope alone, and at a loss to know what help to give her. Eventually, Ruth asked the family general practitioner for help. She suggested that Ruth phone a local voluntary bereavement counselling service. After a few visits from a trained counsellor, Ethel began to come to terms with her husband's death. Although she knew that her life would no longer be the same without her lifetime partner, she realised that she had to make a new beginning for her own and her family's sake. Ruth was relieved that her mother was now able to resume some of the hobbies she used to enjoy, and her own life at university became happier.

 STOP THINK Write down the factors you think might have influenced the way Ethel reacted to Jack's death. Think about how you would cope with Ethel if you were Ruth.

PATHOLOGICAL GRIEF REACTION

Pathological grief reactions occur when the bereaved person is unable for some reason to express or work through their grief, which prevents their recovery from the loss and adaptation to life without the deceased. Such reactions can be classified as delayed, chronic, masked or exaggerated grief.

Delayed grief

The bereaved person is unable to mourn the loss. This may be conscious, when the bereaved person's situation makes it difficult for them to grieve freely, for example in the case of a mother who carries on normally for the sake of her children. It can also be unconscious, when the bereaved person does not believe that the death has occurred, for example when there has been no definite confirmation as in the case of soldiers missing during a war. This may be called absent grief (Faulkner 1995). Delayed grief reactions are often triggered by other losses occurring a long time after the death, e.g. a later divorce or other unrelated loss (Worden 1991).

Chronic grief

The bereaved continues to experience the immediate pain of the loss months and even years later. They therefore are unable to move on in the grieving process and adapt to life without the deceased. Usually chronic grief reactions occur in people who have had ambivalent relationships with the deceased (Parkes 1975).

Masked grief

The grief reaction is masked by the development of physical or somatic symptoms which appear to the bereaved to be unassociated with the loss. Often these are physical symptoms which replicate those experienced by the deceased and these commonly appear on the anniversaries of the loss (Worden 1991).

Exaggerated grief

The grief reaction is excessive and intense. In these cases the bereaved's experience may develop into a serious psychiatric illness, e.g. clinical depression or an acute anxiety state (Worden 1991).

OTHER LOSSES

Persons may react to other losses or illnesses in the same way as they would to a bereavement through the death of a loved one. Examples that doctors may come across include amputation, miscarriage, still births, physical dependency, marriage, divorce, unemployment or even relocation to a new town or city. With these losses the grief experienced and exhibited by the person may be as intense and as debilitating as grief expressed at a death. For these reasons health professionals may miss or fail to appreciate the extent of a person's distress. This may mean that the person experiencing the loss is not offered the help that they need to come to terms with it.

BEREAVEMENT CARE

The amount of support available for the bereaved often varies greatly according to the setting where they or their relatives are cared for. It is usually uncommon for doctors working in general hospitals to have the time or the resources to follow up carers during the bereavement. Often this is done by general practitioners or community nurses who are able to visit the bereaved or telephone them at home. Sometimes they or staff from specialist settings will also run a bereavement support group which the bereaved can attend and meet others in a similar position to themselves. Some settings will send cards to relatives on the anniversary of the death, acknowledging the date and inviting the bereaved to make contact again if they wish. These types of interventions help staff to monitor the bereavement outcome and reassure the bereaved person that he/she is still cared for. However, not every bereaved person will either want or need professional support at this time. The majority of people rely on family and friends or find their own ways of coping. However, in cases where the grief reaction is problematic the doctor should recognise his/her own limitations and summon the help of someone who is specially trained in bereavement counselling. In some extreme cases, it may also be necessary to refer the person on to a psychologist or psychiatrist.

Death and bereavement

- Bereavement refers to the situation of someone who has experienced the loss of a loved one and grief is the emotional response to the loss.
- Normal grief can be described as a series of stages a person must work through until they adapt to life without the deceased.
- The way people react to a loss will depend on their past experiences and present circumstances.

WHAT IS PERSONALITY?

Most people would agree that everyone has a unique personality. This is another way of saying that there are individual differences in behaviour. Personality is difficult to define but many psychologists would agree that it is made up of stable internal factors that are relatively constant over time and that account for individual differences in behaviour. Some characteristics, like shyness, are more obvious at certain ages, and young teenagers may be especially shy about talking about their developing bodies. It is suggested that something within us determines our behaviour but, as we shall see, external circumstances are also powerful. If someone behaves 'out of character', we should look for causes that might be related to health, such as drug abuse, the onset of dementia, or a break-down in a relationship.

There are many different personality theories and these influence how behaviour is viewed. For example, patients who complain about minor symptoms may be regarded as having a low pain threshold. But patients may also complain because they have learned that complaints are rewarded by attention from professionals and family. Complaints might also reflect unconscious conflict. None of these approaches is right or wrong but must be seen as a more or less useful way of looking at individual differences.

One view is that people have a fixed personality that is deep inside but covered up like layers of an onion skin. If only we could strip away the layers we would uncover the 'real' person lying within. The layers give colour or characteristics to a person. This is sometimes known as trait theory.

TRAIT THEORY

Individuals are thought of as having many different traits. These traits can be described by different sets of adjectives relating to behaviour. Cattell made a list of 4500 words in the English language that are used to describe personality. He reduced these to 160 trait words which were used to produce a Sixteen Personality Factor Scale. Some of these factors are correlated with each other, and Hans Eysenck and colleagues used factor analysis (a statistical technique that investigates correlations between different variables, and looks for clusters of association which suggest an underlying structure) to identify two main super factors (Fig. 1):

- **Introversion–extroversion**. People who score highly in extroversion are sociable, lively, assertive, in contrast to introverts who are more retiring and controlled.
- **Neuroticism–stability**. Those who score highly on neuroticism show anxiety proneness, guilt feelings, have low self esteem and experience low mood.

They then added a third dimension, psychoticism, which can be considered as being at right angles to the other two in Figure 1.

- **Psychoticism-impulse control**. Those scoring high on psychoticism are aggressive, cold, and lack empathy.

These trait theories describe differences but we also want to know why they are different and if these descriptions allow us to predict behaviour. Eysenck argued for a genetic determinism and attempted (rather unsuccessfully) to find a physiological basis of these personality types.

In practice there is probably no such thing as the 'true' person because we all perceive people in different ways and we all behave differently to different people. Some of our behaviour is determined by our social role. If you are trying to behave like a responsible doctor you may exhibit one pattern of behaviour, but when celebrating your birthday with friends you may show quite another.

Contrast your behaviour as a student and as a son or daughter. Are they different? Are your views of yourself different from those of your parents?

This exercise stresses the importance of the situation in determining personality. The correlation between personality and actual behaviour is actually low. This ties in with the social learning theory approach (see pp. 20–21).

A patient who seems very timid and anxious when consulting a doctor may be dynamic and forceful at home or at work. This may be because the sick role encourages subservient behaviour and deference to doctors.

We do not always agree with everyone about the characteristics of a person. Consider your reaction if you were told that you were unpunctual. Would this be a fair comment? You might feel that you were always on time for appointments with patients and always turned up in time for ward rounds. However, you might realise that your time keeping at lectures was not so good and that your partner had complained that you were unreliable. Mischel (1968) suggested that far from having consistent traits that are stable over time and situations, we behave in particular ways according to the situation.

IS IT THE PERSON OR THE SITUATION?

The answer is neither one alone but most likely personality results from an interaction between the two. It is hard to imagine an extroverted personality appearing as a shrinking violet, but among people who know you well there will be some common agreement about the kind of person you are.

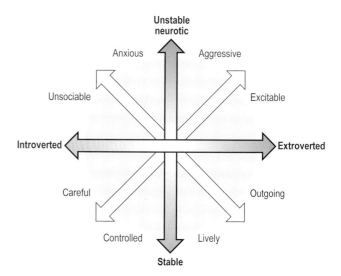

Fig. 1 **Dimensions of personality based on Eysenck's theory.**

Life events including illness can have a marked effect on the way people behave. The threat of a second myocardial infarction may change a person's approach to life. Disfigurement of the body, especially of the face, can lead to a loss of self esteem and lack of social confidence.

 STOP THINK To what extent do you think that people's physical appearance influences their personality?

TYPES OF PERSONALITY THEORIES

Some theories are known as '*ideographic theories*' because they seek to identify an individual's unique characteristics. These are more often used in clinical contexts. They contrast with '*nomothetic theories*' such as the trait theories. These consider that people differ in a number of different traits or characteristics common to everyone. These are often used in large scale research studies.

PSYCHODYNAMIC THEORY

The approach taken by Freud and psychoanalytic theory is ideographic. Freud described three components or mechanisms which interact and mediate behaviour.

His theory is based on the assumption that behaviour is influenced by the unconscious mind. Using an iceberg analogy he described the part above water as representing the conscious experience, and the bulk below as representing the unconscious experience. The unconscious is accessible through the technique of free association and is revealed in dreams and memories of early childhood.

Freud's theory of personality describes three major systems. The *ego* is conscious and is in touch with the real world. The *id* is childlike and demands that its needs be fulfilled. The *super ego* is the individual's conscience and tends to be authoritarian. The three work together but may also be in conflict. The ego has to reconcile impulses from the id and the super ego. There are no actual physiological systems or parts of the brain that correspond to these systems, but Freudians use them to explain individual behaviour.

There are many scientific arguments against the acceptance of Freudian theory of personality. There is little scientific data, no statistical analysis, and the theory is based on patients who were rich middle class women living in Victorian Vienna.

However, it has intuitive meaning, some doctors find it clinically useful and it is important to be aware of psychodynamic theories. They have also been influential in modern literature!

It is not possible to test Freud's theories and most evidence comes from retrospective accounts. There is little evidence to suggest that early potty training is really crucial, but his suggestion that early experiences shape later ways of behaving has found general acceptance. Therapists often look for difficulties in early relationships to explain adult behaviour. We now accept that defence mechanisms such as denial, another aspect of Freud's theory, often explain illness behaviour, or reactions to diagnosis.

VULNERABILITY TO SPECIFIC DISEASES

Personality differences may predict people's behaviour to illness but there has also been much interest in the relationship between individual differences and vulnerability to specific illnesses. Lively controversies have arisen over the relationship between psychosocial and organic factors in cancer and cardiovascular disease. It has been suggested that some people have particular personality characteristics that make them more prone to cancer. Gossarth-Maticek et al (1984) assessed a sample of 1353 elderly Yugoslavian patients and monitored them over ten years. Significant characteristics of those dying of cancer included 'rational and anti-emotional behaviour' and a high level of 'traumatic life events involving chronic helplessness'. Gossarth-Maticek does not define these terms and they are difficult to interpret. This study and other studies have been severely criticised by Pelosi and Appleby (1992). The definition of personality types is imprecise, and the methodology and analyses are unclear. The numbers in the studies are very high and in the Yugoslavian study a 100% follow-up was claimed after ten years. Some of these criticisms have been addressed by Eysenck (1992), but the link between cancer, personality and therapy remains unclear.

Behaviour patterns may be linked to heart disease and a pattern of behaviour known as Type A has been associated with risk of heart attacks (see pp. 104–105). Feelings of hostility appear to be most closely associated with increased risk of heart attacks but the claims are contentious. Although Type A and Type B have been described as personality types, they are better thought of as behaviour patterns that can be modified by interventions. Changing Type A behaviour is often incorporated into rehabilitation programmes following mild heart attacks.

Case study

Mr McDuff was very competitive at work and worked hard to become the top salesman in his area. He drove aggressively and always appeared in a hurry. He was impatient of others and many people thought that his manner to his colleagues was unnecessarily rude. At home he was quiet and never raised his voice, although he had young teenagers in the house. He visited his mother who lived nearby twice a week and she regarded him as quiet, home loving and dominated by his wife. Why does this description sound rather unconvincing? Which aspect of his behaviour would be associated with vulnerability to heart disease?

What is personality?

- There are many different personality theories but they should not be seen as being either right or wrong but as different in their approach.
- Trait theory suggests that behaviour is determined by personality traits which may cluster into factors such as extroversion.
- The situation may influence behaviour more than individual characteristics.
- Freudian psychoanalytic theory suggests that our behaviour is influenced by unconscious motives and these develop during our childhood.
- Individual differences in Type A behaviour may be related to vulnerability to heart disease.

HOW DO WE LEARN?

Learning is not just about acquiring facts or knowledge. Social skills, beliefs and values are also learned. We learn how to respond emotionally, how to recognise symptoms and, as children, we learn appropriate (and inappropriate) ways of behaving (Fig. 1). If we understand how behaviour is learned we may be able to change it. We may wish to change to a more healthy life-style, to learn how to monitor our own glucose levels, or to overcome a phobia. Understanding learning has been of central concern to psychologists, and the source of much debate (Eysenck 1996).

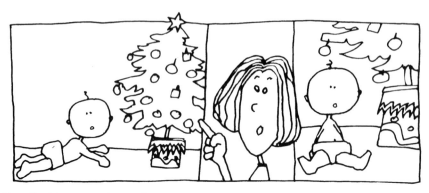

Fig. 1 **If an infant approaches the Christmas tree decorations it will be restrained: this will decrease the frequency of approach.** In practice punishment is a very poor way of changing behaviour and often it arouses emotional responses. What does the baby do when it is not allowed to touch the tree (or approach medical equipment)?

Learning can be defined as a relatively permanent change in behaviour. Behaviourist theories of learning assume that there are laws of learning that are fundamental to all animals, and that humans are no different in this respect. Behaviourism suggests that learning results from stimulus–response associations. A stimulus can be any change, such as the sight of food or a moving ball. A response is a reflex action such as salivation, or a muscular response such as catching the ball. Of course much learning is cognitive — such as the acquisition of knowledge and concepts that is taking place as you read this book.

THEORETICAL BACKGROUND

Operant conditioning

One kind of learning, known as operant conditioning, was described by an American psychologist, B. F. Skinner. In operant conditioning, the likelihood of a response occurring again is increased if the behaviour is followed by a reinforcement. Thus, the behaviour is controlled by its consequences. The principles of operant conditioning have been established through experimentation on animals such as rats and pigeons, as well as humans, and are shown in Table 1.

If a goal results from an accurate kick, then the motor responses leading up to the kick will be reinforced. In this case the reinforcement would be in the form of satisfaction and approval by the team and fans. Success in walking following an amputation would be rewarded internally by feelings of mastery and enhanced self efficacy, and externally by the approval of others. Praise (especially from medical staff) can be a very powerful reinforcer.

Classical conditioning

Operant conditioning is contrasted with classical conditioning described by a physiologist, I. Pavlov. In classical conditioning an initially neutral stimulus becomes associated with an involuntary response by its association with a previously conditioned stimulus. Pavlov worked with dogs, who naturally salivate at the sight of food. After pairing a bell with the food, the dogs learned to salivate at the sound of the bell alone. These principles were later tested with human emotional responses.

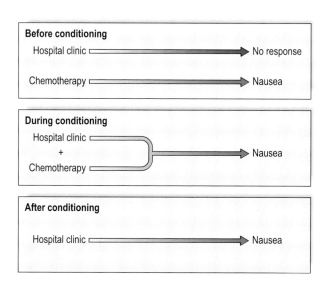

Fig. 2 **Classical conditioning applied to nausea and chemotherapy.**

Watson and Raynor (1920) used classical conditioning to produce a phobia in a 9-month-old child known as Little Albert. Before the experiment he had no fear of white rats but was frightened by loud noises. In the experiment the loud noise was

Table 1 **Principles of operant conditioning**

Principle	Definition	Effect on behaviour	Example
Positive reinforcement	Provides positive, pleasant consequences	Increases probability that the response will occur again	Verbal praise in rehabilitation
Negative reinforcement	Removes unpleasant conditions	Increases probability that response will occur again	Adjusting gait to avoid pain in walking
Punishment	Removes a positive reinforcer or applies an aversive stimulus	Decreases the probability that response will occur again	Vomiting after eating poisonous fungi
Extinction	Removes positive reinforcer	Decreases the probability that response will occur again	Ignoring tantrums in waiting room
Shaping	Reinforces successive approximations to the one required	Gradually increases approximation to desired behaviour	Teaching someone with a learning disability how to feed themselves

paired with the presence of a white rat. After six pairings Albert showed a fear response in the presence of the white rat alone. Fear had now become a response conditioned to the previously neutral stimulus of the white rat. Moreover the fear generalised to other furry animals. White rats and loud noises are not an everyday occurrence but white coats may be associated with painful injections. The fear of pain may become associated with the white coat (and its wearer) and generalise to white coats worn by any staff.

Some patients may develop conditioned responses to the sight or smell of hospitals. If hospital treatment has been associated with nausea, as for example in the case of chemotherapy for cancer, the mere sight or smell of hospital can induce nausea or even vomiting (Fig. 2).

In practice, operant conditioning and classical conditioning probably both occur in many learning situations. Food elicits salivation but also acts as a reinforcer.

STOP THINK
- Does the behavioural approach reduce people to passive objects being manipulated by health professionals?
- What reinforcements do you think would be appropriate for medical staff to use in a hospital setting?
- If someone is on a medically advised weight-reducing diet, success will be reinforced by praise from doctors, family and friends. Why is this not an effective reinforcer and why is it so hard to resist eating crisps and chocolate?
- If playing a fruit machine (or the National Lottery) gave too few prizes, people would soon stop playing. Why?

OBSERVATIONAL LEARNING

This model suggests that behaviour patterns can be learned by watching other people's behaviour. Many clinical skills are learned in this way. Both voluntary and involuntary responses can be learned by modelling.

Children who were going to be admitted to hospital were shown a film of an unstressed child going into hospital, undergoing surgery and going home. Compared with others who were shown an unrelated film they showed less anxiety both before and after the operation (Saile et al 1988). The closer in age and sex the model was to themselves, the more imitation took place. However, the films may have reduced the anxiety of the parents as much as the children so that the child had a very powerful model of an unanxious parent to imitate as well! In the same way, anxiety or embarrassment shown by a doctor will be quickly picked up and learned by a patient. Doctors and medical staff are powerful models.

PRACTICAL APPLICATION

Behaviour therapy has been widely used to modify undesirable behaviour patterns.

Systematic desensitisation
Systematic desensitisation or graded exposure would treat a phobia such as Albert's learned fear of furry animals by gradually exposing the person to the feared object while replacing the anxiety with a relaxed condition. This can be achieved by reassurance or relaxation training. In a diabetic outpatient clinic someone with a needle phobia might be treated by such methods so that they can tolerate injections. Initially this might be done by imagination alone, by visualising the object, and once this is achieved without fear, the syringe could be introduced in the form of a picture. Later it might be shown in vivo, firstly at a distance and then gradually brought nearer (see p. 113).

Token economies
Although used successfully in institutions in the past, token economies have now been questioned on ethical and health grounds, but the approach has been adapted for other health problems. Tokens are given for specific behaviour patterns such as feeding and washing and these can be exchanged for cigarettes or sweets. Children who manage their own diabetic monitoring and diet management may be rewarded using a system of treats.

Learning factual material
Medical students find that they have to learn and recall difficult material (see pp. 26–27). Various strategies have been proposed to help this. *Mnemonics* can be associations of two words or letters, or a word and a visual image. *Rehearsal* can establish words in long term memory, and this is most effective if they are *organised*. Many students make lists, or maps of a topic.

Case study

Night waking in children can be a problem for both child and parents. An otherwise healthy and happy child of age 2 woke up regularly at night, and early in the morning. His parents were becoming exhausted because of broken sleep; they were becoming irritable with each other and their work was suffering.

The parents were asked to monitor their behaviour when the child woke up. They described how they gave the child a drink, read him a story and sometimes took him into their own bed to settle him. It was pointed out that these were acting as reinforcers, as well as the drink filling his bladder causing soaking nappies in the morning.

The parents then left him to cry for longer before responding and gave him minimal attention in the night. Reinforcers were given for sleeping through the night such as giving cuddles and toys in his own bed, not the parents'. Within a few weeks the broken nights were fewer and the child's behaviour was further reinforced by having happy, rested parents.

How do we learn?
- Learning is a relatively stable change in behaviour and may occur by operant conditioning, classical conditioning or observationally.
- Operant conditioning has been used to change health behaviour and is based on principles of reinforcement, punishment, extinction and shaping.
- Principles of learning have been used in behaviour therapy to modify undesired behaviour patterns.

PERCEPTION

Why do we perceive what we do? How does the brain process information so that what we see or hear is what we create, not what is actually 'out there'? This spread shows how perception is not a passive process, but is active, creating and constructing our world. Whereas *sensation* (the stimulus which impacts upon the sense organs) provides the raw data about the environment, it is *perception* which provides meaning.

The main emphasis in this spread will be on visual perception, but these points also apply to other types of perception such as auditory, olfactory or tactile perception.

THE MAIN FEATURES OF PERCEPTION

- **Perception is knowledge-based and partly learned**. For example, early works of art show that artists (and young children) have to learn about perspective; likewise, your perception of pathological signs on a slide under a microscope improves with medical education.
- **Perception is inferential**. When we see part of an object, like the top half of a person sitting at a table, we perceive them as a 'whole' person, not half a person.
- **It is categorical**. We tend to categorise what we see, so that a variety of clinical signs are perceived as a disease in a patient, even though they may not in fact be related.
- **Perception is relational**. What we perceive as small or large depends on context. A 2 cm flesh wound on an adult is seen as less serious than the same size of wound on a child.
- **Perception is adaptive**. We tend to perceive significant things better than insignificant things. For example, we notice a car which is moving more than we notice a stationary vehicle: this is more important for our survival.

WHAT ARE ILLUSIONS, AND WHY ARE WE SUBJECT TO THEM?

Illusions demonstrate how creative a process perception is, because the stimuli are ambiguous, or presented in a context which distorts our perception. Figure 1 (a, b) illustrates this.

We are subject to illusions, not because we are unintelligent or not paying attention, but because the brain interprets reality in the light of our prior experience.

HOW DO WE RECOGNISE WHAT IS PERCEIVED?

Recognition is organising what is perceived into something meaningful by using past experience. A number of theories exist to explain how this is done:

- **Bottom-up processing**. The perceptual system is assumed to analyse a stimulus into a set of features and then the brain matches it to other sets already existing in the brain. If a match occurs, then recognition occurs. For example, in examining a rash, a general practitioner takes note of the shape, type, size, colour and distribution of spots on the skin, then matches them, for example, to previous cases of measles that he has seen, or the colour illustration and description of measles that he has seen in a textbook.
- **Top-down processing**. The context creates expectancy and sets up what is known as 'perceptual set'. If some stimuli are presented, we 'see' what we expect, or want to see, and recognition occurs. For example, the general practitioner learns from the patient that he has been in contact with someone suffering from German measles. This creates an expectancy, and a perceptual set when examining the patient's rash. It can sometimes lead to misdiagnosis when the expectancy is strong.
- **Both mechanisms together**. In trying to read a page of poor handwriting we may use both processes: puzzling out what each letter looks like, as well as guessing meaning from the context. Figure 2 shows how you do this.

(a) Ponzo

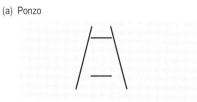

(b) Muller–Lyer

Fig. 1 In these two figures, the sets of horizontal lines are the same length, but we see them as differing lengths according to the rest of the drawing.

 STOP THINK What factors may help to explain why one 45-year-old man perceives his symptoms of dyspepsia as severe and serious, whereas another similarly aged man perceives them as trivial? (See also pp. 86–87)

HOW DO WE INFLUENCE PERCEPTION?

We control our perception by paying attention to different aspects of our environment. Attention is the directing and focusing of perception. It may be:

- **Selective**. We attend more to stimuli that are changing, repeated, intense and personally meaningful. For example, the cocktail party phenomenon: we can hear our own name spoken across a crowded noisy room, although we cannot hear anything else. Certain words catch our attention, for example our names, words connected with significant interests, or important concerns such as words like 'sex' (this phenomenon is used by advertisers to draw our attention to their products!).
- **Divided or focused**. Our ability to divide attention is limited, although it can be improved with practice. It is easier to divide attention if two different types of stimuli are used. For example, you can probably look at pictures and listen to music simultaneously, but it is hard to read and listen to someone talking at the same time.
- **Negatively affected by stress and fatigue**. When we are tired, or when there are more demands being placed

What does this squiggle mean?

Analysis of features alone will not tell you.

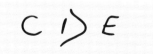

Context is also needed.

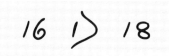

Fig. 2 **Interpretation in context.**

upon us than there are resources to meet those demands, our attention may decrease. This can have disastrous results. Tired doctors are more likely to make errors because they are no longer able to pay full attention to all the details of a particular set of diagnostic signs.

THE RELEVANCE OF THE PSYCHOLOGY OF PERCEPTION TO MEDICINE

The brain is an active component of the perceptual process. Brain damage will result in perceptual distortion, hence an early indicator of organic damage may be perceptual disturbance.

There is often no such thing as the 'correct' way to perceive something: perceptions vary because the perceptual process is a creative one. Obviously most of the time we do not notice this, but sometimes the differences are critical. A pathologist may carry out a post-mortem examination for the police, with an assumption about the cause of death. It may lead them to seek, identify and report an incomplete set of evidence. A second pathologist may discover another, highly significant sign which can change the course of the police enquiry completely.

We are prone to see what the context indicates we should see. Given ambiguous cues we 'recognise' things according to our expectations. A set of ambiguous symptoms presented by a patient will be perceived differently according to our expectations and past experience, not 'objective' reality.

Attention can be divided, with practice. When you start to acquire a skill (e.g. taking blood from a patient, fitting a contraceptive coil) it is almost impossible to do anything else at the same time, such as talking reassuringly to the patient. In time, however, the skill of attending to both aspects of the patient encounter simultaneously can be learned. Stressed and tired doctors become progressively less able to attend appropriately and to do more than one thing at once.

SOCIAL PERCEPTION

Past experience

We may be influenced by our previous experience when making a diagnosis (see Case study). Our perception of people may also be influenced by our past experience. For example, we tend to be more positive towards physically attractive people. In studies of social perception people were asked to choose the company

Case study
We see what we expect to see

A junior doctor, just starting in obstetrics and gynaecology, admitted a pregnant woman late one afternoon. She was complaining of stomach pains. The doctor had herself been in hospital on and off during her pregnancy with a series of minor complaints. She carried out a physical examination, as well as asking the patient for an account of her symptoms, and then recommended bed rest. A second junior doctor was covering the ward at night and was asked to check the patient. His aunt had recently been admitted for an ectopic pregnancy. He immediately suggested an ultrasound scan, although the scanning unit was closed for the night. As a result, a life-threatening ectopic pregnancy was detected, and a successful operation was immediately carried out.

with whom they would prefer to watch television. Most expressed a preference for people who were not physically disabled. In many cases this may be due simply to a lack of experience with disabled people. Congenital deformities may, at first, seem distressing but as you become familiar with such patients you will find that the deformity becomes less distressing and less pertinent. In a sense you no longer 'see' the deformity. Instead you are able to see past these to the people within.

Cognitive constructs

Our impression of people depends on our cognitive constructs. These include sociability, likeability and intelligence. The constructs that we use depend on the context and the people. You will use different constructs when forming impressions of people that you meet at party from those that you use when seeing patients in an outpatient clinic. Sometimes we make errors in assuming that the behaviour of hospital patients is because of their personality rather the situation of being ill in hospital (see pp. 98–99). On the other hand you may also attribute a patient's behaviour to having a particular disease rather than the fact that he/she really does behave in that manner.

SCHEMAS

We have many expectations of other people's behaviour. These are called *schemas*. For example, we expect certain behaviour from waiters in a restaurant, students expect certain standards of behaviour from their lecturers and doctors expect certain behaviour patterns from their patients. Schemas influence what we see even if the behaviour has not occurred. The diagnostic process may involve schemas When you make inferences you may fill in the gaps about the relationship between symptoms. You use schemas in order to do this. The trouble

is, you can make inferences which are in fact not true. You may assume that a patient from a certain part of the country will have certain characteristics which may not be the case, or you might assume that because someone is of a particular sex that individual will behave in certain ways. For example, because you are talking with a young mother you might assume that she is not working outside the home and can therefore attend the clinic at any time with her children. In fact, she may well be a single mother in full-time employment.

We also have schemas about ourselves, called *self schemas*. We retain information about ourselves and this may influence our selective perception.

Patients have schemas too. For example, anxious patients may have a belief that they are unable to cope. Depressed patients may have negative self schemas in which they view themselves as inadequate, hopeless and worthless. These schemas influence what they see, think, feel and do. For example, patients who are depressed will be much less able to solve day to day problems than other people because they do not believe themselves capable of doing so. Telling them to pull themselves together would be pointless. They have no belief in their ability to be competent.

Perception
- Perception is an active, creative process.
- Perception depends on the brain's ability to interpret the senses.
- Attention is part of the perceptual process, and it too can be affected by a variety of psychological factors such as previous experience, motivation, and fatigue.

WHAT IS EMOTION?

Any attempt to understand the psychological reactions of patients to physical disease will involve the study of emotional experiences. The very process of going to see a doctor often generates emotions which may in turn influence the patient's behaviour in a variety of ways; for example, anxiety or embarrassment may obscure symptom reporting, or it may affect retention and understanding of information given (see pp. 112–113).

For many years emotions were considered beyond scientific analysis because they are not overt behaviours. Now researchers in many different disciplines are studying the links between emotions and other psychological processes.

Emotions are:

- transient, subjective experiences
- intentional, evaluative states, i.e. they relate to or are directed at an object and are either positive or negative
- not initiated but 'happen' to us and depend in part upon our cognitive appraisal of a situation and its personal relevance
- accompanied by facial and bodily responses, for example changes in heart rate, sweating.

In humans, facial expressions play a major role in communicating emotions and it is estimated that there are 6000–7000 different facial responses. Certain emotional expressions (for example, a smile or an 'angry' face) seem to be universal because these expressions can be found across different cultures and do not need to be 'taught' (Fig. 1). Facial expressions communicate emotion and may also play a role in affecting the *strength* of emotional experience; asking people to exaggerate their facial expressions to emotional stimuli increases the intensity of the emotions they report.

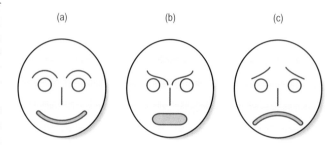

Fig. 1 **Universally-recognised facial expressions of emotion. (a)** Happy; **(b)** angry; **(c)** sad.

far away, as excitement or surprise). The act of labelling a pattern of arousal is dependent upon an 'attribution', which can be defined as a belief about the cause(s) of an event. A medical example would be a patient's belief that their symptoms are due to side-effects of a medication they are taking, rather than illness-related.

More recent theories of emotion have placed particular emphasis on cognitive appraisal as a necessary condition for emotional experience. Lazarus (1991) believes that emotions are determined by the way in which we evaluate and interpret a situation. One possible reaction to the detection of a breast lump is denial, which would clearly influence the emotion experienced.

THEORIES OF EMOTION

One of the earliest theories of emotion, the **James–Lange theory**, held that bodily responses are central to the experience of emotion. Using the example of coming across a bear in the woods, William James asked the question, 'Do we run because we are afraid, or are we afraid because we run?'. He argued that the latter was true. In other words he suggested that bodily responses *precede* the experience of emotion. A medical analogy to the bear example is a woman who detects a lump while carrying out breast self-examination. According to this theory, the woman will first notice bodily changes such as her heart beating faster or trembling, and her perception of these changes will cause her to feel afraid.

An alternative to this is the **Cannon–Bard theory**, which fits in more with the 'common sense' view that there is a direct *central* experience of emotion. According to this theory, in the case of the woman who detects a lump in her breast, the brain registers this information and directly generates the emotion of fear, independently of any peripheral bodily responses that may or may not occur. Early versions of this theory which held that this central brain process occurred in the thalamus have been discredited. More modern views are that different parts of the central nervous system may be involved in producing different emotions.

A third theory by **Schachter and Singer** emphasised the role of perception and cognitive labelling of bodily responses. The perception of a bear triggers physiological arousal, this arousal is noticed by the individual and, *in the light of the situation*, the emotion is labelled as fear (or, if the bear is sufficiently

> **STOP THINK**
>
> Consider the range of possible emotions different hospital in-patients about to undergo minor surgery may experience (see pp. 100–101). For some, this situation may arouse intense feelings of fear, whereas for other patients, the experience might be one of relief (for example, that after months of being on a waiting list, the operation is finally being done!). Now consider some other factors which might influence how this situation is understood/perceived. Past experiences in hospital, personality factors and beliefs about possible 'risks' are important as well as desirability, control, reactions of hospital staff and importance of the outcome of surgery.

EVIDENCE

Figure 2 outlines the different theories of how emotion is caused. The James–Lange theory would predict that each emotion should be associated with different patterns of autonomic changes. This is supported by the observation that while anger and fear both cause heart rate to rise, anger increases, whereas fear reduces, blood flow to the hands and feet (hence the expression 'getting cold feet'). An implication of this theory is that if a person does not receive feedback of peripheral bodily changes, then they should not experience emotion. The effects of beta-blockers, which reduce physiological arousal and may also reduce the experience of anxiety, are consistent with this view. Patients with spinal cord injuries experience the full range of

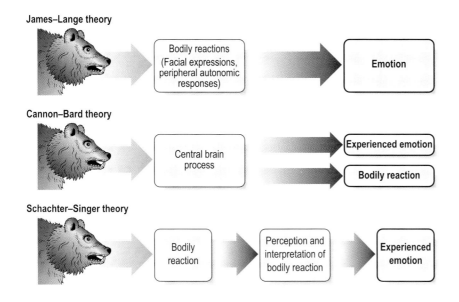

Fig. 2 **Theories of emotion.**

emotions, but often with diminished intensity. Moreover, the higher in the spinal cord the damage occurred (and therefore the less sensory feedback of the autonomic system to the brain), the greater the reduction in the intensity of emotion experienced. Although there is some evidence for the James–Lange theory, many psychologists maintain that in addition to different patterns of autonomic arousal, our interpretation of the situation is important in differentiating emotions.

There is growing evidence for 'updated' versions of the Cannon–Bard theory, that emotions occur through activation of specific parts of the central nervous system; this evidence is also not consistent with the other theories of emotion. For many years attempts have been made to locate areas of the brain responsible for 'producing' emotion. Recent research suggests that the frontal and temporal lobes, and part of the limbic system, play an important role. There is also evidence that our perception of emotions may be more dependent upon the right than upon the left cerebral hemisphere.

The Schachter–Singer theory predicts that if emotional arousal is attributed to a *non-emotional* cause, then the intensity of the experienced emotion should be reduced. Studies have tested this hypothesis by manipulating the way in which people interpret their physiological arousal in order to test whether this affects the kind of emotions they reported.

In a well-known study by Schachter and Singer (1962) (Fig. 3), subjects were injected with adrenaline to produce physiological arousal. One group were told

about the drug's likely side-effects; other subjects were either told to expect 'false' side-effects, or were given no information about the drug's effects. Each subject was then placed in a situation intended to induce different emotions. This was done by having another 'subject', who was actually a confederate of the experimenter, act in either an 'angry' or 'happy' way in front of the subject. According to Schachter's theory, the group who were correctly informed about the side-effects of the drug should be less affected by the confederate's behaviour because they have already had an explanation for their physiological arousal. On the other hand, the group receiving no information about the drug's effects would be most likely to be affected by the situational 'cues', labelling their emotion as either 'happy' or 'angry', depending on the confederate's behaviour. The results largely supported these predictions, although later attempts to replicate these findings have been unsuccessful.

Other research has demonstrated that increased physiological arousal, regardless of how it comes about, can intensify emotional experiences. For example, studies have shown that physiological arousal induced by physical exercise results in subjects reporting more intense feelings of like or dislike when meeting members of the opposite sex.

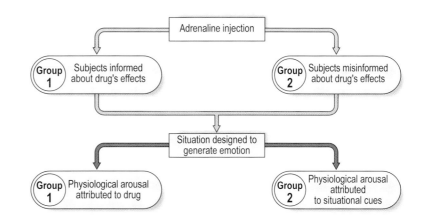

Fig. 3 **Schachter and Singer's (1962) experiment.**

What is emotion?

- Emotions are transient, subjective experiences which include the following components: internal bodily responses, facial expression, a belief or 'cognitive appraisal' that a particular situation is positive or negative.
- Facial expressions are the primary means by which we communicate our emotions to others. Certain facial expressions appear to be universal, found in cultures across the world.
- Theories of how emotion is caused usually focus on the feedback from bodily reactions (James–Lange theory), on the activation of parts of the central nervous system (Cannon–Bard theory), or on the cognitive appraisal or interpretation of a situation (Schachter–Singer theory).
- The frontal and temporal lobes, and parts of the limbic system, have been implicated as important regions of the brain for producing emotion. The right hemisphere is considered to play a more important role than the left hemisphere in our perception of emotion.

MEMORY AND FORGETTING

We are all familiar with lapses of memory — not being able to put a name to a face; forgetting to keep an appointment; poor recall during an exam. Psychologists have learned a great deal about the process of memory this century both through laboratory-based experiments and by studying patients with brain damage which results in unique forms of memory loss. Although a very simplified view, the diagram outlined in Figure 1 is a useful summary of a widely-held model of memory. Items are initially held in a short-term memory (STM) store and whether they become permanently represented in a long-term memory (LTM) store will depend on a host of factors such as how important and interesting they are, and whether we engage in active rehearsal strategies to encode items into permanent memory.

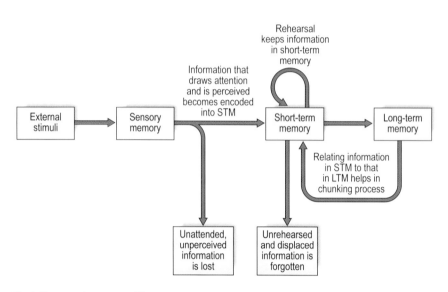

Fig. 1 **Memory: short-term and long-term storage.**

STAGES OF MEMORY

If we listen to a list of unrelated words read out to us, and then are required to recall the words immediately, items presented either first or last are better remembered than those in the middle. This better recall for the more recent items is because we are retrieving them directly from the short-term memory store. If we were to delay recall of the word list by 30 seconds, then this recency effect disappears (Fig. 2).

Even items which do successfully enter into long-term memory may not be recalled when we need them, but are recalled much later. This illustrates the problem of *retrieval*. When a book has been stored in a library, if we lose the catalogue slip, then the book is very difficult to find. This problem of memory loss is clearly very different from being unable to locate the book because it was never stored correctly in the first place. A good practical illustration of this distinction is the difference between testing your knowledge about anatomy by *recall* (describe the structure of the brain) and *recognition* (which of the following is part of the limbic system — medulla, amygdala, motor cortex?). Multiple choice exam questions have already carried out the retrieval part of remembering, leaving only the recognition component to be necessary.

When we consider the problems of forgetting and the poor memory of head-injured and elderly patients, and we are trying to devise methods to aid recall, we need to have clear ideas about the stage at which the process is disturbed. Is it the initial learning which is defective or do those with poor memories simply forget more quickly?

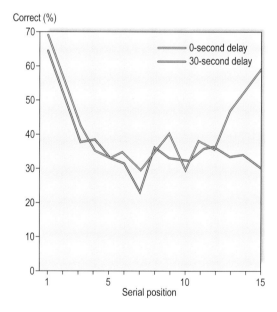

Fig. 2 **The recency effect and short-term storage.**

HOW MUCH CAN WE REMEMBER?

Realising that we have seen a film previously, but only about 10 minutes before its end, or revisiting a childhood home and having a flood of forgotten memories, are powerful experiences which may tempt us into thinking that we do indeed store all events, and given the right conditions, could retrieve such memories. Although there are well-documented cases of people with exceptional memories (one fascinating account is provided by the Russian neuropsychologist Luria), there is no scientific evidence to support this 'videotape' view of memory. To acquire permanent representation in memory we need to organise the new material and establish connections with the existing LTM store. Hence the use of mnemonic techniques which rely on devices such as learning a list of items in relation to an easily-remembered rhyme, or first letter mnemonics such as Richard Of York Gave Battles In Vain for the colours of the visible spectrum. Memory 'tricks' like this should not be scoffed at and have proved useful in helping elderly patients remember people's names.

STOP THINK
- Can you recall the moment you first encountered a younger sibling? Your first day at school? Why are such memories more enduring?
- What were you doing on March 15th last year?

HELPING PATIENTS TO REMEMBER BETTER

When patients have been asked to recall what they have been told during a consultation, they have been found to forget almost half (see pp. 90–93). Memory for medical advice as opposed to diagnostic information can be particularly poor especially in the case of highly anxious or elderly patients. Statements made early in the consultation are more likely to enter LTM (the primacy effect) and those at the end are remembered better initially but then tend to be forgotten (the recency effect). General or abstract statements are more difficult to remember than more specific concrete suggestions. Researchers have concluded that patient recall is aided by following some simple rules:

- Give the most important information early in any set of instructions.

- Stress importance of relevant items (e.g. by repetition).
- Use explicit categorisation under simple headings (e.g. 'I will tell you what is wrong … what treatment you will need … what you can do to help yourself').
- Make advice specific, detailed and concrete rather than general and abstract.

MEMORY AFTER TRAUMATIC BRAIN INJURY

Memory problems often follow accidental trauma from a closed head injury. In their most dramatic form, the patient may be unable to recall not only the events leading up to the accident, but for many years prior to that. This memory loss extending backwards in time is known as retrograde amnesia, as distinct from the inability to form new memories which is known as anterograde amnesia. Such a patient may well report themselves as 10 years younger than they are, and be unable to recall all the events of those 10 years such as marriage, birth of children, employment, etc. At the same time, they will repeatedly need to be told why they are in hospital, and the names of the nurses and doctors caring for them. Eventually these years of memory loss will be recovered, indicating that the problem was difficulty of retrieval, but they may be left with enduring deficits of memory which may be secondary to attentional or concentration difficulties. The exact nature of the deficit will require extensive testing by a neuropsychologist. (A collection of essays dealing with the effects of brain damage can be found in Sacks 1986.)

Case study

HM is an engineering worker who in 1953, in his late twenties, was operated upon in an experimental procedure intended to relieve his incapacitating and worsening epileptic seizures. The operation involved a radical bilateral medial temporal lobe resection, destroying the anterior two-thirds of the hippocampus, as well as the uncus and amygdala. It was successful in alleviating the epileptic symptoms, but left HM with a profound memory impairment. Although he can remember events he experienced and facts he acquired up to 2 years before his operation, he can remember essentially nothing that has occurred since. He recalls nothing of day-to-day events in his own life or the world at large. He does not know what he had for lunch an hour ago, how he came to be where he is now, where he has left objects used recently, or that he has used them. He reads the same magazines over and over again. He has learned neither the names of doctors and psychologists who have worked with him for decades nor the route to the house he moved to a few years after his surgery. Yet despite such difficulties he is not intellectually impaired. His language comprehension and production and conversational skills are normal, he can reason competently and do mental arithmetic. His IQ measured in 1962 was an above average 117 — higher than the 104 measured pre-surgery in 1953. This neurological dissociation supports the idea that the temporary retention of information in working memory and the permanent storage of new information depend on different brain mechanisms (for a more lengthy account of HM's problems see Hilts 1995).

STOP THINK
- How would you set about establishing the extent of retrograde amnesia in a patient for whom you have no autobiographical information?

ORGANIC AMNESIA

Permanent memory loss is a very serious problem necessitating continuous care of such patients. These instances of organic amnesia may be due to long-term alcohol abuse and development of Korsakoff's syndrome; to the brain damage from viral encephalitis; or to other surgical interventions. In all such cases where the memory loss is primary and not secondary to other cognitive deficits, patients are likely to have suffered damage to components of the limbic system, with the hippocampus being a key structure. One such case has been very widely reported in the scientific literature (see Case study).

Memory and forgetting

- The distinction is clear between registration, retrieval, recall, and recognition processes in memory.
- Different kinds of memory mechanisms underlie STM and LTM, as shown by the serial position effect and the nature of the amnesic syndrome in brain-damaged patients.
- Improving memory recall by means of mnemonic aids is especially useful for unconnected items and events.

HOW DOES SEXUALITY DEVELOP?

Sexual identity and sexual behaviour are fundamental in the development of the person and the relevant influences are diverse and complex. The nature of sexuality is such that it has an important effect on health and well-being, and is in turn strongly influenced by these factors. For this reason, it is helpful to understand the development of sexuality.

GENDER IDENTITY

Biological influences

Gender identity (whether you feel male or female) usually coincides with sexual identity indicated by chromosomes, hormones, and sexual organs, but this is not always the case. Biological indices can occasionally be abnormal so that gender may be ambiguous or contradictory.

The sex chromosomes determined at conception, and the subsequent hormonal activity in the fetus, set the pattern for development of the internal and external sex organs, and the sexual differentiation of the brain. There are exceptions. For example, abnormal chromosomes may give rise to a definite gender identity, but altered sexual organs and atypical social and sexual behaviour; or a fetus with normal chromosomes may be exposed to unusual levels of hormones in utero. Some mothers given progestogens to prevent abortion had daughters who developed genital abnormalities and atypical sexual and social behaviour.

Cultural factors

During puberty, gender identity becomes linked to sexual activity. There is often a period of sexual experimentation before individuals feel confident of their orientation. In the development of homosexual orientation, there is some evidence for a genetic factor: monozygotic twins show higher concordance than dizygotic twins, but cultural factors and individual learning experiences will also determine attraction to a partner.

Social and cultural influences

Psychological influences on gender start at birth with the family, where interactions are determined by the perceived sex of the baby (Fig. 1). This process quickly extends to peers, school and the media. It is thought that a core gender identity is fixed by about the age of four.

Cultural pressures may delay the acceptance of sexual identity, since in many societies variations from the norm are not accepted. It may take a long period of adjustment and considerable courage to 'come out', accepting one's own sexuality and letting others know. Fear of one's sexuality being discovered may lead to secretive or reclusive life-styles and can be the source of enormous distress.

STOP THINK Transvestism (most commonly males dressing in female clothing) has always taken place in many societies, either as entertainment for others or in secret. Many cross-dressers have no wish to change their sexual identity, but get pleasure from cross-dressing. Sexual excitement is sometimes involved, but at other times cross-dressing is done in private to comfort the individual and to relieve stress. What does this say about society's sex-role stereotypes and expectations of men?

THE DEVELOPMENT OF SEXUAL ACTIVITY

Although some sexual behaviour (genital play and stimulation) is seen in infants, the level of activity rises before puberty and this takes the form of sexual play with other children or solitary genital stimulation (masturbation). Peers are the major source of knowledge about sexual behaviour.

The age at which sexual intercourse first takes place varies not only from culture to culture, but across time and according to class. The average age of first intercourse has fallen in the last 40 years in the UK from 21 to 17 (see Table 1). In the 1960s, surveys in Europe showed that sexual activity including intercourse took place at an earlier age in working class males and females than amongst the middle classes. By the 1970s, the differences were disappearing. Whether this was due to greater awareness of sexual issues, the contraceptive pill, or changes in class structure is not clear.

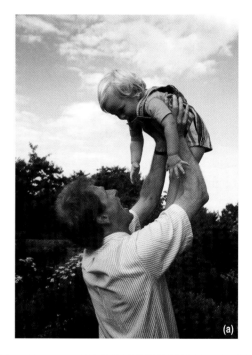

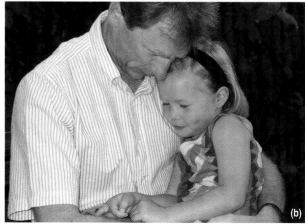

Fig. 1 **Parents play with their offspring in different ways according to the child's gender.** More 'rough and tumble' games with boys (**a**); more talking and cuddling with girls (**b**). This difference can be seen from the baby's birth onwards.

Table 1 **Age at first sexual intercourse by age at interview**

Age at interview	Women		Men	
	Median age at first intercourse	% (No.) reporting first intercourse before age 16	Median age at first intercourse	% (No.) reporting first intercourse before age 16
16–19	17	18.7 (182/971)	17	27.6 (228/827)
20–24	17	14.7 (184/1251)	17	23.8 (271/1137)
25–29	18	10.0 (152/1519)	17	23.8 (268/1126)
30–34	18	8.6 (116/1349)	17	23.2 (235/1012)
35–39	18	5.8 (73/1261)	18	18.4 (181/982)
40–44	19	4.3 (55/1277)	18	14.5 (150/1042)
45–49	20	3.4 (37/1071)	18	13.9 (115/827)
50–54	20	1.4 (13/933)	18	8.9 (61/684)
55–59	21	0.8 (6/716)	20	5.8 (35/603)

Analysis was based on weighted data.

(Source: Wellings et al . BMJ 311: 417–420, 1995)

Apart from the variations in sexual preferences, e.g. homosexuality, the most common pattern of long-term sexual partnership is heterosexual monogamy. Although in many human societies polygamy is part of religious and cultural structures, in practice many men do not take more than one wife at a time, either through lack of availability or resources. Worldwide, the pattern of human attachment is often serial monogamy (one partner after another) rather than lifelong monogamy. The high rates of divorce in the developed world are one example of this.

Sexual activity continues through adulthood into old age (see pp. 14–15). While the sexual behaviour of young adults and those in middle age are written about, discussed, and form the subject of films and plays, the needs of the elderly are seldom portrayed. Sexual interest continues in this age group although functioning changes: for example in post-menopausal women, reduced oestrogen may cause thinning and dryness in the vagina, making intercourse more painful. In men, ageing is associated with increased time to achieve an erection, longer refractory periods and increased need for tactile rather than psychic stimuli. For men these changes are most marked after the age of 70 or so. It may be difficult for the elderly to discuss sexual problems with a doctor because their interest in sex is sometimes seen as inappropriate.

SEXUAL PROBLEMS

Sexual difficulties can arise through problems in functioning (e.g. erectile difficulties in the male, or failure to achieve orgasm in the female); incompatibility (differences in appetite or style of sexual activity); problems of fertility (inability to conceive, or fear of conception); psycho-social problems arising through sexual behaviour (e.g. problems of sexual identity or problems with the law); and sexually transmitted diseases. A number of medical conditions give rise to sexual problems. Most common among these are multiple sclerosis, cardiovascular disease, diabetes, epilepsy, and renal disease. A person who has become dependent on alcohol is also likely to experience sexual problems, and there are prescribed drugs which carry loss of interest, or problems in functioning, as unwanted secondary effects. For example, drugs given to reduce blood pressure may cause erectile and ejaculatory difficulties in men. Psychological factors, especially anxiety and depression, frequently affect sexual interest and performance (see pp. 112–115).

Sexual problems arising from medical conditions or their treatment may be overlooked by doctors through their own embarrassment or that of their patients. Yet many sexual problems can be effectively treated by a combination of approaches: medical interventions (e.g. changing a drug, the use of hormones), surgical interventions (e.g. vascular surgery); or counselling (see pp. 126–127). Counselling can take different forms: examining relationship difficulties; education; reassurance; and behavioural psychotherapy, first expounded by Masters and Johnson (1970). In this approach a couple will tackle a problem in a series of behavioural targets, reviewing progress and discussing difficulties at each session. This has been developed subsequently by the authors and others, and has been extensively evaluated.

Case history

A 29-year-old woman came to see her general practitioner because of infertility. Karen stopped the contraceptive pill 2 years ago but had not conceived. She was well, and reported no relationship difficulties. Her 34-year-old husband, Chris, was a marketing manager on a short-term contract.

Before referral to the infertility clinic, the GP wanted more information and asked to see each partner separately. Both partners said that the frequency of sexual intercourse was low. Karen assumed that this was due to her husband's tiredness through overwork and did not want to add to this by putting pressure on him. Chris acknowledged that he was very anxious about work, had resumed heavier drinking again with a recurrence of gastritis, and was experiencing erectile difficulties. Afraid of impotence, he did not initiate sex, but wished that Karen would do so sometimes. He said that he was too embarrassed to say this to her.

Instead of referral for infertility, they went to a sexual problems clinic for five sessions. There was a ban on intercourse at first to take the pressure off both partners. With the therapist as intermediary, they began to communicate honestly about their own worries and expectations of sex. Chris was given advice on anxiety management and targets for reduced drinking. In their homework, goals were set for increasing sexual activity, which was to be non-threatening but included Karen taking the initiative sometimes. By the fourth session, Chris was drinking 10 units or less per week, and the frequency of intercourse had increased to two or three times per week. Karen conceived 7 months later.

How does sexuality develop?

- Sexual development is influenced by biological, social and cultural factors.
- Difficulties can arise in sexual function, compatibility, fertility, psycho-social function, or as a result of sexually transmitted disease.
- Medical and psychological disorders can interfere with sexual function.
- Sexual problems can be effectively treated by medical or surgical interventions, or by counselling, particularly behavioural psychotherapy.

INTELLIGENCE

Variability in intelligence is one of our most basic human characteristics. Malnutrition, head injury, poor ante-natal and obstetric care, disease, chromosomal abnormalities and ageing can all affect the ability to learn and cope with life. Communicating effectively requires taking into account patients' ability to comprehend medical information. Defining a patient as 'bright' or 'dull' can have important consequences for that individual. (Likewise, whether or not your teachers define you as clever or not will have important consequences for your future!) Intelligence is a value-laden term, which we often use to explain behaviour, but which we have difficulty in defining.

What is intelligence?

A common answer to this question is that intelligence is what intelligence tests measure! Intelligence is a 'construct' — it is not something we can see or touch. Intelligence can only be inferred from behaviour which we think of as 'intelligent'.

Psychologists commonly think of intelligence as consisting of two types of mental ability: fluid intelligence and crystallised intelligence (Cattell 1991). Crystallised intelligence is thought of as acquired capacity, i.e. diverse skills and knowledge acquired in a particular culture. Fluid intelligence, on the other hand, is conceptualised as an unspecialized mental ability. Fluid intelligence enables us to learn from experience, and experience enables us to use fluid intelligence more effectively.

Performances on different kinds of intelligence tests are often highly correlated, which is why psychologists use the term 'general intelligence'. The term 'g' refers to the hypothetical general or common factor which underlies performance on the different types of intelligence tests.

- Are you clever because you are healthy, or healthy because you are clever?
- Do you think you will become more or less intelligent as you age?

How is intelligence measured?

Fluid intelligence is assessed by tasks that measure speed of mental processing, abstractions and generalisation, and relational thinking, as well as the management of large amounts of information over time. Crystallised intelligence is assessed in terms of general knowledge, vocabulary, attainment at school and learned mental skills.

Nowadays performance on intelligence tests is usually scored with 100 as the mean for a given age range. People with an IQ (intelligence quotient) over 130 represent the top 2.5% of the population. An IQ of 148 is required in order to become a member of Mensa, the society for intellectually gifted people.

Those scoring less than 70 (2 standard deviations below the mean) are classified as 'mentally impaired', 'mentally handicapped' or, in the United States, 'mentally retarded'. Terminology has changed over the years in an attempt at destigmatisation. Although it was not always the case, there is now greater recognition that it is unwise to make major educational decisions using a cut off of 70 IQ points.

Are men and women equally intelligent?

Intelligence tests have been constructed so that there are few differences between males and females in test performance. When intelligence tests were first being devised females tended

to perform better. Questions which led to marked male–female difference were removed because it was believed that there were no differences in intelligence between females and males.

Overall equivalence on test performance does not, however, imply equal performance on every type of ability. Males consistently outperform females on visual–spatial tasks such as mental rotation and spatio–temporal tasks, such as tracking a moving object through space. Males also score higher on tests of proportional and mechanical reasoning and on many quantitative abilities. On verbal tasks females tend to outperform males. There are also marked sex differences in dyslexia, with males more likely to be diagnosed with dyslexia or other types of reading disability.

Is it true that there are racial differences in intelligence?

See if you know the answers to the questions in the box below — the answers are at the end of this spread. (Don't cheat and look at the answers before trying the questions!)

Aboriginal IQ test

1. As wallaby is to animal, so cigarette is to _____.
2. Three of the following items may be classified with salt-water crocodile. Which are they? Marine turtle, frilled lizard, budgerigar, black snake.
3. You are out in the bush with your children and you are all hungry. You have a loaded rifle. You see three animals, all within range: a young emu, a large kangaroo, and a small female wallaby. Which should you shoot for food?

Most people in the UK get the answers 'wrong'. This test — The Original Australian Test of Intelligence — provides a good demonstration of the difficulty of developing culture-free intelligence tests. This test was developed for use with Aboriginal people in Australia (Saunders et al 1983).

Many of you will be aware that there are numerous studies showing that Black people, i.e. people of African-American origin, do less well on intelligence tests than White people (Howe 1997). Were you also aware that Oriental or Asian people often do better than White people on intelligence tests? It is curious that whenever the media calls attention to studies or controversies about racial differences on intelligence tests they fail to mention the better performance of Asians and Orientals.

How large are the racial differences in test performance? Most of the research has been done in the United States, where Black Americans score on average 10–15 points lower than White Americans. This fact is not debated; the controversy revolves around interpretations of the difference. Some argue that the difference in test performance is due to group differences in inherited ability. Others point out that the difference can be attributed entirely to environmental and cultural differences.

Is intelligence inherited?

One of the biggest issues which has taxed researchers in the field is the extent to which intelligence is inherited. Most researchers think there is some genetic component, but how much? On average people from the same family have similar IQs. The children of intelligent parents do well on IQ tests, and the children of those who have low IQ scores have lower than average scores. This suggests that intelligence may be, at least partially, inherited.

Most research seems to suggest that between 50–70% of the variability in IQ test scores can be attributed to genetic differences (Chipuer et al 1990).

Does stimulation increase intelligence?

Rats raised in stimulating or even relatively 'normal' environments grow more neurones in the brain than those in deprived environments. It is not known if babies raised in especially stimulating environments grow more neurones. Nevertheless, it is widely believed that stimulation is beneficial (see Case study).

Are there links between health and intelligence?

Intelligence and social class are highly correlated. Those in Social Classes I and II perform, on average, better on intelligence tests than those in Social Classes IV and V. Social class is also associated with health. Mortality and morbidity rates are inversely related to social class (see pp. 44–45) So, yes, there is an association between intelligence and health. The question is whether or not being healthy makes you more intelligent or whether being intelligent helps in some way to make you healthier.

It is not perhaps too difficult to imagine that intelligence and educational level might be related to healthy eating and healthy life styles, which would themselves influence health. It is also not difficult to see how poor health might affect intellectual functioning.

It is now fairly well established that malnutrition and exposure to toxic substances result in lowered intelligence under some conditions. Prolonged malnutrition appears to have long-term effects on intelligence. Intervention with dietary supplements can, however, also have long-term beneficial effects. It is worth noting that the effects on intelligence may be indirect. Malnourished children are less motivated to learn, less responsive to

adults, and less active in exploration than more adequately nourished children.

Toxic chemicals also lower intelligence. Lead has a well-established negative effect, as does extensive ante-natal exposure to alcohol. Ante-natal exposure to aspirin and antibiotics has also been found to be linked to lower IQ (Zigler, Valentine 1979).

Does intelligence decline with age?

For a long time it was thought that intelligence did decline with age. Cross-sectional studies of people of different ages showed fairly large differences between younger and older subjects, with younger people performing much better on intelligence tests. However, the findings from longitudinal studies showed a rather different pattern. On many of the types of intelligence tests, especially those of crystallised intelligence, IQ increased with age, peaking in the mid 50s (Schaie 1990).

Tests of fluid intelligence revealed patterns of performance which are more complicated, and which do show some decline in test performance with age. Tests of fluid intelligence are frequently timed and the much slower reaction times of older people impairs tests performance. Given unlimited time to solve test problems the performance of older and younger people on tests of fluid

intelligence are frequently quite similar. Nevertheless, there is evidence that over time fluid intelligence declines (Fig. 1).

It is the association of speed of information processing with intelligence test performance that has caused some researchers to conceptualise intelligence as merely information processing speed. The idea is that people whom we label as intelligent are those who can process information quickly. Others can learn the same things, but it might take them much longer.

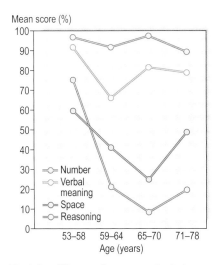

Fig. 1 **Age differences in scores on the factor components of the Primary Mental Abilities (PMA) Test.** (Adapted from Schaie et al 1990).

Case study

The Head Start pre-school programme in the United States which started in the 1960s was designed to provide a stimulating nursery education to children from deprived backgrounds (Neisser et al 1996). Few of the Head Start programmes were properly evaluated so the evidence as to their effectiveness is hard to assess. Some programmes achieved remarkable success, with those participating in the programme scoring 6–10 IQ points higher on entering school, compared to those of a similar background who were not in the Head Start programme. One study found that the gains were still there 12 years later. Some studies, however, indicated that any gains made were quickly lost.

Answers to Aboriginal IQ test

1. The right answer is 'tree'. The Community's earliest contact with tobacco was in the form of a 'stick' tobacco, so it is classified with 'tree'.
2. Crocodiles, turtles, lizards and birds are all classified as minh (animals), while snakes, along with eels, are classified as yak (snake-like creatures).
3. 'Small female wallaby' is the right answer. Emu is a food which may be eaten only by very old people. If parents and children both eat kangaroo, the children will get sick — everyone knows that!

Intelligence

- Intelligence, though hard to define, is conceptualised as being of two types: fluid and crystallised.
- Crystallised intelligence does not appear to decline with age, but fluid intelligence does.
- Asian and Oriental people do better on intelligence tests than Whites and Whites do better than Blacks. Controversy surrounds suggestions that this could be due to genetic differences rather than cultural or environmental differences.
- Men outperform women on tests of spatial ability and women outperform men on tests of verbal reasoning.
- Health and intelligence are highly correlated, but causality is uncertain.
- Providing a stimulating environment to babies and pre-school children appears to increase intelligence, though the effects are not always long lasting.

LEARNING TO SPEAK

Although most children learn to speak at least one language remarkably rapidly and without being explicitly taught, some children do experience difficulties. These difficulties may be either specific to language or associated with other problems, such as a general cognitive delay or a socio-emotional disorder. Health care professionals can help to identify these children so that appropriate interventions can be arranged (usually through referral to a speech and language therapist). An understanding of the ways in which children's language typically develops is essential to effective developmental surveillance. Also, even when language development is progressing normally, children do not always use and understand language in the same way as adults. Knowing about the nature of children's language abilities can help doctors to communicate with children.

THE NATURE OF LANGUAGE DEVELOPMENT

Language is a complex system which is structured on several levels. Children have to acquire several types of abilities in order to produce and understand spoken language.

Phonological development

Children's early attempts at producing language are often idiosyncratic and may differ not only from adults' language but also from that of other children. Individual children sometimes have their own pronunciations for particular words. At around the age of 18 months children usually show evidence of beginning to develop a *phonological system*, in that the way their pronunciations differ from adults' pronunciations can be described by a set of rules known as *phonological processes* which apply to classes of sounds (see Table 1). However, children vary in the extent to which they use phonological processes and in the particular processes used. For instance, one child may show a fronting process, while

another may show deletion of final consonants and another may show a combination of both these processes. In all three cases, there is a system underlying the child's speech, but the nature of the system differs from child to child. Therefore a young child's speech may be difficult for a stranger to understand and yet may be quite readily comprehensible to someone familiar with the child who has had the opportunity to adjust to that particular child's phonological system.

Grammatical development

Children show a tendency to move from producing and comprehending language in unanalysed chunks to developing a more analytical, rule-based system. This shift is illustrated by the stages which children typically go through in acquiring the past tense forms of verbs.

- *Stage 1:* correct uses of both regular (e.g. *walked*) and irregular (e.g. *went*) past tense forms.
- *Stage 2:* overgeneralisation of regular past tense form (*-ed*) to irregular verbs (e.g. *goed*).
- *Stage 3:* correct uses of both regular and irregular past tense forms.

It is generally argued that at Stage 1 children are imitating individual past tense verb forms as unanalysed wholes, whereas at Stage 2 they have abstracted out the regularity that *-ed* refers to the past but are applying this too generally, until at Stage 3 they have identified the exceptions to the general rule. The occurrence of overgeneralisation errors (often beginning at around the age of 3 years) suggests that children are not simply imitating adults' speech (since adults do not typically make such errors) but rather that they are actively working out the rules and regularities which underlie language use, even though they are not necessarily conscious of these rules. This also shows that a child who makes errors is not necessarily less advanced developmentally than one who produces correct linguistic forms — the nature of the

child's underlying linguistic system must be considered.

Semantic development

Research on children's semantic development indicates that children are actively testing out hypotheses about the meanings of words and that their hypotheses are sometimes incorrect. Children sometimes begin to use a particular word in their own speech before they have a full understanding of its meaning. This gives rise to various types of errors:

- *Overextensions* occur when the child uses a word with a meaning which is more general than the meaning which adults would give it. Overextensions are particularly common between the ages of about 2 and 3 years.
- *Underextensions* involve the child using a word with a meaning which is more specific than the meaning which adults would give it.

Sometimes children appear to understand words which they do not use themselves. However, such understanding may draw heavily on non-verbal cues (for example gestures and facial expressions) rather than purely on knowledge of the words' meanings, especially in children younger than about 7 years. Therefore, a child who appears to understand a particular word in one context will not necessarily be able to understand the same word in a different context. Conversely, in cases where non-verbal cues conflict with the spoken message, young children will often respond to the message which is being conveyed non-verbally and thus may appear to have misunderstood the spoken message. For example, a child is unlikely to be reassured if a doctor says 'There's nothing to worry about,' while at the same time looking anxious.

Pragmatic development

Children are usually first introduced to language in contexts where they are communicating with familiar adults about the 'here and now'. Bruner (1983) describes how language is initially used as a tool for talking about activities that an adult and child are engaged in together and for directing one another's attention to aspects of the immediate situation (e.g. while looking at picture books together or playing ritualised games such as peek-a-boo). Ultimately, though, one of the most powerful features of language is the ability which it gives us to communicate about topics divorced from the immediate

Table 1 **Examples of phonological processes**

Process	Description	Examples	
		Adult	**Child**
Cluster reduction	Where several consonants occur together, the cluster is simplified by deleting one or more consonants.	*Crisps* *Stop*	*Cips* *Top*
Final consonant deletion	Consonants are deleted from the ends of words.	*Car* *Sweet*	*Ca* *Swee*
Fronting	Consonants which are pronounced at the front of the vocal tract are substituted for those pronounced at the back of the vocal tract.	*Coat* *Game*	*Toat* *Dame*

Case study

Tim is four years old and has recently been diagnosed as suffering from asthma. Consider the following conversation in which Tim's GP is trying to communicate with him about how to control his asthma.

GP: *Do you know what this is?* (holding up an inhaler)
Tim: *Yes.*
GP: *What is it?*
Tim: *A puffer.*
GP: *Yes, but its proper name is an inhaler. When should you use your inhaler?*
Tim: *Don't know.*
GP: *Well, you should use it when you are feeling wheezy or when you are going to do something that usually makes you wheeze, like running or stroking a cat. Can you tell me when you should use your inhaler?*
Tim: *Before I stroke the cat.*
GP: *Good. Does stroking the cat make you wheeze?*
Tim: *No.*

This GP's style of conversation has many of the characteristics of school talk. Contrast this with the following conversation in which another GP, talking to a similar child called Kate, uses a style of communication which aims to mimic home talk.

GP: *Now, let's see what I've got here.* (Taking inhaler out of briefcase and handing it to Kate.)
Kate: *A puffer. I've got a puffer too.*
GP: *Yes, I know.*
Kate: *Is that your puffer?*
GP: *Yes, but this one is just to show to people. I don't need to use it. Do you know why you need to use your puffer?*
Kate: *Because I get wheezy sometimes. What's that?* (Pointing at booklet of pictures which GP has picked up from desk.)
GP: *It's a picture book. Let's have a look through it and see if we can find some of the things that make you wheeze. We could take turns to say what is in the picture. Maybe Daddy would like to join in too.* (GP, Kate and her father look through the book together and discuss the pictures in relation to Kate's asthma.)
Kate: *There's some children running in a race.* (Pointing at picture).
Father: *You like running in races, don't you, Kate?*
Kate: *Yes, but when I run fast I sometimes start wheezing and I have to sit down for a rest.*
GP: *Well, you could try using your puffer before you run and that might stop you from getting wheezy.*

What do you think are the main differences between the two conversational styles in the Case study?

context. Therefore it is important that children develop the ability to use language in a range of social contexts.

In particular, when children start attending nursery or school, they will encounter a different style of language use from what they were accustomed to in the home. Tizard and Hughes (1984) found that the communication abilities which 4-year-old children demonstrated when talking to their mothers in the home context were far superior to those which they demonstrated when talking to their teachers in the nursery school context. Furthermore, the discrepancy

in communication abilities between the two contexts was even more marked for children who came from working-class backgrounds than for those from middle-class backgrounds. These findings have two important implications. First, they suggest that social class differences in language use may make the transition from home to nursery/school more difficult for working-class children than for middle-class children. This may be one of the factors contributing to social class differences in educational achievement, which in turn are thought to be related to inequalities in health (see pp. 48–49).

Second, Tizard's findings suggest that one way of enhancing the effectiveness of communication with young children in clinical situations would be to try to incorporate some of the features of home talk. The following characteristics of 'home talk' and 'school talk' have been identified by Wells (1983) and Tizard and Hughes (1984) (see Case study).

Home talk is:

- mostly initiated by the child
- concerned with immediate shared interests and activities
- supported by the shared knowledge and experiences of the participants
- characterised by a sense of reciprocity and by the joint negotiation of meaning and purpose between the child and the adult.

School talk is:

- mostly initiated and controlled by the teacher
- concerned with the teacher asking questions for the child to answer to display his or her knowledge
- less supported by shared knowledge (since the participants are less familiar with one another)
- characterised by an emphasis on explicit, grammatically correct language.

PRACTICAL IMPLICATIONS

Communication with young children can usually be enhanced by:

- using a conversational style which mimics home talk
- working closely with someone who is familiar with the child and so is likely to be used to any idiosyncrasies in the child's linguistic system
- using non-verbal communication (for example, demonstrations with toys, pointing to pictures/objects) to support and reinforce spoken messages
- ensuring that verbal and non-verbal messages are not in conflict.

Learning to speak

- There are four main aspects of language development: phonological, grammatical, semantic and pragmatic.
- Children's uses of language are influenced by their underlying linguistic system, which sometimes differs from that of adults and other children.
- Young children's linguistic abilities are very context-sensitive.

HOW DOES THINKING DEVELOP?

Do children simply know less than adults or do children and adults think in qualitatively different ways? For example, are children just as capable as adults of understanding why they are ill or why they should take their medication, if they are presented with the relevant information? Or do children under a certain age lack the necessary concepts to make sense of such explanations? Questions like these are addressed by psychological research into cognitive development, which investigates age-related changes in intellectual abilities.

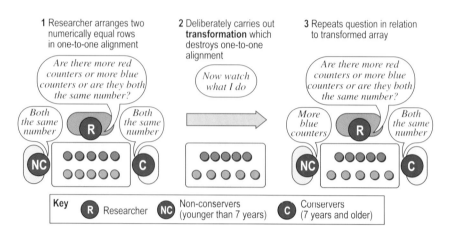

Fig. 1 **Conservation of number task.**

DIFFERING VIEWS OF COGNITIVE DEVELOPMENT

Jean Piaget (1896–1980) revolutionised the study of cognitive development by arguing that young children do not just know less than older children and adults, but that they view the world in radically different ways. For example, on the basis of his research findings, Piaget argued that until the age of about 7 years, children are not able to reason logically and lack fundamental concepts in such areas as number and causality.

Most researchers agree with Piaget's general claims that:

• Cognitive development is influenced by an interaction between biological and environmental factors.
• Children play an active role in acquiring knowledge and making sense of their world.
• Children's thinking is sometimes qualitatively different from adults'.

On the other hand, many researchers (e.g. Donaldson 1978) have challenged certain aspects of Piaget's views and have argued that he has tended to underestimate:

• young children's logical competence and conceptual understanding
• the influence of contextual factors on children's performance
• the extent to which children's performance depends on their familiarity with the specific content of reasoning tasks.

To illustrate these differing views, we will consider two aspects of cognitive development: understanding of number and of causality.

UNDERSTANDING OF NUMBER

To investigate children's ability to reason about numerical relationships, Piaget used tasks like the one in Figure 1. He found that children younger than about 7 years typically changed their answer when the question was repeated after the transformation, and he described these children as 'non-conservers'. In contrast, children of about 7 years and upwards typically succeeded on the task and were therefore classed as 'conservers'. Piaget interpreted young children's failure to conserve as being symptomatic of their inability to reason logically: they lack an understanding of general principles, such as that the number of objects in a set is independent of their spatial arrangement.

However, other researchers have found that young children's performance on conservation tasks can be improved by modifying the way the task is presented. For example, when the transformation was carried out by a 'naughty teddy' character who likes to 'mess up games', many more 4- to 6-year-old children responded correctly than when the transformation was carried out deliberately by the researcher (Donaldson 1978). In interpreting this finding, Donaldson argues that the deliberate nature of the transformation in Piaget's version of the task misleads children into inferring that it is relevant to the question which follows it, and thus into misinterpreting the question as referring to length. This type of reasoning is characteristic of what Donaldson terms *embedded* thinking, in which the child actively attempts to make sense of the total situation by attending to non-verbal cues as well as to what is said and by making inferences about other people's intentions. Young children, according to Donaldson, are capable of reasoning logically, but they are most likely to demonstrate this in contexts where they can exploit their understanding of human purposes and where non-verbal cues support the spoken message.

UNDERSTANDING OF CAUSALITY

With respect to children's understanding of causality (see Donaldson and Elliot 1990), Piaget argued that until the age of about 7 years children show:

• an inability to distinguish appropriately between causes and effects
• a tendency to 'psychologise' by inappropriately explaining physical and logical phenomena in terms of human motives and intentions.

For example, when they were asked to complete sentences, they tended to reverse the order of the cause and effect, as in: *That man fell off his bicycle because … he broke his leg.* Also, when Piaget interviewed children about the causes of various phenomena (such as dreams, the movement of the clouds, and the workings of a steam-engine), they gave explanations which were not simply incorrect but were of the wrong type, in that they tended to explain physical phenomena in psychological terms, for example: *Why do the clouds move across the sky? … Because they want to.*

However, the phenomena which Piaget asked children to explain were ones for which information about causal mechanisms was not directly accessible to them, so it may be that they psychologised as a last resort rather than because they really believed that physical phenomena in general have psychological causes. Several studies have shown that when children are presented with demonstrations of physical phenomena involving familiar principles (e.g. that an object will fall if a supporting object is removed), even 3-year-olds tend to give explanations in terms of physical causes. Similarly, when they are explaining events with which they are directly involved, children as young as 3 years show an ability to distinguish appropriately between causes and effects. Thus, it appears that young children do have a basic understanding of causality, but that their ability to apply their understanding depends on the context and on their knowledge of specific causal phenomena.

UNDERSTANDING OF ILLNESS

How do these findings and arguments relate to children's understanding of illness? Some researchers have argued that children's developing understanding of illness is consistent with Piaget's account of the development of causal reasoning (see Table 1).

It is important to be aware of the types of explanations of illness that are typically given by children at particular stages of development, since this can be helpful in anticipating and alleviating misunderstandings and anxieties (see pp. 92–93). For example, young children who believe that all illnesses are caught through contagion or contamination may be anxious

Table 1 Developmental changes in understanding of causes of illness

Approximate age	Explanations of illness
4–7 years	Contagion: illness caused by proximity to ill people or to particular objects Illness viewed as punishment for own misbehaviour
7–11 years	Contamination: illness caused by physical contact with ill person Illness caused by germs
Over 11 years	Internalisation: processes (e.g. swallowing, inhaling) through which external causes influence internal bodily processes Psychological factors can influence physiological processes Multiple, interacting causes

Based on studies by Bibace and Walsh 1980 and Kister and Patterson 1980

about coming into contact with children with non-infectious illnesses, such as epilepsy or leukaemia.

On the other hand, the typical stages in understanding the causes of illness may not represent the limits of children's ability to understand explanations of illness. Since most young children do not receive much tuition about the causes of illness and since the underlying mechanisms are not directly observable, it may well be that the typical stages merely reflect what they have had the opportunity to learn through experience. For example, most of the illnesses which children experience in early childhood are infectious so it is perhaps hardly surprising that they tend to overgeneralise the concepts of contagion and contamination.

Furthermore, although the stages outlined in Table 1 are based on the typical answers given by a particular age group, there is considerable variation among individual children. In order to communicate effectively with a child about illness, it is therefore important to try to establish the nature of that individual's understanding. It seems plausible that at least some individual differences in understanding of illness will be related to differences in the extent to which a child's previous experience has included relevant concepts and explanations.

 STOP THINK What would you do/say to help a 4-year-old child who was worried about catching appendicitis from the child in the next bed?

Case study
Children's understanding of their blood

When a 3-year-old girl with leukaemia joined a playgroup, the staff were concerned about how to explain her illness to the other children, and a group of researchers decided to investigate this topic (Eiser, Havermans and Casas 1993). They interviewed healthy 3- and 4-year-old children about their knowledge and experiences of blood, and then gave the children an explanation of the functions of different types of blood cells, illustrating their explanation with drawings. Although on the whole the children had difficulty understanding the explanation, the children who showed most understanding were those who had mentioned a personal experience involving blood.

The researchers also interviewed the 3-year-old girl with leukaemia. In the course of her treatment, she had received more extensive and more frequently repeated explanations about blood than the healthy children had, and these explanations obviously had clear personal relevance to her. Her knowledge of the structure and function of blood was found to be much more advanced than that of the healthy children: "she knew that blood … is full of red cells which make new blood, white cells which fight infection, and platelets which stop bleeding. 'Sometimes the platelets don't come and then you keep bleeding.' About the leukaemia, she said that she was 'full of bad cells — they just come'. Doctors took the blood out of her body to get rid of the leukaemia cells. Then they took an enormous syringe and put new blood in" (Eiser et al 1993, p. 535).

Although this explanation includes some misunderstandings and some of the phrases may be simple repetitions of adults' speech without full understanding, and although we do not know how typical the explanation is of other 3-year-olds who are receiving treatment, it is nevertheless extremely impressive for such a young child and it suggests that young children's ability to understand explanations of illness may be much greater than has often been supposed.

How does thinking develop?

- Young children do not simply know less than older children and adults: they sometimes think in qualitatively different ways.
- Piaget's view that these differences reflect an inability in children younger than 7 years to reason logically and to understand fundamental concepts (such as those of number and causality) has been challenged.
- Young children's cognitive abilities depend not only on their underlying concepts but also on the context in which tasks are presented.
- Although children do not *simply* know less than adults, the quality of their reasoning is influenced by the extent of their knowledge in a specific domain, such as illness.
- Children are most likely to understand explanations which:
  – take account of their existing level of understanding
  – are linked to their own experiences and immediate concerns
  – are presented with appropriate non-verbal contextual support.

UNDERSTANDING GROUPS

The effectiveness of medical staff depends on team work. No doctor works completely alone. So, if doctors are going to act competently, they need to know how groups can be used to best advantage. Groups can also have negative effects which can be controlled, if understood, and groups can influence our social and personal identity. Becoming medical students, and eventually joining the medical profession, results in more changes in people than just occupational category: they become different people, with different identification, interests and loyalties.

WHAT ARE GROUPS?

Groups are essential and pervasive. We all belong to groups of different kinds. It has been estimated that we each have membership of about 100 groups, ranging from our family, our nationality, or our professional group, to the gang of personal friends. A group can be broadly defined as a system whose parts interrelate, or with reference to people, as two or more individuals having a collective identity and goals.

FEATURES OF GROUPS

Conformity

In groups we all tend to be conformists. Most ordinary people will usually conform to group opinion, despite having private reservations. Conformity is sometimes seen as negative: for example it can be as a result of real or imagined pressures. A conformist might also be defined as a person who has managed to avoid being defined as a deviant. Yet conformity can be important and valuable. To an extent we all conform when we learn professional skills. We do as others do when we learn to become a competent professional, but there may be negative influences, as for example when we fail to challenge an incorrect but popular opinion.

Factors that are known to increase conformity:

- Having lower status in the group
- Having an authoritarian personality
- Being part of a mixed sex group
- Having a high level of commitment to the group
- Rating the group as 'attractive'
- Believing the group to be competent
- Being in a group with no other dissidents.

Obedience

Most people obey authority. In one well-known psychology experiment, carried out by Milgram, subjects were asked by a respectable-looking experimenter to administer electric shocks to volunteers. The prediction was that 1/1000 would obey. However, in fact two thirds did as requested. (The shocks were not in fact real!)

Factors which influence the likelihood of obedience are not only similar to those affecting conformity, but also include the perceived benefit of obeying the person in authority.

Many human systems depend upon obedience to authority, e.g. the armed services. To some extent hospital medicine relies on obedience to authority to ensure that there is a clear and appropriate understanding of responsibility for patients. If consultants are ultimately responsible for patient care, they must be able to trust that junior medical staff will carry out instructions. Automatic obedience, however, is not wise. Occasionally, senior staff make errors in their instructions, and young doctors need to think critically as they work, and be courageous enough to question a wrong decision.

Deviance

Groups do not tolerate people who do not belong. Dissenters are:

- normally unpopular, because they threaten the cohesiveness of the group and challenge its opinions
- likely to be rejected by the group because they are threatening and produce feelings of discomfort for others
- usually seen as particularly valuable by the group if won over
- need one another to survive the hurt of rejection by a group, possibly by setting up a new group of their own.

GROUP STRUCTURE

Groups which function well have:

- a shared goal, which may be formal or informal (for example to administer treatment, to have a good night out)
- a structure and set of roles (for example leader and led)
- norms or general rules about the right way to behave (for example the type of clothes worn, the style of language used)
- a sense of belonging

- both social and 'task' aspects, that is, there is a social, interpersonal aspect to the group as well as its formal, stated objective or 'task'; a group which only completes tasks may seem efficient, but it engenders little loyalty and does not survive long.

 Consider groups in places where you have been, for example in a tutorial or work group. Most groups or teams tend to show the above features, especially if the team has worked together for a long time. You may also have noticed that group members tend to do different things to keep the team functioning (Fig. 1). Also, different people tend to behave fairly consistently in one group, but may also behave differently in another group. For example, a nurse may be the task leader at work who always generates new ideas, but at home is the one who keeps the peace.

Which one are you? Have you noticed that your role changes depending on what group you are in? Why?

GROUP DEVELOPMENT

Groups do not just gel instantly; they take time to form before they can work together effectively. They appear to pass through noticeable stages before becoming a proper group. It is sometimes hard to go through these stages because they often appear unproductive but they are important in the long term. It appears that there are four main stages in group development:

- *Forming:* when members first gather together.
- *Storming:* when the rules and roles are disputed.
- *Norming:* when the rules and roles are agreed upon.
- *Performing:* when the group eventually starts to work together.

INTER-GROUP CONFLICT

Sometimes groups conflict with one another. Inter-group conflict is very common and occurs between rival football clubs, different schools, NHS professional groups, and nations. While competition may be healthy, if it escalates, conflict can lead to serious disputes, even war, and eventually genocide. This can happen when one group thinks itself so superior to another that total annihilation of the other group is legitimate. This stems from all the above features of groups. 'In-groups' and 'out-groups' are formed where the 'in-group' feels good about itself and simultaneously superior to, but persecuted by, the 'out-group'. Perhaps the 'out-group' consists of deviants who were rejected by the 'in-group' because they would not or could not conform. Alternatively they may have disobeyed the leader of the 'in-group', or be different in some way, for example by racial origin or sex.

One notable feature of inter-group conflict is stereotyping, whereby members of the 'out-group' are lumped together and seen as all bad, weak or aggressive, or as possessing admired but feared characteristics such as intelligence, cunning or sexuality. Individual differences between people are minimised: hence all white people are seen as mean, all women are seen as petty, all football supporters are seen as hooligans, and so on.

GROUP THERAPY

Therapy is often carried out in groups. Obviously if many people can be helped by one trained professional, instead of individual half hour sessions, this has economic benefits. Membership of groups has also been shown to have psychological benefits. Support from other people may come from self help groups (see pp. 96–97) but there may also be more formal groups set up in hospital or general practice. The first account of creating a group for a specifically therapeutic purpose was published in 1907, when an American internist, Joseph Pratt, set up groups to provide support and encouragement for patients with tuberculosis (Hajek, 1997).

Group therapies may take one of four basic approaches or a combination which may be pragmatically chosen on the basis of the composition of the group. The *analytical approach* might analyse motives for the group members' behaviour; an *interpersonal approach* might provide an opportunity for social learning; an *experiential approach* might generate emotional experiences; and a *didactic approach* might impart new information and teach new skills.

No two groups will be the same and identifying the treatment approaches may be difficult. Group therapists become very skilled at facilitating. In a group therapy for women suffering from post-natal depression women are encouraged to discuss their experiences and they learn from each other. Group members might share their doubts about their ability to be a good mother (analytical); share anxiety and feelings of inadequacy (experiential); share ways of coping with the demands of the new baby, mother-in-law problems or partner relationships (interpersonal); and learn from the therapist about realistic expectations of babies' behaviour and early mothering (didactic).

The evidence for the benefits of group therapy compared with individual therapy is positive. Membership of a group increases the chances of stopping smoking, and membership of cardiac rehabilitation provides social support which increases the likelihood of adhering to a programme.

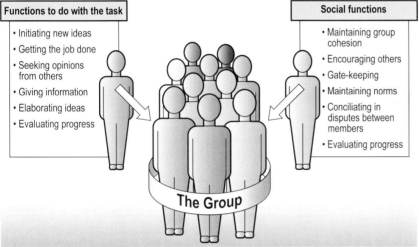

Functions to do with the task	Social functions
• Initiating new ideas • Getting the job done • Seeking opinions from others • Giving information • Elaborating ideas • Evaluating progress	• Maintaining group cohesion • Encouraging others • Gate-keeping • Maintaining norms • Conciliating in disputes between members • Evaluating progress

Fig. 1 **Typical roles in a group.**

Case study

The medical staff of a large inner city general practice decided to establish an asthma clinic in order to respond to the increasing numbers of patients coming to the surgery for help. Part of the strategy of the clinic included the assessment of patients within their own home environments, which would be carried out by the community staff in the practice. The medical staff then announced the plan to the Health Visitors and District Nurses, without consulting them about the feasibility of the assessment procedures. Some nurses tried to carry out the assessments as requested, while others declared the whole strategy to be unworkable given other time constraints. One of the nurses who was eager to implement the strategy was criticised heavily by the others, and soon afterwards gave in her notice. Some of the medical staff felt some sympathy for the nurses and suggested that the plan had been implemented too hastily, but they were accused by the others of being behind the times. Each group of staff considered the other group to be thoughtless, unprofessional, selfish and lazy. The atmosphere in the practice became unpleasant and hostile, so that even the patients began to notice it. Only the appointment of a practice manager who agreed to review the whole issue allowed the situation to calm down and return to normal again.

Understanding groups

- People take on a role when they join a group often without being aware of it.
- Groups encourage conformity and give us a sense of belonging.
- Groups may punish non-conformers by making them feel odd, unwanted and rejected.
- Groups can be a force for good, encouraging patriotism, team-work, loyalty and identity.
- Inter-group conflicts also underlie most forms of industrial dispute, religious and political rivalry, war and even genocide.

CONCEPTS OF HEALTH, ILLNESS AND DISEASE

Medicine is particularly concerned with identifying and treating diseases. This model of disease is called biomedicine, drawing as it does on medical sciences with an emphasis on biological abnormality. Biological abnormalities are not found for all diseases (e.g. some mental illness), and biomedicine is only one way of looking at the ill-health which people experience. It is also important to understand how people feel when they are ill, and what their own interpretations of their symptoms are. In this way, health care can be provided more sensitively, doctors can get a fuller picture of what ails their patients, and patients can be part of the process of identifying what is wrong with them and what can be done about it.

Health has also become an important concept in recent years, especially through an increasing emphasis on promoting well-being as well as preventing illness. However, health is not easy to define. Health, illness and disease mean different things to different people. Definitions and understandings change over time and vary according to social group and individual experience. We will consider the extent to which these concepts are as much social (that is to do with society) and personal as they are to do with biology.

- What does being healthy mean to you? What do you think it may mean to someone who is 75 years old?
- What impact might defining something as a disease have on a patient?
- Why is it important to understand the patient's own beliefs?

DISEASE

Defining disease may at first seem to be quite straightforward. However, changes in medical knowledge may alter our understanding (e.g. many diseases are now thought to have a genetic component) or new symptoms and diseases may appear (e.g. HIV/AIDS). Typically, in Western medicine, disease refers to pathological changes diagnosed by signs and symptoms: it is considered to be objective and defined by doctors. Yet, as the above examples show, definitions are not fixed but change over time in the light of new knowledge and experience. Disease, then, is defined within particular social contexts and historical periods. Homosexuality used to be defined as a disease but is now much more socially accepted as a lifestyle choice; alcoholism used to be seen as immoral, but it is now often typified as a disease. Heart disease, while existing before the twentieth century, was seldom considered a specific cause of death until this century. We are increasingly being able to define disease at earlier and earlier stages, or even identify risk factors for disease. This can lead to many more people being defined as diseased, even in the absence of any symptoms. It is possible to feel quite well but for disease to be present.

Armstrong (1994) has argued that normality plays a crucial role in how medicine defines disease. If the definition of normal relates to what is statistically normal, or an average measure, it is not always clear-cut where the normal becomes the abnormal or pathological. What is normal for one person may not be normal for another, or whole populations may display some kind of pathology which, while representing disease or risk of disease, is normal in some sense. Normality can also be seen as being

socially rather than biologically defined. Here, normality is viewed more in terms of what is considered acceptable or desirable. Mental illness, for example, is very much rooted in culture, and what is considered abnormal behaviour varies. An extreme example would be the labelling of political dissidents as mentally ill, as occurred in the former Soviet Union. Some disabled people also challenge the medical definitions of their conditions and argue that it is society which disables them (see pp. 116–117), and that there should be greater acceptance of difference and variation between people.

Biomedicine is only one way of understanding disease. Humoral theories, elaborated by Hippocrates, understood disease as an imbalance between four humours. Echoes of such understandings are still present today, for example in the promotion and use of cough expectorants and laxatives. Other systems of medicine, such as Indian Ayurvedic medicine or Chinese medicine, also stress the importance of balance. These are complex, professionalised systems used in other cultures to explain disease (as well as health and illness) and organise health care.

In practice, it is important for doctors to be aware of the limits of their own definitions of disease, to have some understanding of the factors involved in changing definitions, and to consider also their patients' own views.

ILLNESS

Illness is a subjective experience and as such will be defined and responded to differently by different people. How people interpret bodily experiences may have no direct relationship with the presence of a medically defined disease. It is possible to feel quite unwell, but to have no detectable disease. People's own experience, as well as their wider knowledge, is drawn from their own culture (their 'lay referral network') and from other sources of knowledge — the media, their doctors. People's own beliefs are important to understand as these may influence whether they seek health care, the type of health care they seek, and also their reasons for seeking professional advice (see pp. 84–85).

When people try to make sense of what is wrong with them, they may interpret symptoms as normal: we all expect to experience headaches from time to time and may just accept that as inevitable. They may also have an explanation for a symptom which serves to normalise it even if it is out of the ordinary, say feeling queasy the morning after a party. At different stages of the life cycle, people may interpret symptoms and illness differently — aches and pains in joints may be seen as an

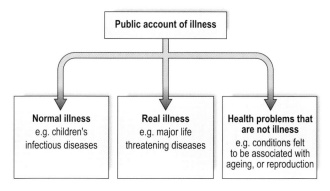

Fig. 1 **Public accounts of illness (After Cornwell 1984).**

inevitable part of ageing, but greater attention might be paid to symptoms which could indicate something more serious, such as chest pain.

Importantly, illness can be thought of as a moral category and, especially in a society which emphasises personal responsibility for health, people would like to describe themselves as healthy. Research, such as Cornwell's detailed study conducted in the East End of London (Cornwell, 1984), has found that many people consider that having the right attitude is important in preventing illness and maintaining good health, and that one should not 'dwell on illness'. She found that people produced what she termed 'public accounts' when she first started interviewing residents. Because of the moral imperative to be seen as healthy, when people first spoke about illness they would prove its legitimacy by describing illness as normal, real or a health problem which was not illness (Fig. 1).

As her study continued, she found that people were much more prepared to talk about a whole range of experiences which they felt had affected their health. It is important for those involved in preventing disease and caring for those who are ill to understand this process of legitimising illness. Getting behind these 'public accounts', Cornwell found that people discussed their experience of illness as part of their everyday lives, affected by their social roles (work, domestic commitments) and their experience of health services. She termed these 'private accounts'. Since doctors often only have a short time with their patients, it is important that they allow for the tendency of people to provide 'public accounts', and that they realise that patients' underlying concerns and worries may be much less clearly and openly expressed (see pp. 86–87).

HEALTH

A negative view of health would define it as the absence of disease. However, the World Health Organisation (1946) offers a more positive definition: a 'state of complete physical, social and mental well-being and not merely the absence of disease or infirmity'. This recognises the important social aspects of health. The Health and Lifestyle Survey, conducted in England and Wales (Blaxter 1990), found this holistic view of health was often echoed in what people said about being healthy. However, concepts of health differ across the life course. The survey found that younger men thought of health as physical fitness,

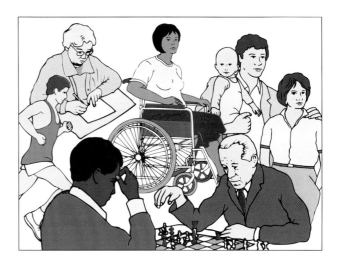

Fig. 2 **Health means different things to different people as it is not just the absence of disease.**

while younger women emphasised energy and coping. In middle age the emphasis moved towards notions of mental and physical well-being, while older people stressed the ability to do things, as well as contentment and happiness (Fig. 2).

Both large scale surveys such as this and other smaller, in-depth studies have found that people define themselves as healthy despite experiencing symptoms. In other words, they have quite functional definitions of health. Judgements are made about what is normal for someone of a similar age or with similar experience. A study of working-class women in the North East of Scotland (Blaxter and Paterson, 1982) found that the grandmother generation (average age 51 years) had low expectations of what good health was — it was being able to carry on and being able to work, despite experiencing disease and illness.

PRACTICAL APPLICATION

Within society and between cultures, there are varied concepts of health, illness and disease. All concepts are inherently social, and it is important to recognise this in practice. Doctors and patients may have competing views, and patients may not reveal their subjective experiences in the belief that these are not important. However, if medicine is to deal seriously with the patient in the context of his or her family and social relationships, then listening to and understanding his or her perspective becomes a prerequisite for good practice. It is inappropriate to consider lay concepts of health and illness as wrong, while claiming that medicine's view of disease is objective and right.

Case study

In a project conducted in Scotland on people in their middle years, participants were encouraged to talk in-depth about their health and concerns about illness. Often health was seen in functional terms, as expressed by this 53-year-old woman, who said that health was:

'Just being able to face the day, get up and get out and get on wi' ma hooswork or eh, just being able to be fit, just being able to cope wi' everything'.

Health was also seen as being related to having a positive attitude, and to an element of good luck or chance. The research participants described the ageing process as affecting health — for example this 56-year-old man said of minor ailments: *'I think you don't shrug them off the same'.* Another 45-year-old man said *'the health starts to deteriorate a little bit'.* (Cunningham-Burley, Milburn 1995)

Concepts of health, illness and disease

- Health, illness and disease are social concepts.
- Health and illness are defined differently by different social groups.
- Someone can perceive themselves to be healthy yet at the same time experience illness and disease.
- People initially provide 'public' accounts of their experience and concepts of illness in contrast to more 'private' accounts as their trust in the interviewer/doctor grows.
- Doctors play a crucial role in defining disease, but these definitions change over time.

MEASURING HEALTH AND ILLNESS

The measurement of health and illness has become increasingly important as doctors, researchers and funders have tried to evaluate the relative contributions of biological, psychological, social and environmental factors in the causes of illness and the outcome of treatments. However, measuring health and illness is often rather more problematic than one might expect.

MORTALITY

All deaths (and all births) in all developed and in many developing countries are required to be registered so that, together with census data, accurate counts can be made of the number of births and deaths and of changes in population size. Mortality rates, particularly infant and maternal mortality rates, are often used as proxy measures of a country's health and development (see pp. 42–43).

In order to take account of differences in population size between countries or regions and changes over time, *crude death rates* are calculated by dividing the raw number of deaths by the number of people in the population.

However, because the chances of dying vary by age and sex (older people and men are more likely to die over a given time-period than younger people and women), allowance is normally made when making comparisons between areas, regions and countries for the age and sex of the population. *Age/sex specific death rates* calculate the proportion of deaths in a particular age group specifically for men, or women.

Life expectancy is an attempt to derive a summary figure of mortality in an area or country and approximates to a measure of average length of life. Figure 1 summarises overall life expectancy for selected countries.

Cause-specific death rates are also available using cause of death entries on

death certificates. However, studies on the accuracy of cause of death entries reveal errors arise from changes in medical knowledge and fashion, from different reporting procedures in different countries, and from coding errors. (Cause of death is coded using the International Classification of Diseases [ICD] which is regularly updated.)

Standardised Mortality Ratios (SMRs) are commonly used to compare death-rates for specific subgroups in a population. An SMR is the ratio of the number of *observed* deaths to the number of *expected* deaths (which would have occurred if the study population had experienced the same mortality as a reference population — allowing for age and sex differences), and is usually expressed as a percentage. An SMR of 100 indicates that observed deaths equals the expected number of deaths (average mortality). An SMR > 100 indicates observed deaths exceed expected deaths, and an SMR < 100 indicates observed deaths lower than expected deaths. For example, Figure 2 shows that in England in 1991–93 men aged 20–64 in social class III non-manual had average 'all cause' death rates, whereas social class I and II men were about 30% below average, social class III manual and IV men were about 17% above average and social class V men were 89% above the average for men in this age group (Drever et al 1996).

SMRs are useful summary indicators of mortality in a sub-population or specific social group, and social scientists

have used it particularly to investigate social inequalities in health (see pp. 44–45). However, it is important to remember that disease-specific SMRs are subject to the errors outlined above, and that SMRs by social class are subject to other errors, for example incorrect reporting of a deceased relative's occupation. Recent studies suggest that this is not as serious a problem as first thought (Drever et al, 1996).

MORBIDITY

Whilst death is (generally) a certain and countable event, mortality rates do not tell us much about illness or health in a population. Illness, morbidity and health are, however, considerably more difficult to define, and hence to measure, than death.

STOP THINK

How would you measure the health of people being treated for:

- angina?
- depression?
- eczema?

Can you think up one 'instrument' that would work for all three?

SELF REPORT MEASURES OF ILL-HEALTH AND HEALTH

The *General Household Survey (GHS)* is a national sample survey of UK households conducted once a year. It routinely asks two questions: one about chronic and one about acute illness. Figure 3 shows how responses have changed over the last 20 years. Whilst the GHS provides a regular picture of ill health in the UK, and has been shown to be generally valid and reliable, the sample size makes it difficult to examine differences in morbidity at regional or district level, or other sub-samples.

A large number of self-report instruments have been developed to measure the impact of specific diseases on health (Bowling 1995), most of which incorporate a variety of scales designed to assess the physical, psychological and social effects of disease. There are also a number of instruments designed to measure health and well-being, in contrast to disease and illness (Bowling, 1997). These instruments, however, find it difficult to

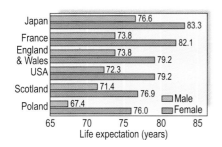

Fig. 1 **Life expectancy at birth (1993).** (Source: WHO 1996 World Health Statistics Annual 1995. WHO, Geneva, Table B-3.)

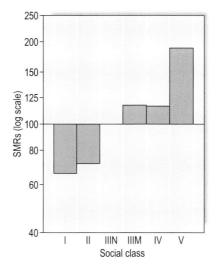

Fig. 2 **SMRs from all causes by social class (based on occupation) for men aged 20–64, England and Wales 1991–1993.** (From Drever et al 1996)

operationalise the concept of health without reference to concepts of illness — pain, disability and mental distress. Thus, for example, the *Nottingham Health Profile (NHP)* covers six dimensions of health and asks the respondent to agree/disagree with statements like: 'I'm tired all the time' and 'I have unbearable pain'. A more recently developed instrument is the *SF-36*.

Care should be taken not to assume that these instruments measure health or ill-health comprehensively: they are summary indicators. Furthermore, care should also be taken when comparing the results of studies using different instruments.

Sickness absence rates are another way of measuring self-reported (and doctor certified) ill-health, but their usefulness is limited by different national reporting requirements, exclusion of non-working people and reasons other than illness for going 'off sick'. Thus, sickness absence may also be an indicator of low morale rather than significant physical or mental illness.

HEALTH SERVICE USE MEASURES

Consultation rates with a doctor are sometimes used as a proxy measure of illness in a population. Measured as the number of consultations with a doctor in a defined time-period in a given population, consultation rates suffer from a number of limitations. In many countries (but not the UK) it may be difficult to define and measure the denominator population. Use of a doctor is strongly influenced by availability of doctors in a particular area/country, and psychological, social and cultural factors strongly influence people's decision to consult a doctor (see pp. 84–85), and these may change over time.

Community morbidity rates are also calculated in the UK using survey data collected in general practice on reason/diagnosis for the consultation. Such data can reveal changing trends in morbidity, but similar caveats need to be borne in mind as outlined for GP consultation rates. GPs also vary considerably in their tendancy to diagnose particular diseases.

Similarly, *referral rates* to hospital and *hospital admission rates* provide some information on patterns and trends in morbidity, but they too vary considerably by referrer practice, supply of hospital services and admission and discharge practice. Beale's study of the ill-health effects of factory closure makes particularly interesting use of health service use data (see pp. 60–61).

QUALITY OF LIFE

A number of instruments have been developed to measure quality of life, and some of these have then been used to 'adjust' years of expected life for the quality of the years: quality

Case study

Fitzpatrick (1994) has illustrated the problem of measuring changes in the health of people with rheumatoid arthritis. Four different instruments were used to measure the degree of change in dimensions of health (Table 1).

Table 1 **Degree of change indicated by four different health status instruments***

Dimension	Effect Size**	Dimension	Effect Size**
Mobility		*Mood/Emotions*	
AIMS	0.43	AIMS	0.83
HAQ	0.38	NHP	0.59
NHP	0.27	FLP	0.61
FLP	0.69		
Pain		*Social*	
AIMS	0.73	AIMS	0.06
HAQ	0.53	NHP	0.24
NHP	0.38	FLP	0.60

AIMS = Arthritis Impact Measurement Scales; HAQ = Health Assessment Questionnaire; NHP = Nottingham Health Profile; FLP = Functional Limitations Profile
*From a sample of patients with rheumatoid arthritis considered to have improved over a three-month period.
**Effect size = difference between mean score at time 1 and mean score at time 2, divided by standard deviation at time 1. Effect size of 0.20 or less considered small, 0.50 moderate, and 0.80 or higher, large.
(Adapted from Fitzpatrick R, 1994)

The NHP reveals little change in mobility, pain, or social well-being, whereas the FLP shows high change in mobility, mood, and social well-being. The AIMS reveal little change in social well-being, but considerable change in pain and mood. Which instrument is to be preferred?

adjusted life years (QALYS). Thus, for example, five years of life with no pain or disability may be valued as equivalent to seven years of life with some pain or not being able to walk. Considerable controversy currently exists as to the validity and reliability of the scales used to measure and *value* 'quality of life', but there are increasing pressures to develop such instruments and techniques to assist in the allocation of scarce health service resources (see pp. 144–145).

It is important to be clear about the purpose for which an instrument has been designed and how this relates to its use. Care should be taken when thinking of using instruments for different purposes, for example — for clinical care, for screening, for evaluation, or for prioritisation or rationing services.

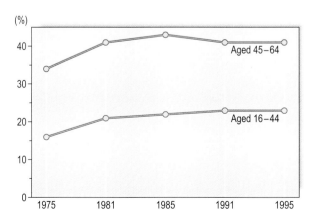

Fig. 3 **Percentage of persons aged 16–64 reporting longstanding illness.**
There is little difference between males and females. (From: Living in Britain 1995, Office of National Statistics, Crown copyright 1997)

Measuring health and illness
- Mortality rates are useful indicators of a country's overall health and development.
- Mortality rates need to be adjusted for the age and sex of the population.
- Disease-specific mortality rates can reveal trends in specific diseases, but tell us little about illness or morbidity in a population.
- Morbidity measures range from instruments asking for self-reported perceptions of illness, through more complex self-report measures of health, well-being and functional ability, to measures of health service use.
- Most morbidity measures suffer from problems of validity and reliability, and should be used for the purpose for which they were designed.

CHANGING PATTERNS OF HEALTH AND ILLNESS

Births and deaths in Britain are officially recorded and analysed by the Registrar General. The data provided on birth and death certificates are compiled by the Office of Population Censuses and Surveys which publishes annual reports showing the incidence of disease and deaths due to specific causes and a variety of statistics relating to use of hospital and outpatient services. These reports, which are public documents and can be consulted in libraries, provide an important source of information about changing patterns of health and disease.

CHANGES IN LIFE EXPECTANCY

Over the last century there has been a marked decline in premature death throughout the developed world. In 1888, a newborn baby in England and Wales had an average life expectancy of just over 40 years. By 1930, average life expectancy at birth had risen to just over 60 years and by 1988 it had reached nearly 80 years (Fig. 1). However, if a child survived into middle age, life expectancy even in 1888 was quite high. A 45-year-old woman in 1888 could on average expect to live to nearly 70 years of age, in 1930 she could expect to live to just over 70 and in 1988 she had an average age expectancy of nearly 80 years. These increases in life expectancy are perhaps the clearest indicator of the improvement in public health to occur over the last hundred years.

The major cause of this increase in life expectancy is a dramatic fall in the death rate for infants during their first year of life. In 1888 in England and Wales, out of every 1000 infants under the age of 1 year 145 died. By 1930 this figure had been more than halved to 68 infant deaths for every 1000 and the rapid decline continued until the present-day rate of nine infant deaths per 1000. The single factor which most accounts for our improved life expectancy at birth is that at the end of the twentieth century almost all new-born babies can expect to live through childhood. In many developing countries in the world, life expectancy at birth remains below 50 years of age because of high rates of infant mortality.

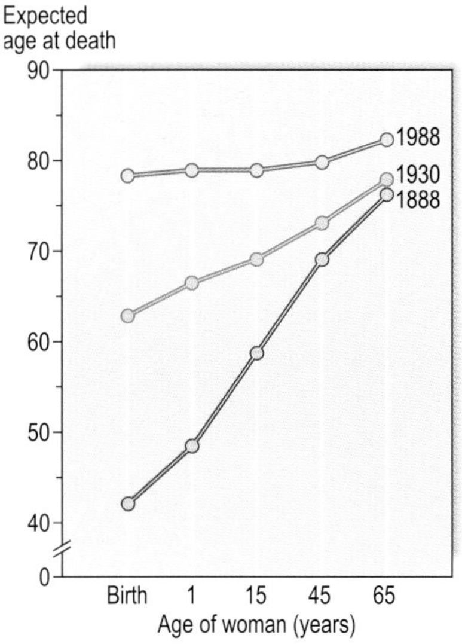

STOP THINK If you were going to practise medicine in a developing country today, what sorts of ill health would you expect to encounter and what sorts of intervention would you become involved in?

According to McKeown (1979) the most important factor leading to changes in infant and child mortality has been a dramatic improvement in child nutrition and maternal nutrition over the past 100 years. Improved maternal nutrition has led to higher birthweight babies, and the availability of hygienic weaning foods such as milk improved the chances of babies surviving once they stopped breastfeeding.

DISEASES WHICH HAVE DECLINED

Another way to look at the changing nature of health and illness is to compare rates of death due to particular causes over the years. In order to examine the relative importance of different diseases over time we need to take account of the fact that the population structure might also have changed over time. For example, cancers are more common in the older age groups and if the proportion of older people in the population has increased whilst the actual rate of cancer has stayed the same, we are likely to make the mistake of assuming that the rate of cancer is increasing. This could be very misleading and might lead to an unnecessary investigation into the causes of the apparent increase. In order to calculate real changes in the rates of different diseases over time we can calculate what are called Standardised Mortality Ratios (SMRs) (see p. 40). These enable us to examine changes over time and consider the possible causes of these changes (Table 1). Over the past century, death rates due to nearly all causes have declined. The most striking changes in death rates have occurred for tuberculosis and influenza. SMRs for tuberculosis have changed from 867 in the period 1891–1895 to 4 in 1986–1990. Similarly, standardised mortality ratios for influenza have changed from 514 in 1891–1896 to 7 in 1986–1990. These changes suggest that a very important improvement in health has been due to our ability to control the spread of infectious disease and fight it more effectively when we are infected.

An important debate surrounds the explanation of changing rates of infectious disease. A great deal of medical research effort has been devoted to the identification of viruses and bacilli and to the development of vaccines and cures during the last 100 years. For example, the tubercle bacillus was first identified in 1880. However, the introduction of the BCG vaccination to prevent infection did not take place until the 1950s. It can be seen from Table 1 that deaths due to

Expected age at death

Fig. 1 **Average life expectancy for a woman at different ages in 1888, 1930 and 1988 (England and Wales).** (Registrar General's Mortality Statistics 1994)

Table 1 **Standardised mortality ratios for selected causes of death, 1890 to 1990 in England and Wales**

Cause of death	1891–1895	1921–1925	1946–1950	1961–1965	1986–1990
Tuberculosis	867	393	157	20	4
Influenza	514	359	57	36	7
Digestive diseases	750	263	114	75	79
Diseases of the respiratory system	526	250	93	94	60
Diseases of the genitourinary system	309	226	113	60	35
Diseases of the skin, subcutaneous tissue musculoskeletal system and connective tissue	671	381	127	97	182
Malignant neoplasms	–	–	96	103	115
Diseases of the heart	–	–	93	89	63
Cerebrovascular disease	–	100	92	95	60
Suicide	137	125	106	112	74

Source: Registrar General's Mortality Statistics, HMSO

tuberculosis had dropped dramatically long before the introduction of the BCG suggesting that some other factor, such as improved nutrition, public health measures and housing conditions, or changes in the nature of the bacillus, must have contributed to the decline (McKeown 1979). (See also Fig. 1, p. 64.)

STOP THINK Bearing in mind the impact of immunisation on death rates from tuberculosis, speculate on how important vaccination against HIV will eventually prove to be (Fig. 3).

Deaths due to some causes have not changed a great deal over the years. The SMR for diseases of the heart, cerebrovascular disease and suicide have shown a steady but undramatic downward trend over the last 50 years. Although the rate for suicide has gradually declined over the years it reached an all-time high during the years of the economic depression, 1931–1935, with an SMR of 150. The only cause of death to show an upward trend over all the years it has been recorded is malignant neoplasm or cancer. Over the last 20 years, death rates amongst women from cancer of the trachea, bronchus and breast have increased steadily, whilst amongst men death rates for cancer of the prostate have increased steadily.

COMMON DISEASES AT THE END OF THE 20TH CENTURY

Whilst standardised mortality ratios are very useful for examining upward and downward trends in the rates of disease over time, if we want to know which are the most common causes of death in a population we need only examine the rates per head of population. In 1991, the five most common causes of death for both men and women were diseases of the circulatory system, neoplasms, diseases of the respiratory system, accidents including violence and suicide and diseases of the digestive system (Table 2). In 1991, deaths certified as due to disease of the circulatory system accounted for 45% of all male deaths and 46% of all female deaths. Treatments for these conditions are an important area of medical research and practice and survival rates are improving. However, an understanding of the causes of heart disease and cancer remains important and they have been linked to a variety of socioeconomic, cultural and behavioural factors. For example, Figure 2 shows recent

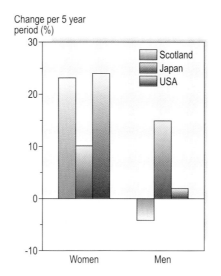

Fig. 2 **Change in lung cancer incidence 1972–1987.** (Registrar General's Mortality Statistics 1994)

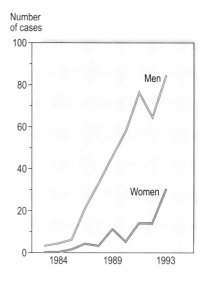

Fig. 3 **Incidence of HIV infection registered in Scotland 1984–1993.** (Registrar General's Mortality Statistics 1994)

Table 2 **Death rates per million population in England and Wales in 1974 and 1991 by cause of death**

Cause of death	Men		Women	
	1974	1991	1974	1991
Diseases of the circulatory system	6118	4533	6149	4570
Neoplasms	2771	2833	2244	2559
Diseases of the respiratory system	1816	1043	1458	1054
Accidents, violence and poisoning	496	427	379	223
Diseases of the digestive system	292	285	309	361
Diseases of the nervous system	126	203	132	213
Diseases of the endocrine system	113	170	178	200
Mental disorders	28	145	47	282
Diseases of the genitourinary system	179	97	153	115
Diseases of the musculoskeletal system	30	44	83	135
Diseases of the blood	27	38	47	45

Source: Registrar General's Mortality Statistics, HMSO

changes in the incidence of lung cancer amongst men and women in Scotland, Japan and the USA. These changes may be closely linked to changes in the tendency of men and women to smoke cigarettes, which may in turn be related to cultural changes in the past 30 years.

An important consequence of increases in life expectancy and in the prevalence of diseases for which cures are unknown is that medical practice is increasingly concerned with the management of chronic ill health and the prevention of disability amongst a population whose average age is on the increase.

STOP THINK What implications do the changing patterns of mortality have for the demographic structure of the population and health care over the next 50 years?

Changing patterns of health and illness

- The single factor which most accounts for our improved life expectancy at birth in the UK is that at the end of the twentieth century almost all new-born babies can expect to live through childhood. This has occurred largely as a result of improvements in nutrition.
- Over the last century infectious disease has declined dramatically. This may be a result of a) changes in people's susceptibility to infection; b) changes in the nature of the biological agents; c) the introduction of medical treatments.
- In 1991, diseases of the circulatory system accounted for 45% of all deaths. Malignant neoplasms accounted for 25% of all deaths.

SOCIAL CLASS AND HEALTH

In clinical practice, we are particularly concerned with the health of individual patients. When clerking a patient we ask about occupation with an expectation that what we are told — bus driver, publican, lawyer, computer programmer, cleaner — will tell us something about the risks associated with work. We may also make an instant appraisal of their life-style and material circumstances. Whilst there are significant differences between individual bus drivers and individual lawyers, there is also strong evidence that people's health is closely associated with their occupation, their occupational group and their social class.

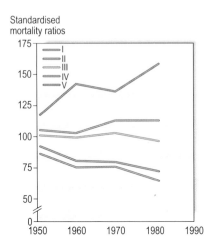

Fig. 1 **Trends in mortality by occupational class for men aged 15–64 years (1950–1980).** (Registrar General's Decennial Supplements and Mortality Tables. HMSO, London)

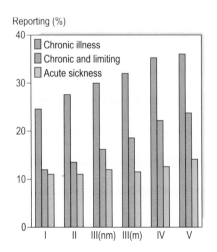

Fig. 2 **Morbidity in Great Britain by socio-economic group, 1991.** (General Household Survey 1993, OPCS, HMSO, London)

THE RELATIONSHIP BETWEEN SOCIAL CLASS AND HEALTH

Since the turn of the century there have been great improvements in the health of the UK population (see pp. 42–43). Inequalities between different sections of the population still exist, however, and one form of disparity which has received particular attention is social class inequality in health. For most of this century, death rates for the UK can be calculated for occupational classes by combining data collected on birth and death certificates with occupational data collected at the Decennial Census. Social class is a general measure obtained by combining occupational groups roughly equivalent in skill and 'general standing in the community' to form occupational classes; these can be seen as an indirect indicator of education, income, standards of living, environment and working conditions. The Registrar General's classification (Table 1) is the most commonly used in health research even though it does have some flaws — for example it does not include people who are unemployed (see pp. 60–61), or deal adequately with women's occupations (see also pp. 46–47).

If we consider social class differences we find the following. Both **reproductive** and adult mortality rates increase regularly, and often sharply, with falling occupational class, and this disparity has existed, although to differing degrees, for many decades. Figure 1 illustrates the persistence of the gradation in all-cause standardised mortality ratios (SMRs: see p. 40) from social class I through to social class V since the 1950s. Class differentials exist in each of the 14 major cause-of-death categories used in the International Classification of Diseases.

When married women are classified according to their husband's occupation, similar if smaller differentials also appear. Only one cause of death for men, malignant melanoma, and four for women, including breast cancer, show a reverse trend.

In general the evidence suggests that disparities in illness, and especially chronic illness, are at least as wide as disparities in death (Fig. 2). These facts are not challenged; controversy lies in their interpretation and in the implications of different interpretations for policies of preventive or corrective action. Four major theoretical explanations were presented by the influential Research Working Group on Inequalities in Health, The Black Report (Townsend et al 1992).

STOP THINK

Do you think that in countries with greater social security and welfare provision than in Britain the mortality gap between the non-manual classes and manual classes will be narrower?

Why should it be that the social class mortality gradient for breast cancer and melanoma is reversed?

EXPLANATIONS FOR THESE RELATIONSHIPS — THE FOUR HYPOTHESES

Cultural/behavioural explanations

These explanations stress individual or life-style differences, rooted in personal characteristics and levels of education, which influence behaviour and are therefore open to alteration through health education inputs leading to changes in personal behaviour. Cultural and behavioural explanations suggest that low socio-economic status, low pay, and insecurity produce inadequacies in diet and dietary values, lack of knowledge, and lack of long-term goals, giving fewer possibilities of making maximum use of health and other services and of taking preventive health measures (see p. 50). Their main focus has been on the health-related behaviours of cigarette smoking, diet and lack of exercise:

- There are higher rates of smoking among manual groups, which will contribute to ill-health.

Table 1 **The Registrar General's social class classification**

Social class	Description	Examples	% of population
I	Professions Business	Lawyers Large employers	5
II	Lesser professions Trade	Teachers Shopkeepers	20
III (nm)	Skilled non-manual	Clerical workers	15
III (m)	Skilled manual	Electricians Lorry drivers	33
IV	Semi-skilled manual	Farm workers Machine operators	19
V	Unskilled manual	Building labourers	8

- There is lower consumption of vitamin C, carotene and fibre along with a higher dietary sodium/potassium ratio among the manual occupational classes.

Materialist or structuralist explanations

These explanations emphasise the role of economic and associated socio-structural factors, for example the labour and housing markets, in the distribution of health and well-being. Proponents of this explanation believe that social structure is characterised by permanent social and economic inequality which exposes individuals to different probabilities of ill-health and injury:

- Poor-quality and damp housing has been shown to be associated with worse health and particularly with higher rates of respiratory disease in children (see pp. 56–57).
- All-cause mortality has been shown in one study to be directly related to income, with the age-adjusted relative rate of the poorest group of subjects being twice that of the richest group. The rate increased in a stepwise fashion between these extremes (Davey Smith et al 1990; see also pp. 58–61).

Social selection

These explanations argue that the occupational class structure is seen to act as a filter or sorter of human beings, and one of the major bases of selection is health: physical strength, vigour, or agility. In this hypothesis, health determines social class.

- Illsley found that women who were taller and in better health than the other members of their class of origin were both more likely to marry into a higher social class and have lower rates of prematurity, stillbirths and first-week infant deaths. He concluded that class differences in these health indices were due to health-related social mobility at marriage, rather than to factors associated with the mother's social class.

Case study
Health and environment — findings from a study of men's health beliefs

Respondents discussed environment when they spoke of health. They separated environments into those which were healthy and those which were unhealthy. Environments referred to were their places of living or work. As one respondent said:

R362: *'I think a lot of illness is self-inflicted through the style of life of the occupation or the environment ... people in, who are working in industries where there are a lot of fumes, em, dangerous chemicals, things like this.'*

With regard to the home environment respondents spoke of differences between residential areas and living conditions.

KM: *'Are there things about your life now that you would say have a good effect on your health?'*
R306: *'I suppose the environment I live in. I have a back and front garden and a reasonably contented family. I suppose these things contribute to it.'*
KM: *'In what ways do you think they contribute?'*
R306: *'Well, it helps to make you feel more settled, this is going back to a sort of mental attitude. If you have that sort of mental attitude I think you can help yourself.'*

Reproduced with permission from Mullen 1993.

- Goldberg and Morrison (1963) reached a similar conclusion in the case of schizophrenia. They found that while the fathers of schizophrenics had the same social class distribution as that of the general population, patients with schizophrenia were disproportionately concentrated into social class V, and had been downwardly mobile for periods of time ranging from a few weeks to several years.

Artefact explanation

This suggests that both health and class are artificial variables produced by attempts to measure social phenomena and that therefore the relationship between them may itself be an artefact — an accidental effect — of little causal significance.

- Errors may be produced when two different data sets (e.g. death certificate and census data on occupation) are combined in order to calculate mortality rates for social classes.
- The failure of health inequalities to diminish in recent decades may be counterbalanced by the reduction in the proportion of the population in the poorest classes as a result of increased upward social mobility.

PRACTICAL IMPLICATIONS AND CONCLUSION

Each of the above theories has practical implications as to what would need to be done to reduce social class inequalities in health. Cultural/behavioural theories lay stress on health education. Social selection theorists believe that since the inception of the National Health Service health inequalities have been reduced, but that such improvement has been masked by health selection over the life course. Supporters of the materialist theory call for more radical approaches involving structural changes to our society and the redistribution of wealth. The artefact theory does not directly lead to specific interventionist policy implications.

In general, following the Black Report's own conclusions, recent research has tended to favour the materialist/structural hypothesis. This has partly been supported by the discovery of similar socio-economic differentials in health and mortality in European countries, as well as in the USA and Australia. The developing consensus does, however, make some concessions to the cultural/behavioural thesis, but in a modified form. Proponents are willing to accept that cultural influences could be at work, but only if any behavioural differences are linked to sub-cultures directly related to social classes. There is also some evidence for indirect health selection, via differences in nutrition and other behaviours and attitudes, though less for direct health selection.

Social class and health

- Although the mortality levels in our society continue to decrease, social class differences persist.
- Cultural/behavioural explanations stress individual and life-style influences on health.
- Materialist/structural explanations emphasise the role of economic factors in maintaining discrepancies in health.
- Social selection theorists state the converse view that health directly influences social position.
- Artefactual explanations suggest that the observed differences are the result of the way we measure social class and mortality.
- Recent research favours a combination of materialist and behavioural approaches, where healthy or unhealthy life-styles are seen to be linked to people's social positions.

GENDER AND HEALTH

Gender is one of the important dividing elements of social life, along with social class and ethnicity. Gender patterns from wider society are reflected in medicine. People working in the health services need to understand gender differences and their implications for health and health service uptake, in order to provide the most appropriate and acceptable care to their patients.

GENDER AND SEX

This chapter refers to gender differences as opposed to sex/biological differences between women and men. Social scientists make the distinction between sex and gender, whereby 'sex' refers to physical and biological differences and 'gender' refers to the social definitions of how women and men should behave under certain circumstances. Society 'prescribes' how the biological sex is transformed into the social gender. Thus biological men learn to behave in a male way and to carry out male tasks. The French philosopher Simone de Beauvoir (1960) summarised this transformation in the phrase: 'One is not born, but rather becomes, a woman.' Every society produces norms, rules, expectations for each gender and these differ from place to place as well as over time. Consequently, what is regarded as male behaviour in one time and place can be seen as female behaviour in another. Thus society as a whole produces women and men.

 Women live longer than men but are more likely to be ill. What explanations can you give for this paradox?

DIFFERENCE IN MORTALITY AND MORBIDITY: MEN AND WOMEN

Women in most countries live longer than men, with the exception of a small number of the least developed countries (see Fig. 1). Men are more likely to die compared with women in the same age group, from the day they are born. Table 1 clearly shows some gender differences in Scottish mortality statistics. The perinatal mortality rate indicates that in any one year baby boys are more likely to die than girls. This pattern is the same for any other age group in Scotland and for other industrialised countries, and many developing countries.

Morbidity statistics for Scotland (Table 1) indicate that for all discharges from hospital, excluding psychiatric and obstetric specialties, women stay in longer than men do and their average bed occupancy rate is also higher. However, there is little difference in the number of discharges per 100 000.

 Why are women more likely to be residents in mental institutions than men are?

Possible explanations for gender differences in health

Some of the gender differences in mortality, especially in babies and infants, are related to 'natural' differences in biological and genetic make-up. However, as boys grow up to become men, social causes of death, especially those related to lifestyle, become more important. Men are more likely to suffer fatal accidents at work and during their leisure time. Men are more likely to be exposed to a hazardous environment than women, and many hazardous occupations in Britain are male dominated: e.g. mining, fishing, and construction work. Generally, men are more likely to display more dangerous behaviour — to drink, to drive too fast, to use illegal drugs, or be involved in dangerous sports such as boxing or motor racing.

At the same time many diseases which do not in themselves kill but are often chronic and disabling affect more women than men. Approximately two-thirds of the disabled population of 4 million in the UK are women, and a large proportion of that inequality is due to age difference (see below). However, not all differences in this respect between men and women can be traced back to social factors. Some of the difference between male and female mortality and morbidity in coronary heart disease can be linked to the contraceptive pill and hormones (Committee on Health Promotion 1996).

MEN AND WOMEN AS CONSUMERS OF HEALTH CARE

Women are not only more likely to be ill, they are also more likely to use health services. Figure 2 illustrates that both poor

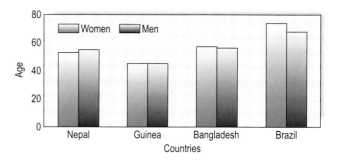

Fig. 1 **Life expectancy rates for selected developing countries.** (Most recent estimates for the World Bank 1987–1992.)

Table 1 **Selected mortality and morbidity rates for men and women, Scotland 1995**

		Measure	Female	Male
Mortality	Perinatal mortality rate	Rate[1]	9.2	10.1
	Under 1	Rate[2]	6.0	6.4
	15–24	Rate[2]	0.4	1.0
	45–54	Rate[2]	3.4	5.5
	85 and over	Rate[2]	171.9	210.6
Morbidity (per 100 000 population)	All discharges[3] mean stay in hospital	Days	9.8	6.9
	All discharges[3] average occupancy bed rate	Rate[4]	432	308
	All discharges[3] hospital inpatient	Rate[4]	16 071	16 289
	Mental illness: hospital inpatient admissions	Rate[4]	589	557
	Mental illness: hospital inpatient residents	Rate[4]	266	227

1. Rates per 1000 total births including stillbirths and deaths up to 7 days after birth
2. Rates per 1000 population
3. Excludes psychiatric and obstetric specialties and excludes day cases
4. Rates per 100 000 population

(Source: ISD 1996: Tables 1.6; 1.8; 4, 3; 4.5; 4.9)

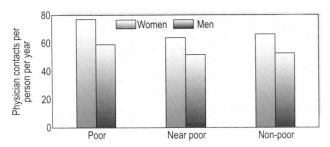

Fig. 2 **Physician contracts, according to sex and poverty status: USA 1991.** (National Center for Health Statistics 1995, Table 77. Poor persons are defined as below Bureau of Census poverty threshold. Near poor persons have incomes to less than 200% of poverty. Nonpoor have incomes of 200% or greater than poverty threshold.)

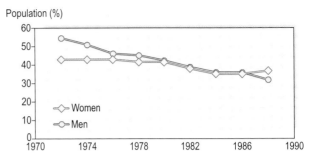

Fig. 3 **Smoking prevalence in Scotland among ages 16 and over.**

and rich American women consult their doctor more often than men do. This pattern holds for the UK and other industrialised countries as well as the USA.

Women visit the doctor more often than men even if one ignores the consultations related to child-bearing (Miles 1991: 63), but the hospitalisation rate is higher for men than for women, when maternity and gynaecological cases are excluded (Leeson and Gray 1978), except for mental illness (see Table 1).

Differences in illness patterns of women and men will lead to different needs for health care provision. Women live longer than men, so consequently a large proportion of the elderly population is female. The overwhelming majority of hip fracture patients are elderly people, hence the majority of patients with a hip fracture are female, and they are more likely to occupy a bed in an orthopaedic ward. Moreover, the uptake of health care is not only determined indirectly through morbidity, but also directly by social and cultural factors. Two main factors are highlighted below:

- What is defined as illness in women is often a social definition instead of the purely scientific exercise of diagnosis and treatment. Pregnancy and childbirth, for example, help to define women as being ill, because of their biological role.
- Women consult family doctors more often than men do, not only for themselves but also for their children and elderly relatives.

The first explanation is related to the fact that all societies make assumptions about what is appropriate gender-related behaviour. This is often referred to as sexual stereotyping. One aspect of this in western cultures is that female socialisation makes it more acceptable for women to adopt the 'sick role'.

One of the possible explanations is that women are less likely to be in full-time employment, therefore they are likely to lose less income than men when they take on a sick role. There is also evidence that doctors give different emphasis to the 'same' symptoms, according to gender. For example, men's 'back troubles' are regarded more seriously, being seen as directly caused by heavy work. Women's 'back problems' are often labelled as part of women's general gynaecological condition. Similarly, mental health problems in women are seen to be internally caused, and thus subject to medical intervention, while in men these are seen as caused by external factors. In other words, men's problems are seen to be related to what they do, and women's problems are related to what they are.

SMOKING PREVALENCE: SOCIAL AND HEALTH PROBLEMS

Smoking illustrates the importance of gender for the medical profession for two quite distinct reasons (see pp. 80–81). First and foremost, smoking is seen as the most important cause of preventable death. Secondly, patterns in smoking prevalence between men and women have been changing over the past three decades. It also shows that differences between men and women in health behaviour, in this case smoking, are not static. Forty years ago it used to be 'normal' among men from all social classes to smoke, whilst at that time only a small proportion of women smoked. Smoking prevalence among adults has fallen steadily since 1972. However, whilst the proportion of men who smoked regularly dropped, the proportion of female smokers increased in the same period. In the 1980s the proportion of women taking up smoking in their teenage years increased rapidly. Figure 3 indicates that smoking levels in Scotland have declined faster amongst men than women. In 1988 the proportion of Scottish women smoking was, for the first time ever, greater than that of men. The reason for this change has been sought in women's emancipation, advertising, and health promotion.

Furthermore, the incidence of lung cancer is increasing among women, and this is closely related to the social changes in smoking prevalence.

Case study

M. is an obstetrician who visits the family doctor because of sleeping problems. During the consultation the doctor asks him about factors that might have an influence on getting to sleep. He mentions the following: the heavy work load in the maternity hospital, drinking a little too much in order to deal with stress and sleeplessness, the frequent quarrels with his partner for no apparent reason, having two noisy children (under five) at home, and living a long distance away from elderly parents. Do you think the family doctor would advise this patient differently if you were told that obstetrician M. is a woman rather than a man?

Gender and health

- At any age men are more likely to die, but women are more likely to be ill.
- Gender differences have a greater impact on health and health care than differences in biological sex.
- Women consult doctors more often than men do.
- Medical professionals have different expectations of and ways of dealing with male and female patients.

ETHNICITY AND HEALTH

The World Health Organization's programme *Health for all by the year 2000* emphasises the importance of equity of access to good health and good health care. There is now a lot of research suggesting that good health and good health care is not as accessible to people in minority ethnic groups as it is to other groups in most societies. It is important for health professionals to consider their roles in developing and delivering equitable and appropriate health services for all ethnic groups in the countries in which they work.

'RACE', RACISM AND ETHNICITY

Ethnicity or 'race' are increasingly used as key variables in health research; however, the terms 'race', 'ethnicity', and 'ethnic group' are often used loosely, and the meanings underlying their use have often been ignored.

The concept of 'race' does not exist in any biologically meaningful way. There is more genetic variability within than between so-called 'racial groups'. Although there are clear differences in physical characteristics between people whose ancestry lies in different parts of the world (eye colour, skin colour, hair colour), these characteristics are of no importance to health. Physical characteristics are only important when values are attached to them in a society, so that one group defines another group as 'different' and assumes them to have particular behavioural characteristics because of the way they look. This can result in negative discrimination, usually called racism.

The term 'ethnic group' is used to denote groups of people who share similar histories and cultural characteristics which give them a distinct identity. Thus we all have 'ethnicity', whether we consider ourselves to be 'Scottish', 'Australian', 'Maori', 'Bangladeshi' or any combination which describes the national and cultural background to which we feel we belong.

MEASURING ETHNICITY

Not only have the terms 'race' and 'ethnicity' been used very loosely in the past: the way they are used has been hotly contested. Most research on the health of minority ethnic populations has relied on place of birth as a proxy for ethnic group.

 STOP THINK What may be the effect of using the health of migrants as a proxy for the health of minority ethnic groups?

Other approaches ask people to assign themselves to particular categories, as in the 1991 Census in Great Britain (see Table 1). This type of categorisation conflates skin colour (e.g.

'white'), with nationality (e.g. 'Bangladeshi') with presumed ethnic identity (e.g. 'Black – Caribbean' compared to 'Black – African'). However, all of these approaches show that the categories used are constructed by researchers themselves rather than being real. This means that it is important to think about the way in which measurement of 'ethnic groups' influences research findings and what they mean.

In the British 1991 Census, about 94% of people described themselves as 'white' (including people born in Ireland, as well as people of Turkish, Greek, Cypriot and other European origins). Thus about 6% of the population described themselves as one of the other categories, about 44% of whom were born in Britain. These overall statistics mask a residential concentration of many minority ethnic groups; for example in Spinney Hill ward, Leicester, 61% of residents described themselves as 'Indian', whereas 16% described themselves as 'white' (Smaje 1995).

SOCIO-ECONOMIC INEQUALITIES BETWEEN ETHNIC GROUPS IN BRITAIN

Unemployment rates for most minority groups are considerably higher than those for whites, particularly amongst young people (see pp. 60–61). Although national data on average income are not routinely broken down by ethnic group, a recent survey by Leicester City Council provides relatively up to date evidence of lower incomes amongst people of Asian origin in Leicester: the gross median weekly earnings of 'Asian' men and women were just 82% of the earnings of 'white' people.

VARIATIONS IN MORTALITY BETWEEN ETHNIC GROUPS

All-cause mortality statistics for 1979–83 show wide variations in the standardised mortality ratios (SMRs) between people born outside the UK.

Table 2 shows that in 1990 the stillbirth and infant mortality rates for babies whose mothers were born in the 'New Commonwealth' were 40% higher than those for babies whose mothers were born in the UK. However, there were considerable variations within this group, and between rates of stillbirth, neonatal and post-neonatal deaths.

Table 1 **The British 1991 Census question on 'ethnic group'**

'Ethnic group — please tick the appropriate box'	
White	Pakistani
Black — Caribbean	Bangladeshi
Black — African	Chinese
Black — other (please describe)	Any other Ethnic Group (please describe)
Indian	

If the person is descended from more than one ethnic or racial group, please tick the group to which the person considers he/she belongs, or tick the 'Any other ethnic group' box and describe the person's ancestry in the space provided.

Table 2 **Stillbirth and infant mortality rates by mother's country of birth, England and Wales 1990.**

Mother's country of birth	Stillbirths[1]	Neonatal deaths[2]	Post-neonatal deaths[2]
All	4.6	4.5	3.2
United Kingdom	4.4	4.3	3.2
Irish Republic	5.1	3.7	3.4
'New Commonwealth'	**6.9**	**6.1**	**3.7**
Bangladesh	8.6	3.9	1.6
India	5.3	5.1	2.2
Pakistan	9.1	7.8	6.4
East Africa	6.9	5.6	2.0
Rest of Africa	7.6	7.1	2.8
Caribbean	5.7	8.4	4.2

[1] Rate per 1000 total births
[2] Rate per 1000 live births
Definitions: Stillbirths, late fetal deaths after 28 weeks gestation; Neonatal deaths, deaths at ages before 28 days after live birth; post-neonatal deaths, deaths at ages 28 days or over but less than one year.
Source: Parsons, Macfarlane and Golding 1993.

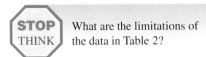

STOP THINK What are the limitations of the data in Table 2?

Other data show that death rates for coronary heart disease are higher among people born in the Indian sub-continent and among men born in the African Commonwealth, whilst those for cerebrovascular disease are higher for people born in Ireland, in the Indian sub-continent, in the Caribbean and in the African Commonwealth. People born in the Indian sub-continent, in the Caribbean and in the African Commonwealth also have higher rates of death from diabetes (Smaje 1995). However, these three groups also show low rates of death from some (though not all) cancers.

There are some diseases that, whilst they are of low overall prevalence, have a specific impact on some minority ethnic groups. Sickle cell disorders and thalassaemia are examples of this. They are both inherited disorders of the red blood cells which mainly (but not exclusively) affect black and ethnic minority groups (see pp. 68–69). A recent estimate suggests that there will be up to 6000 cases nationally by the year 2000 (Smaje 1995), which is a similar figure to the number of individuals affected by haemophilia and cystic fibrosis (Anionwu 1993).

No single explanation will clarify these varied and complex patterns. For example, genetic distribution may explain higher prevalence of sickle cell disease amongst people with origins in Africa and the Middle East, but cannot explain higher or lower rates of infant mortality or coronary heart disease. Cultural explanations are often used by medical researchers but they tend to 'blame the victim' by locating specific health problems within individuals' behaviours. They are also often based on stereotypes of the 'culture' of minority ethnic groups, which assume that everyone of a particular colour or ethnic origin has the same cultural values and behaves in the same way. Explanations which point out the impact of socio-economic inequalities and racism are used less often by medical researchers, but used more often by people in minority ethnic groups themselves.

Despite the importance of understanding these variations, and explanations which might account for them, it is important to remember that the same diseases kill people in minority and majority ethnic groups. Thus cancer prevention and treatment is as important an issue to groups of people with origins in the

Case study
Lack of services for sickle cell disease in the UK

Services for sickle cell disease, although improving, are lagging behind the numbers of cases arising in the UK. Major obstacles to progress are the inadequate education of health care professionals, disadvantage within the black community and institutionalised racism.
Consultant haematologist writing in 1990, quoted in Anionwu 1993

I was hearing that not enough money goes to research on sickle cell. It's not a disease of the white people and they don't know much about it...
Blacks and Laws 1986, quoted in Anionwu 1993

They know that I have got the disease but they don't really know too much about it, and I don't think, this is my personal view, I don't think they're interested because it's not a white man's disease, and I mean, from once it's not a white man's disease, and I can't see them really digging into this thing to get any knowledge out of it, because it is black people, and it's black people's problem.
Debbie, 17, 2 years before she died, quoted in Anionwu 1993

Indian sub-continent as it is to people with origins in Europe, despite slightly lower overall death rates amongst the former.

UNEQUAL AND INAPPROPRIATE PROVISION OF HEALTH CARE

Despite the WHO's commitment to equity of access to health and health services, it is often suggested that many health services are inappropriate to the needs of minority ethnic populations. For example health services have been concentrated on issues which are seen by health professionals to be of special relevance to particular ethnic groups, whereas people themselves may not attach such significance to them. In Britain this led to health education on such issues as rickets or fertility control, whereas the prevention of coronary heart disease or screening and services for sickle cell disease have been largely ignored (see Case study). This issue is neatly summarised as 'birth control for white women, fertility control for black women' (Stubbs 1993).

The other criticism of health services for people in ethnic minority groups is that the methods by which health issues are brought to the attention of minority groups is often inappropriate, and interventions are therefore often unsuccessful. For example, recent Government policy on food has resulted in many campaigns to increase the proportion of fruit and vegetables and fibre in the population's diet, and decrease the proportion of fat. Yet all too frequently the kinds of foods often eaten by minority ethnic groups are not mentioned in advertising campaigns.

Ethnicity and health

- The concept of 'race' does not exist in any biologically meaningful way.
- Thinking of people as belonging to different ethnic or racial groups can lead to direct and indirect discrimination.
- Every indicator of poverty shows that black people and other ethnic minority groups are at increased risk of being poor, principally through the effects of racism and negative discrimination.
- Mortality statistics show wide variations between people born in different countries, but death rates are not always worse amongst ethnic minorities in Britain. Medical researchers often use genetic and cultural explanations for the differences but material explanations, and the effects of racism, are also likely to be important.
- There is evidence of unequal and inappropriate provision of health services for people in ethnic minority groups.

PERCEPTIONS OF RISK AND RISK-TAKING BEHAVIOURS

The identification of risk factors for disease is important for prevention of ill-health and the promotion of good health. We know that social factors are implicated in the patterning of ill-health. However, there is also increasing emphasis on the importance of lifestyle and the role of health-related behaviours for certain diseases. These behaviours can be termed risk-taking behaviours, because of the known risks they pose for an individual's health. Often, these are seen as being within a person's control, and in recent years there has been a growing emphasis on an individual's responsibility for their own health and the promotion of behaviour change to reduce an individual's risk of disease and ill-health.

This has brought with it an emphasis on self control, on moderation in behaviour, and on the provision of information to inform people of the risks to health attendant with certain lifestyles. This implies that individuals are interested in and able to control their lives in this way and tends to promote a sense of rationality which often does not fit well with how people actually lead their lives. Individuals' potential for control over lifestyle and health is limited by the social circumstances which shape people's lives, as well as exerting their own effect on health (see pp. 44–45). These circumstances can restrict the choices that people make, and help to explain why some people still take risks with their health. Understanding people's own perceptions of risk and the contexts within which their risk-taking behaviours occur is important for doctors and others who may be assessing a patient's risk of disease and encouraging a more healthy lifestyle.

- Why might knowledge of risk factors for ill-health not influence an individual's behaviour?
- In what ways are individuals constrained in their actions?
- Think of one 'unhealthy' behaviour that either you or someone you know does. How much of this do you think can be explained by social context?

PERCEPTIONS OF RISK

Ignorance is often considered to be a major barrier to following lifestyle advice, although there is much evidence to suggest that the lay public are well aware of the publicised risks to health, such as the relationship between smoking and lung cancer or the range of risk factors associated with heart disease. Knowledge itself is not a powerful predictor of behaviour. Differences between lay and expert perceptions of risk in relation to health can be better understood when lay knowledge is viewed as part of a much broader consideration of people's lives and experience. It is important that lay perceptions of risk are not just seen as wrong or based on ignorance, but rather as embedded in particular social and cultural circumstances, as examined in the following research example and the case study.

Example 1: lay understanding of heart disease

Heart disease is a major cause of death in many industrialised societies, and preventing it is important in reducing the disease burden for both individuals and society. Much of the emphasis, in terms of prevention, has been on lifestyles: individuals are encouraged to adopt healthy behaviours in order to reduce their risk of heart disease.

A large, in-depth study of people living in South Wales investigated lay understanding and explanations of heart disease. This research took place during a large campaign to prevent heart disease (Davison et al 1991). The results showed that people had their own explanations for the causes of heart disease which drew on, yet differed from, the publicised lifestyle risks. In this 'lay epidemiology', people drew on a range of knowledge and experience to explain who was a 'candidate' for heart disease (Table 1). This included lifestyle factors, heredity, social environment such as work, physical environment such as climate, and a degree of randomness attributed to luck and chance.

This demonstrates that people understand the risks associated with heart disease and, in fact, draw on risk factors beyond those just associated with lifestyle. However, people were also well aware, from their personal observations, that people at high risk of getting heart disease do not always suffer from it, and that sometimes those at low risk do. People know that predicting who will get ill is difficult in multifactorial conditions. Any attempt to oversimplify this with an emphasis on risk-taking behaviours is

likely to be sceptically received, as lay people's own experience and knowledge tells them that the process is more complicated and less certain than such an emphasis implies.

RISK TAKING BEHAVIOUR

Just as it is important to understand lay perceptions of risk, risk-taking behaviour must also be examined in the context of individuals' lives. Risk-taking behaviours often do not take place in isolation, but in interaction with others. This can explain why some people indulge in behaviours which are considered to be, even by themselves, detrimental to health. Social circumstances may also help to explain such behaviours (see pp. 44–45). Two examples will help to demonstrate the importance of social context in understanding risk-taking behaviour: one considers the practice of unsafe commercial sex between men, the other smoking among women with young children, living on low incomes.

Example 2: unsafe commercial sex between men

A study by Bloor et al (1992) of the risk-taking behaviours of male prostitutes in Glasgow, Scotland, demonstrated the importance of social interaction and social relations in determining behaviour. All but one of the ten male prostitutes they contacted were practising unsafe commercial sex. However, these same

Table 1 **People who may be identified as coronary candidates**

- Fat people
- People who don't take exercise and are unfit
- Red-faced people
- People with a grey pallor
- Smokers
- People with a heart problem in the family
- Heavy drinkers
- People who eat excessive amounts of rich, fatty foods
- Worriers (by nature)
- Bad-tempered, pessimistic or negative people
- People who are under stress from
  – work
  – family life
  – financial difficulty
  – unemployment/retirement
  – bereavement
  – gambling
- People who suffer strain through
  – hard manual labour
  – conditions of work/home
  – excessive leisure exercise
  – overindulgence
    (sex, dancing, drugs, lack of sleep, etc)

Source: Davison C et al 1991

prostitutes knew that this behaviour was risky, especially in terms of HIV transmission, and also knew that they were vulnerable to infection. It was the social circumstances surrounding male prostitution which led to the practice of unsafe sex. Unlike much female prostitution, where negotiation of fee and terms is established by the prostitute at the start of the encounter, the male prostitutes studied were subjected to client control — they themselves had little say over what should happen. This situation can partly be explained by the covert and stigmatised nature of the activity: it is neither legal nor socially sanctioned. The practice of unsafe sex, in this context, can be understood once the social reality of male prostitution is considered. It cannot be explained through lack of knowledge, a sense of invulnerability, or as irrational behaviour.

Example 3: women with young children living on low incomes

Smoking is a major cause of ill-health and death, and its effects are well publicised (see pp. 80–81). A cursory consideration of cigarette smoking would suggest that individuals have considerable control over the behaviour. However, although smoking rates in the UK are generally decreasing, it is a behaviour that is becoming increasingly associated with disadvantage. Smoking rates are not decreasing as quickly amongst those lower down the social scale.

Research by Graham (1989) on women with young children living in low income households in England demonstrates why poor social circumstances may lead to smoking. She found that smoking plays a very important role in the lives of women who are socially disadvantaged. Smoking was a way of coping with living in poverty: it provided a short break from domestic responsibilities and a strategy to deal with things if they got too much (Fig. 1). In the absence of other resources, smoking was the one activity which the women could claim as their own, giving precious time to themselves. Rather than defining such behaviour as irresponsible, Graham notes that it shows a commitment to the overall welfare of the family, enabling life with few resources to be successfully managed.

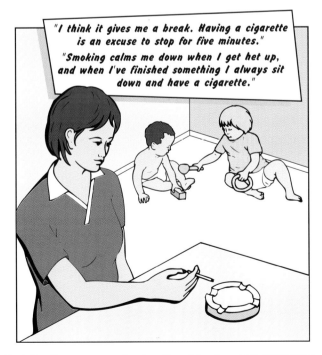

Fig. 1 **Smoking as a means of coping with social and economic disadvantage** (Graham 1989).

Case study
Young people and smoking

In a qualitative study of young people's perceptions of smoking, Allbutt et al (1995) found that those studied were well aware of the risks associated with smoking: indeed some had direct experience of its effects within their own families. However, both smokers and non-smokers discussed the positive aspects of smoking, such as the image, weight loss or relaxation. These are some of the things they said:

- 'It felt good, I felt big.'
- 'It relaxes you, that's why I like it.'
- 'If you've got a drink or a cigarette it's easier to talk to somebody because you can do something with your hands if you're not talking to them.'
- 'It helps me when I'm stressed.'

Smoking itself was experienced as an activity which took place within a group, where friendship is important. These positive aspects may encourage risk-taking behaviour. Attempts to prevent young people smoking must then go beyond the provision of relevant information, and take on board the meaning which the behaviour has for them, in the context of their own lives.

PRACTICAL APPLICATIONS

Recognition of the social context of risk, both in terms of perceptions of risk and risk-taking behaviours, is important for doctors as they become involved in public health and health promotion, and also as they deal with individual patients. It must not be assumed that those engaged in risk-taking behaviours are ignorant of their relationship to health. Doctors should try to elicit people's own explanations and treat these as reasonable, based on their own experience. This should lead to greater understanding and empathy between doctor and patient. Similarly, account must be taken of the circumstances within which people live and how this may influence their behaviour. It is also important to understand the particular contexts within which risk-taking behaviours occur. Doctors must not promote 'victim blaming', where those who engage in behaviours considered damaging to their health are deemed to be irresponsible. Often such behaviour can be considered a rational response to poor social conditions, or the only choice in a situation where the individual has little control.

Perceptions of risk and risk-taking behaviours

- The concept of a risk factor for disease is important for both professionals and the lay public.
- Risk perceptions and risk-taking behaviours are part of a wider social context including both social conditions and social interactions.
- These may constrain the choices which individuals can make; risk-taking behaviours should be seen, at least in part, as being socially determined.
- Promoting healthy behaviours means more than encouraging individuals to change.

STRESS

Stress has been implicated in a wide variety of psychological and physical problems ranging from anxiety states (see pp. 112–113) to some cancers (see pp. 108–109), arthritis, heart disease (see pp. 104–105) and a greater likelihood of getting infectious diseases. Although much research links stress to many illnesses the evidence is correlational and it is extremely difficult to show cause definitively. Medical treatments and procedures, as well as pain and illness, can themselves be stressors.

WHAT IS STRESS?

The word 'stress' is used in many different ways, but it is helpful to separate the causes, 'stressors', from the responses, 'signs of stress or strain'.

Stress occurs when the demands made on a person are greater than their ability to cope. Stressors can be acute or chronic and people show great variation in their response to stressful situations. Even within an individual, responses will vary over time.

SIGNS OF STRESS

- *Biochemical:* alterations to HCTH, endorphin levels.
- *Physiological:* higher blood pressure; rapid shallow breathing.
- *Behavioural:* sleep problems; increased alcohol intake; absenteeism at work; increased errors; loss of sense of humour.
- *Cognitive:* poor concentration; poor memory; negative thoughts.
- *Emotional:* mood swings; feeling weepy; irritability.

Stress is sometimes described as positive ('a challenge') but it is less confusing to find another word (e.g. 'pressure') for this and keep 'stress' to describe a negative condition. The 'positive' aspect of pressure can be seen in Figure 1, the 'arousal curve' which shows how some pressure is needed to encourage optimum performance. It also shows, graphically, how an excess of pressure turns to stress and poor performance.

WHAT CAUSES STRESS?

Stressors can be either internal or external. Internal demands include personal expectations, attitudes and beliefs often arising from past experience, while external demands range from environmental factors (such as overcrowding, see pp. 56–57), to demands from others (to be a good son/daughter), work demands (examinations) (see pp. 58–59) or the social and cultural climate (competitiveness).

Although stressors can be many and varied, there are often two important underlying characteristics of stressful situations: lack of control with a sense of helplessness in the face of events and unpredictability.

- Why might stress be considered positive?
- How does what you think contribute to stress?
- What causes stress in *your* life?

MODELS OF STRESS

There are a number of models of stress, of which we will consider three: one which concentrates on the physiological response, one social model which focuses on the causes of stress and the interaction model which brings the disparate parts together.

General adaptation syndrome (GAS)

This is the oldest stress model, developed by Selye in the 1940s, and is a three-stage model explaining physical stress responses.

- *Alarm stage* — the acute stage (fight or flight) when the body responds instantly to the stress. Visible signs include rapid heart rate, shallow breathing, sweating.
- *Resistance stage* — the characteristic signs of the alarm stage fade and the body appears to 'return to normal'. If the stressor persists, however,

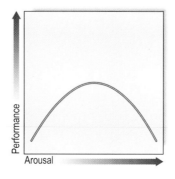

Fig. 1 **The positive aspect of pressure: the arousal curve.**

the body continues actively to 'fight' it and the body's resources (e.g. nutrients, vitamins) are depleted.

- *Exhaustion stage* — new symptoms begin to emerge and the body becomes increasingly susceptible to illness. Although there is some evidence for the physiological changes in both animal and human studies, this model does not explain why some people respond like this, and others are unaffected by the same event.

Life change model

This model focuses on the changes, or life events, for example bereavement or marriage (Table 1), that occur in an individual's life over a given period of time. It is hypothesised that any change (positive or negative, wanted or unwanted, planned or unexpected) requires the individual to readjust to their environment and thus constitutes a stressor. A build-up of life events and constant readjustment is likely to contribute to health problems.

Life events are a common measure of stress in research, partly because the questionnaires are quick and easy to use and many correlations with illness, ranging from heart disease to cancer, depression and schizophrenia have been found. There are a number of methodological problems, however, not least the accuracy of the individual's memory for events and separating cause and effect. For example: did the divorce cause depression, or depression cause divorce, or was it a third factor, long-term unemployment, which affected both?

Table 1 **Selected examples from the Holmes-Rahe Social Readjustment Rating Scale**

Life event	Mean value
1. Death of spouse	100
2. Divorce	73
3. Marital separation	65
4. Jail term	63
5. Death of close family member	63
6. Personal injury or illness	53
7. Marriage	50
8. Fired at work	47
9. Marital reconciliation	45
10. Retirement	45
11. Change in health of family member	44
12. Pregnancy	40
13. Sexual difficulties	39
14. Gain of new family member	39
15. Business readjustment	39
16. Change in financial state	38
17. Death of close friend	37
18. Change to different line of work	36
19. Change in number of arguments with spouse	35

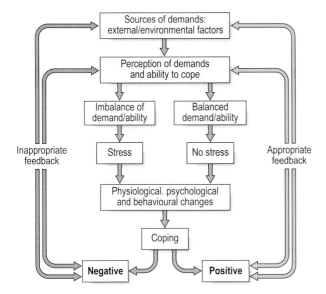

Fig. 2 **The interaction model.**

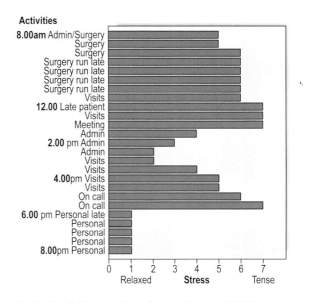

Fig. 3 **GP activities and stress.** (Source: Porter et al 1989)

Interaction model

Interaction models incorporate both response models (e.g. GAS) and stimulus models (e.g. life events) and provide an explanation of stress as an interaction between the person and the environment (Fig. 2). Internal factors such as a person's perceptions, attitudes, emotions, habits and lifestyle interact with external environmental factors. Experience of stressors and the coping strategies adopted influence how such stressors are perceived in the future. These personal factors, or 'mediating factors', can increase or reduce susceptibility to stressors. They include:

- *Social support:* having someone to talk to about problems and who is supportive of you is an extremely important factor in coping with stress.

- *Beliefs and attitudes:* how much do you contribute to stress by irrational beliefs and negative attitudes, e.g. 'I must do everything perfectly or else I am a failure' (see pp. 128–129).
- *Perception:* do you see problems as a challenge or threatening and unfair?
- *Personality:* there is no one personality type associated with stress although much research has been carried out on Type A behaviour patterns. Hostility seems to be the important factor in relation to poor health outcome.
- *Coping strategies:* successful coping strategies reduce the impact of the same stressor (and possibly others) in the future.
- *Certainty/uncertainty:* most people cope better with bad news (e.g. being made redundant, being told their diagnosis) than they do with not knowing what will happen or what is going on. Knowing allows a person to plan and adjust.
- *Lifestyle:* good diet, regular exercise, sufficient sleep mean that the person is physically better able to cope with stress.

Case study

Dr Green is a general practitioner in a large group practice serving a large market town. Figure 3 shows how he spent one day, and his half-hourly pressure scores.

He had been on call the night before and reported that he had not got much sleep. He had received three calls and made three visits between 11.00 p.m. and 7.00 a.m.

He started his 8.30 a.m. open (non-appointment) surgery session in a branch surgery early at 8.10 and was due to finish at 9.30 so that he could get on with home visits. However, the surgery didn't finish until 11.20 — after seeing 19 patients and failing to see three who had left because they couldn't wait any longer. No other GPs and no nurse were at the branch surgery to help out. He reported feelings of maximum stress at noon when he was trying to finish the calls before a meeting he had arranged previously for 1.00 p.m. with the local psycho-geriatrician and geriatrician. After the meeting, he was able to relax a little over some administrative work. He then did 2 hours of home visits, but still had administrative work to do before going home. This made him late for supper and a Christmas function with his wife at 6.30 p.m. When he got there, he relaxed, but he had to return to practice administration again at 10.30 p.m., commenting that routine administration was seldom completed during the working day (8 a.m.–6 p.m.), and that he had worked on administration until 2.30 a.m. on the Monday and Tuesday nights. He had not been feeling 'on top of the world' over the previous 2 weeks, but he was generally feeling positive and reported no negative feelings.

The outstanding feature of this doctor's work was the running late of his surgeries, which also occurred in appointment surgeries where he booked patients at $7^1/_2$ minute intervals but generally took at least 10 minutes. Feelings of stress were particularly acute when other commitments — be they practice or personal — impinged on his ability to be flexible and run late.

(From Porter et al 1989)

Stress

- Signs of stress can be biochemical, physiological, behavioural, cognitive and emotional.
- Stressors can be internal and external
- Models of stress are increasingly interactionist to account for the relationship between individual and environment.

HEALTH BELIEFS AND HEALTH BEHAVIOUR

People's own behaviour can have an important effect on their health. A healthy life-style can reduce the risk of illness through 'preventive health behaviours' (such as not smoking, exercising and eating a healthy diet) and the effects of illness can be minimised by what are called 'sick role behaviours' (such as seeking medical help and complying with treatment, see pp. 84–85 and pp. 90–91). How then can people be encouraged to take care of their health through appropriate preventive and sick role behaviours?

THE HEALTH BELIEF MODEL

In the 1950s US public health researchers began to investigate which beliefs were generally associated with health behaviours. The aim of this research was to identify beliefs which could be targeted by health education programmes which, if successful, would promote health behaviour amongst the general population.

The Health Belief Model (HBM) which emerged focused upon people's beliefs about the threat of ill health and the costs and benefits of health behaviour (see Fig. 1). Threat perception involved perceived *susceptibility* to illness or health breakdown (e.g. How likely am I to suffer from breathing difficulties or contract lung cancer if I smoke?) and the anticipated *severity* of the consequences of illness (e.g. How bad would it be if I suffered from breathing difficulties or contracted lung cancer?). The model also included beliefs concerning the *benefits* or effectiveness of a recommended health behaviour (e.g. If I give up smoking what will I gain?) and the costs or *barriers* associated with the behaviour (e.g. How difficult will it be to give up smoking and what will I lose?). Two other factors were included: *cues to action* which trigger health behaviour when people are aware of a health threat and convinced of the effectiveness of action (e.g. advice from a doctor) and general *health motivation* (i.e. how highly a person values good health).

How useful is the Health Belief Model?

In 1984 Janz and Becker reviewed 46 studies which tested the degree to which the four key beliefs in the HBM were distinguishable among people who adopted or failed to adopt health behaviours. They separated studies of the adoption of preventive behaviours (e.g. breast self-examination) from those of sick role behaviour (e.g. taking medication) and counted the number

in which each of the four beliefs was found to be significantly associated with health behaviour (i.e. correlated with the behaviour to a degree that could not be reasonably attributed to chance). They then calculated the percentage of studies which found each belief to be a useful predictor of health behaviour (see Fig. 2).

This review showed that perceived costs or barriers are especially important, suggesting that minimising the degree to which health behaviours are thought to be painful, time-consuming, expensive or embarrassing will help promote them. Note too how perceived severity is less important in relation to prevention than responses to symptoms or medical advice. This suggests that stressing susceptibility to health problems will be more effective in promoting preventive health behaviour than emphasising the severity of the threat.

Applying the Health Belief Model

Three key applications of HBM are:

- identifying health promotion targets at individual and population levels
- identifying those least likely to comply with medical treatment/advice
- understanding why some people put their health at risk.

Identifying beliefs which might prevent a patient from following medical advice (see pp. 90–91) can facilitate effective health education. A doctor could, for example, discuss a patient's susceptibility to further health problems if they do not follow advice (e.g. to give up smoking) or help them think of ways of minimising the costs (e.g. by seeking support from others and planning substitute pleasures).

Health-related intentions — an extension of the Health Belief Model

King (1982) extended the model in a study of hypertension screening. She designed a questionnaire which included measures of intentions as well as questions based on the Health Belief

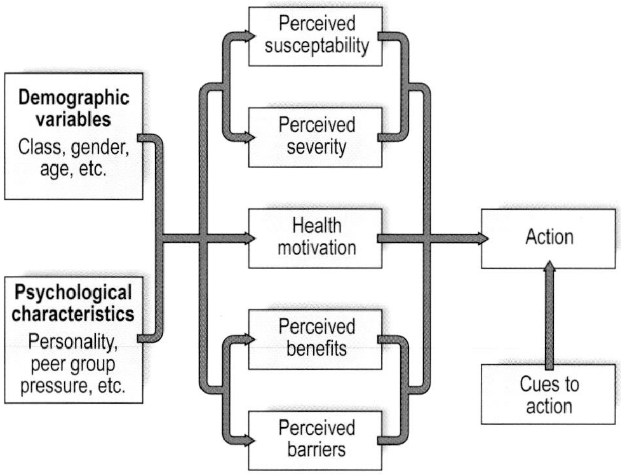

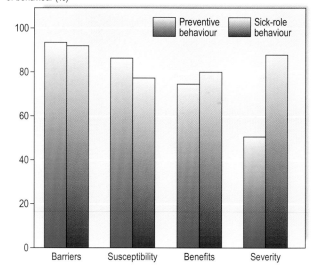

Studies in which health belief was predictive of behaviour (%)

Fig. 2 **Health beliefs and their predictive effects on preventive and 'sick role' behaviour.** (From Janz and Becker 1984.)

Fig. 1 **The Health Belief Model.** (Based on Becker et al 1977.)

Model. Her model correctly predicted whether people did or did not attend later screening, in 82% of cases. Measures of intention were found to be the most powerful predictors of attendance.

Davies (1968) found that 44% of patients who had not followed their doctor's advice had not in fact intended to do so and only 8% of those who had not intended to follow the advice actually did so. These findings strongly suggest that people's intentions are useful predictors of preventive health behaviour and sick role behaviour. Doctors could enhance the effectiveness of their advice by finding out what their patients' intentions are and promoting health-related intentions.

Promoting intentions using subjective norms

Research (e.g. Ajzen & Madden 1986) has shown that, in general, intentions are strongly related to 'subjective norms'.

People's subjective norms refer to their beliefs about the extent to which other people approve of a behaviour and the extent to which they value that approval. For example, people are more likely to change their diet if they believe that their family and friends approve of the change and they feel that this approval is important. Even when patients intend to follow their doctor's advice, their intentions may be undermined if it is disapproved of by valued others outside the surgery. This means behaviour change will be easier for patients who are actively supported by those they are closest to.

Subjective norms can also be targeted in mass media health promotion campaigns. For example, in one HIV-preventive

---

Case study
Health beliefs and condom use

John and Mary are heterosexual teenagers. Both have been reminded of the risk of sexually transmitted diseases, including HIV, through health education campaigns. They are motivated to protect their health, they acknowledge the potential seriousness of sexually transmitted diseases and know that condoms offer good protection.

John believes that only gay men and drug injectors are at any appreciable risk of HIV infection and that other sexually transmitted diseases are not very serious. He has never used a condom and believes that they may reduce intimacy and sensation during intercourse. Consequently, he does not buy or carry condoms.

Mary takes oral contraceptives. She is concerned about her susceptibility to HIV and chlamydia infection and consistently used condoms with her last two partners. She does not find them off-putting and thinks they provide good protection against infection. Mary no longer has a regular sexual partner and does not carry condoms because she is worried that if she is seen carrying them her girlfriends and boyfriends will think she is regularly seeking casual sex and question her morals.

John and Mary become attracted to each other in a night club and go back to John's home because his parents are away. When Mary mentions condoms John rejects the implication he is infected and declares that he 'never' uses condoms. In fact he does not have any and does not know how to use them. Mary is very attracted to him and decides to take a risk rather than lose John's affection. The next day Mary has a hangover and is worried about the risk of infection. John also has a hangover but he is not worried and intends to go 'clubbing' again that night.

---

television campaign in the UK an interview was staged with a woman working in a condom factory. Talking against a noisy background of spinning condom machines, Mrs Dawson explained that her factory had never been so busy. She suggested that this was because young people are buying more condoms and the campaign slogan was 'Keep Mrs Dawson busy. Use a condom'. The implied message was that most sexually active young people use condoms and would approve of the viewer using one (see also pp. 106–107).

 Mr Davidson is a 48-year-old lorry driver who has seen his GP about a series of illnesses over the past 6 months. He always complains of stress and overwork and his GP thinks he needs to take more rest and exercise and reduce his working hours.

How should his GP go about discussing these changes with Mr Davidson? List some helpful remarks the doctor could make that might begin to change Mr Davidson's view of his health (see also pp. 70–71).

Perceived self-efficacy — a further extension of the Health Belief Model

Perceived self-efficacy refers to a person's confidence in their ability to perform a behaviour successfully. Research has shown that those who strongly believe that they can successfully carry out a health-related action are more likely to intend to do so and are more likely to be successful when they try. The body of research supporting these links is so strong that this belief has been incorporated into later versions of the Health Belief Model. Perceived self-efficacy can be increased through encouragement, teaching, demonstration and practice.

PROMOTING HEALTH BEHAVIOUR

A person is more likely to undertake a health-related behaviour when they believe that:

- their health is important
- they are susceptible to a health threat which could have serious consequences
- the proposed action will be effective and does not have too many costs
- others approve of the action and their approval is important
- they can successfully carry out the action.

Finally they are more likely to carry out the action if they intend to do so and are reminded to do so (see also pp.70–71).

Health beliefs and health behaviour

- By identifying beliefs associated with health-related behaviour and seeking to change those beliefs it is possible to promote health-related behaviour.
- The Health Belief Model highlights the importance of perceived susceptibility and severity, perceived costs and benefits of health behaviours, general health motivation and cues to action.
- Intentions are important predictors of future behaviour, and belief in the approval of others promotes intention formation.
- High perceived self-efficacy promotes intention formation and makes successful performance more likely.
- Health beliefs can be targeted in individual consultations to increase patient compliance as well as in mass media campaigns to promote preventive health behaviour.

HOUSING, HOMELESSNESS AND HEALTH

Housing affects health directly and indirectly. Lack of adequate housing causes both mental and physical ill health. It can make existing illness and health problems worse, and can delay recovery from illness and reduce the effectiveness of medical interventions.

HOUSING AND HEALTH

In Victorian Britain, concerns about housing conditions causing ill-health led to programmes of slum clearance. This commitment to improving public health by changing harmful social conditions contributed to the decline in infectious diseases and increases in life expectancy (see pp. 42–43).

The end of the Second World War saw the start of a period of growth in public sector housing which culminated in high-rise housing estates in the 1960s. The shift to quantity rather than quality of housing brought problems such as dampness, lack of sound insulation and privacy from neighbours, as well as social isolation associated with the difficulties of getting in and out of high-rise flats. Although research evidence emerged during the 1970s and 1980s which showed the negative health impact of these 'new' housing problems, the importance of housing was relatively neglected as health policy focused on individual behaviour rather than social conditions as the cause of ill health.

The late 1980s and 1990s saw a decline in the availability of affordable housing in both the private and public sectors and a rise in the numbers of homeless people who were 'roofless' or living in temporary accommodation.

HOMELESSNESS AND HEALTH

Homeless people may be 'roofless', living on the streets, or in temporary accommodation. People who are homeless are frequently exposed to extreme environmental hazards such as damp, cold and noise, as well as overcrowding, risk of violence, risk of accidental injury, poor hygiene, and poor access to health services. Figure 1 shows the main illnesses associated with homelessness. It is difficult to research the health of homeless people and this is a limited picture.

Housed but homeless

Although social policy distinguishes between people who have permanent accommodation and the homeless, it has

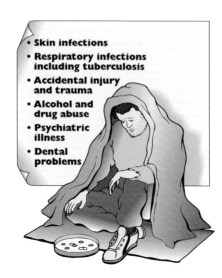

- Skin infections
- Respiratory infections including tuberculosis
- Accidental injury and trauma
- Alcohol and drug abuse
- Psychiatric illness
- Dental problems

Fig. 1 **Illnesses associated with homelessness.**

been suggested that the definition of homelessness should be based on the 'Lack of a right of access to own secure and minimally adequate housing space' (Bramley et al 1987). Under this definition people are also without a home if permanently housed in accommodation which is harmful to health, deprives them of resources which are necessary to maintain or protect health, or presents barriers to their daily activities.

Difficulties in showing that lack of adequate housing has an impact on health: the artefact explanations

Researchers in housing and health, as those in other areas of social inequalities and health, have to rule out the possibility that associations between housing and health occur as a result of other factors. The two most common 'artefact explanations' which have to be ruled out are those of 'confounding factors' and 'downward drift' (see Table 1).

If researchers have sufficient data on other social conditions and past health and housing history, it is possible to use statistical techniques to take these other factors into account and to assess the independent contribution of housing to health.

Table 1 **Key problems in establishing the links between lack of adequate housing and ill health**

Confounding factors
Lack of adequate housing is frequently associated with other factors which are known to cause ill health, such as unemployment or low income

Downward drift
People in poor health 'drift' into poor housing or homelessness because of the consequences of ill health

Table 2 **Lack of adequate housing: effects on health**

Direct effects
- Exposure to physiological effects of the environment or harmful agents fostered by environmental conditions

Indirect effects
- Exposure to poor living conditions in childhood may have consequences for health in later life
- Causes stress or discomfort which increases general susceptibility to physical illness and emotional problems
- Exacerbates or delays recovery from existing health problems
- Undermines social relationships
- Makes it difficult or stressful to get on with the tasks of daily life
- Makes it difficult to access other resources which are necessary to sustain or promote health

How does lack of adequate housing affect health?

The housing environment can affect health both directly and indirectly (Table 2).

- The direct effects of lack of adequate housing can be explained using a medical model of how disease and illness are caused. In this model, specific aspects of the environment have physical effects which lead to specific symptoms or illness.
- Another model of illness is the 'general susceptibility model' in which aspects of the environment act as stressors which make people more susceptible to illness. This model can be used to explain the indirect effects of housing on health. Specific features of the environment are not linked to specific illnesses as they are in the medical model.

These models can be used to guide epidemiological research which attempts to quantify the relationship between different aspects of social conditions and the environment. As well as trying to *quantify* the relationship between housing and health, it is also important to understand the experience of living in inadequate housing, the impact on daily life and the compound effects of different aspects of inadequate housing and other conditions of social deprivation.

'It's very noisy being right by the motorway but we couldn't open the windows anyway, because of all the break-ins. The walls are running with damp and there's mould on our walls, our clothes and shoes. It's freezing cold most of the time and in winter we all huddle into the one room. The kids are always sick and I'm at my wits' end.' (Hunt, 1997)

Overcrowding
- Has a detrimental effect on relationships within dwellings
- Leads to loss of privacy which adversely affects mental health
- Increases the risk of infections particularly where there are shared amenities such as kitchens and toilets

Noise
- Unpredictable intermittent noise (e.g. from noisy neighbours or traffic) has psychological consequences including sleep disturbance, irritability and poor concentration

Dampness
- Causes poor respiratory health
- Acts as a stress which leads to depression, emotional distress and increased risk of physical illness

Cold
- Exposure to cold is a direct physiological stress and source of discomfort which increases general susceptibility to illness
- The elderly, people with an illness, young infants living in cold housing and people who are roofless are at risk of hypothermia

Poor architectural design
- Unsafe building design can increase the risk of accidental injury
- Lack of play space (both inside and outside) for children, dwellings which are easy targets for burglars and vandals, where the design restricts access (dark and threatening stairways or footpaths, high-rise accommodation, accommodation which has too many stairs for the residents) are stressful and affect mental health
- Lack of adequate insulation and ventilation makes dwellings difficult and expensive to heat, leading to problems of cold and dampness

Being roofless or living in temporary accommodation
- Can be a source of disruption and stigma which makes it difficult to get jobs and maintain or access health services

Living in a 'bad' area
- Makes it difficult to access resources which would maintain or promote health, including healthy food, leisure and entertainment facilities, health services and employment opportunities

Poorly constructed houses cost more to heat and are often occupied by people on low incomes who cannot alleviate the problems of dampness and condensation by spending more on heating. The term 'fuel poverty' describes the compound effect of inadequate construction and low income of occupants.

STOP THINK

For a family with young children living in damp and overcrowded conditions, what are the possible consequences for health services of housing-related illness? What are the possible costs to the health service of inadequate housing?

Fig. 2 **Features of inadequate housing which are detrimental to health.**

A range of factors associated with housing have been shown to cause physical illness and discomfort as well as depression and emotional distress (Fig. 2).

For example, dampness can lead to overcrowding when occupants can only afford to heat one room. Dampness and mould can cause damage to property and thus add to the financial burden of replacement or redecoration to those struggling on low incomes. Keeping the house clean can be difficult and visible mould and the smell of dampness may lead to embarrassment about inviting friends and family in. Concerns about the impact of dampness on the health of children can be an additional stress.

Case study
The direct effects of dampness on health

A study in Britain (Platt et al 1989) looked at whether toxic fungal air spores which are present in damp and mouldy houses could explain the association between dampness and respiratory symptoms. The study involved the collection of health information from around 800 respondents. Measures of the internal housing environment were then taken by an independent team of surveyors who were 'blind' to the results of the health survey.

Reporting of respiratory symptoms was higher where the levels of damp and air spore counts were higher, indicating a 'dose–response relationship'. The health survey asked about other factors which might influence respiratory health such as smoking, ownership of pets and the use of indoor appliances as well as other social factors known to be associated with poor health. The relationship between respiratory symptoms, dampness and air spore count remained after all other possible explanatory factors were statistically ruled out.

WORKING IN THE HOME

There are defined fitness standards for formal work environments such as factories and offices (see pp. 58–59), but not for domestic housing. People who are not in formal employment may spend substantial amounts of time in housing environments which would not meet the minimum occupational health standards. Carrying out 'housework' such as child care, cleaning and cooking is particularly stressful in poor conditions.

HOUSING AND HEALTH SERVICES

It is important for health professionals to consider the extent to which patients' illness or distress are the result of their living conditions. Health professionals are sometimes asked to comment formally on this in assessments of medical priority for rehousing or assessments for community care (see pp. 146–147). The moves to day-case interventions and early discharge from hospital make it even more important that health professionals know about patients' housing conditions and ensure that poor living conditions do not exacerbate illness or prejudice recovery.

As more emphasis within the health service is placed on health promotion and illness prevention, an understanding of the impact of inadequate housing on health is increasingly important.

Housing, homelessness and health
- The housing environment affects health directly and indirectly.
- Overcrowding, noise, dampness, cold, poor design and poor neighbourhood are detrimental to health.
- Being housed does not necessarily imply having a home.
- 'Housework' is often carried out in conditions that would not satisfy 'Health and Safety at Work' standards.
- Provision of adequate, affordable housing is an important component of a policy for health.

WORK AND HEALTH

The United Nations Declaration of Human Rights states that 'Everyone has the right to work'. Does this imply that work is 'good' for us and for our health? Is all work good for us? Table 1 summarises some of the characteristics of work which have been identified as important for health, and this spread looks at the nature of, and evidence for, the relationships between some of these characteristics and people's health and well-being.

INCOME AND HEALTH

Economic growth and the creation of national wealth has enabled many people to enjoy higher standards of living than their grandparents or their parents. Until recently there has been a narrowing of incomes for different occupational groups, and overall real average earnings (allowing for inflation) have been rising. However, Figure 1 shows that income inequalities in Britain have been increasing since 1980.

At the simple level, the association between income and health is obvious from the data presented on class and health: class is inversely related to health, income levels are closely related to social class, therefore income levels will be inversely related to health (see pp. 44–45).

Research on the relationship between income and health has been slow to develop, largely because it is difficult to collect reliable data on people's life-time earnings. However, research by Wilkinson (1996) has suggested that, when looking at Western-style industrial countries, those countries which have the widest distribution of incomes typically exhibit the

Table 1 **Characteristics of 'healthy' jobs**

Advantages	High wages Good benefits Security Healthy, safe environment
Demands	Not excessive demands Busy, but not rushed Not conflicting demands Not excessive hours
Skill discretion	Interesting and varied tasks Ability to use skills, be creative Ability to learn new skills
Decision authority (control)	Ability to control how to do the work Participation in decision-making Having a say on the job
Support	Opportunities for social contact Collaboration and collective effort Good relationships with colleagues Good relationships with supervisors Feeling valued Promoting self-esteem Providing status and identity

highest mortality rates (Fig. 2). This is supported by recent British figures on life expectancy which show a fall in life expectancy over the same 10 years that income inequalities have increased.

STOP THINK What do you predict will happen to mortality rates in the former Communist East European states which are likely to experience a widening of income distribution now that they are moving towards a more market economy? What other factors might be important?

A HEALTHY AND SAFE ENVIRONMENT AT WORK

Estimates of the extent of occupational ill health, injury and loss of life vary from country to country and between occupations, and are likely not to be particularly accurate or comparable because of different reporting requirements and conventions, and different health and safety legislation.

In Britain, official estimates include a figure of about 2% of all deaths in 15–64-year-olds directly attributable to work: about 550 injuries and 900 'prescribed' or compensatable occupational diseases leading to death in 1987–88. These overall official figures have been declining over the last 20 years, but are generally regarded as an underestimate of the total amount of occupational ill health.

ACCIDENTS AT WORK

Accidents are the fourth main cause of death and the main cause of admission to hospital, and although accidents at work account for less than 5% of all accidental deaths in the UK, 20% of all accidental deaths to adults occur at work.

From 1971 to 1980, the fatal accident rate fell from 3.5 to 2.3 per 100 000 employees and has subsequently levelled off at this figure. However, the rate for fatal and major injuries per 100 000 employees increased by 8% from 1981 to 1985. The increase was particularly marked for the manufacturing sector (29%), agriculture and fishing (34%) and construction (41%) (Harvey 1988).

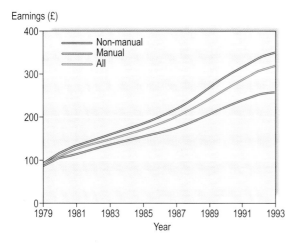

Fig. 1 **Average UK gross weekly earnings, full-time employees on adult rates.**

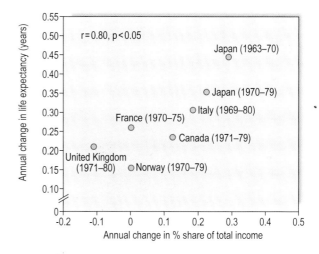

Fig. 2 **Annual change in life expectancy and percentage of income received by least well-off 60% of population.** Two figures for Japan were combined when calculating correlation coefficient. (Wilkinson 1992.)

Factors which have been implicated in the occurrence of accidents at work are:

- payment systems which relate pay to productivity (performance-related pay, piece work or bonus systems) and which encourage people to take risks
- informal work-group pressure to take risks to maintain productivity and pay
- production processes which are psychologically and physically tiring or boring which can result in tiredness or a lack of concentration
- production processes which run faster than the operative can manage safely
- unexpected changes in routine procedures or an unplanned event requiring a fast response (identified in oil-rig accidents)
- exposure to direct physical hazards like dust, smoke, noise, vibration, heat, poisons, ionising agents, and chemicals
- inadequate testing of chemicals
- withholding from workers details of chemicals being used in production
- unsafe design and poor maintenance
- safety measures which hinder communication, or are uncomfortable or slow the worker down
- lack of training and poor supervision; the cost of effective safety measures
- worker collusion for fear of losing their jobs
- accident proneness — the chance of having an accident doubles in the first 6 months after a divorce
- alcohol consumption.

There is an inherent conflict for employers and employees in the implementation of a healthy and safe environment. Creating such an environment is usually costly in terms of both time and design, which can reduce profitability and increase the possibility of job-loss. Two independent studies found that only in about 18% and 11% of cases respectively was the employee responsible for the accident, whereas management were found to be responsible in 68% and 75% of cases respectively.

Factors contributing to the rise in accidents associated with major injury are:

- an increase in the number of self-employed people (who are more at risk of accidents)
- greater propensity to report accidents
- more small firms
- economize over safety
- sub-contracting in the construction industry
- the 'employment' of younger people on short-term training schemes rather than longer-term apprenticeships.

INDUSTRIAL DISEASES

There has been a fall in the incidence of 'prescribed' occupational diseases as a result of progress in the reduction of occupational risks from life-threatening diseases like asbestos-related lung cancer and mesothelioma, and bladder cancer caused by chemicals used in the rubber and dyestuff industries.

STRESS AT WORK

There is now an extensive literature on the relationship between stress and health, but there are problems of disentangling the many confounding factors (see pp. 52–53). One approach, which has recently been applied to a large study of sickness absence records of British civil servants (North et al 1993), has incorporated the theory that stress is the product of (a) the demands of the job and (b) the decision latitude (or decision authority — Table 1) that the worker has over that job. The study reported that men and women in lower-grade jobs were more likely to have higher rates of short- and long-term spells of sickness absence. Smoking and alcohol consumption, low levels of control, little variety in use of skills, fast work pace, low satisfaction and negative support at work, financial difficulties and negative support outside work were the main risk factors which accounted for the differences in absence. However, despite the sophistication of the research methods used, these variables could only explain one-third of the variation in sickness absence rates.

DOMESTIC LABOUR

Over the last 10 years, attention has also focused on the fact that housework, or domestic labour, is routine, boring, unpaid and unvalued. About 75% of women describe housework as 'boring', compared with 64% of operatives' description of working on a car assembly line. Not going out to work is also a significant risk factor for depression in women (see pp. 114–115). The main reasons that women give for wanting to have a paid job are to supplement the family income, to get out of the house to meet people, and to feel valued. However, when they do find a job, it is likely that they will earn less than men doing similar work, despite equal pay legislation.

Case study
Joe's story*

'The rollers stopped and we called out downstairs, "What's going on?" So Joe went to see to save time — but then they stopped the chute as well, see? So now the rollers down here won't start either. The shaker wouldn't start. But then the blokes up there started up the chute and it was all coming down again, see. So Joe climbed across the rollers and pushed the start button. And his finger caught in a roller like that, you see. And as soon as the rollers started up he lost his footing and all his weight came down on the finger and he just dropped and pulled it off like that'.

* From Nichols 1975

Work and health

- There is an inverse relationship between income and health.
- Countries with the greatest inequality in the distribution of incomes exhibit the highest mortality rates.
- Official figures for occupational death, injury and disease underestimate the total amount of occupational ill health.
- Accidents resulting in fatalities have been falling whereas accidents resulting in major injury have been increasing.
- Performance-related pay, production processes, exposure to hazards, insufficient or inappropriate safety measures, recent stressful events and alcohol consumption are among a number of factors associated with accidents at work.
- High job demands and low job control create stress which appears to be associated with ill health.
- Housework is more tedious and less valued than most paid jobs and is a risk factor for depression.

UNEMPLOYMENT AND HEALTH

There is now extensive literature on the relationship between unemployment and health, and a growing consensus has emerged as to the degree and type of health effects produced by unemployment. Although there is closer agreement as to the type of health effects of unemployment, there is still debate over the mechanisms of causality. Unemployment is often viewed as a stressful life event, an event which might produce psychological and financial strain, and a potential contributor to illness susceptibility. Other work has focused on issues round the possible causal link between low income and poor nutrition, while some researchers have been more concerned with the social isolation faced by the unemployed which may lead them to adopt the health-damaging behaviours of increased alcohol and tobacco use, and drug taking (Fig. 1).

THE EVIDENCE
Psychological morbidity

Hill (1973) described three stages of unemployment: an initial stage characterised by denial and a feeling that nothing much has changed, that a new job will soon turn up; an intermediate phase when all job-seeking efforts fail, the individual becomes pessimistic and suffers active distress; and a third stage when the individual becomes fatalistic and adapts himself or herself to a new and more restricted state.

An important series of studies on psychological well-being was carried out by Warr and his colleagues (1978) on different sub-groups of the unemployed. An index of present life satisfaction was found to be strongly negatively associated with unemployment status both for redundant steel-workers and men attending unemployment benefit offices. On the other hand a measure of constant self-esteem yielded no differences between managers with or without a job. A similar pattern emerged for measures of positive well-being, where a person was asked if he/she had experienced positive events in the past few weeks. Positive affect in recent weeks among redundant steel workers was clearly associated with their employment status at the time of interview whereas the index for the more stable self-esteem showed no variation with employment status in two teenage samples.

Indicators of negative well-being, where the interviewees were asked if they had experienced negative events — for example, feelings of loneliness — in the past few weeks, showed the clearest overall relationship with significant differences between employed and unemployed respondents in every case.

This series of studies also threw light on some of the factors which moderated the negative impact of unemployment:

- People who were committed to their work and who became redundant were found to be particularly disadvantaged.
- Age and length of unemployment were likely to be intercorrelated: and so older people were less likely to become re-employed and were more likely to be sick. The middle-aged unemployed, in fact, were found to have the lowest well-being scores.
- Although they found differences between the sexes, with men having higher rates of psychological morbidity than women, this was thought to be related to personal commitment to their work. When the variable of personal work involvement was held constant the sexes were equally affected.
- The results on length of unemployment and psychological well-being emerging from these studies were inconclusive and further research was needed.

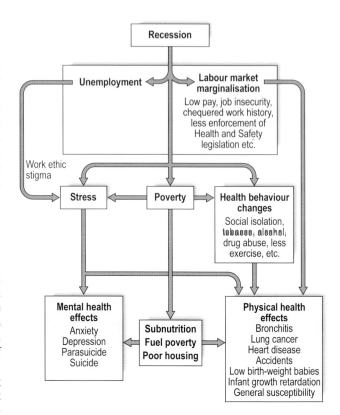

Fig. 1 **How might unemployment lead to poor health?** (Source: Smith 1987)

- Social support and the financial security of the unemployed person were suggested as positive moderators but were not adequately tested.

Physical morbidity

Any cross-sectional analysis comparing groups of employed workers with men and women unemployed shows that employed people are healthier despite occupational hazards. These studies also give us some interesting pointers towards the health condition of the long-term unemployed (for more than 1 year), among whom there are likely to be far more health problems than among the short-term unemployed. Such studies cannot, however, tell us whether these effects are specifically caused by unemployment. Selection processes operate; individuals may have become unemployed because they had health problems to begin with. It is also difficult to separate out the direct effect of unemployment from any indirect effect of poverty, bad housing conditions, geographical location and social class. Although most of the research so far discussed can produce correlations between unemployment and health, the establishment of causality requires studies over time, looking at workers before termination of their employment and following them through and after redundancy.

An important American longitudinal study looked at 100 men and 74 controls before two factories closed and followed the cohort for the next two years. The controls were found to be healthier than the terminees. Myocardial infarction was at the expected level, but the risk of coronary heart disease had increased among the terminees. Research by Beale and Nethercott (1985) on a factory closure in south-west England found increased consultation rates with GPs and increased referral rates to hospital among redundant workers and members of their families compared with controls.

Mortality

Death rates have been found to rise in times of economic depression, unemployed people have higher death rates than the employed, and death rates rise with increasing duration of unemployment. A British study (Moser et al 1984) looked at 5861 men aged 15–64 who were waiting to take up a job or seeking work in the week before the 1971 census. The standardised mortality ratio for 1971–81 for men aged 15–64 at death who were seeking work in 1971 was 136. It was higher in the second half of the decade (144) than in the first half (129) and was raised for all ages, although it was particularly high among those under 54, reaching over 200 in those aged 35–44 (Fig. 2). The causes of death that predominated among the unemployed were malignant neoplasms, particularly lung cancer, and accidents, poisonings and violence, particularly suicide. These findings have been corroborated by findings from the British Regional Heart Study (Morris et al 1994) which, after controlling for social class and health at time of entry into the study, found that unemployed men aged 40–59 were 1.7 times more likely to have died after 5-year follow-up than men who were not unemployed during that time.

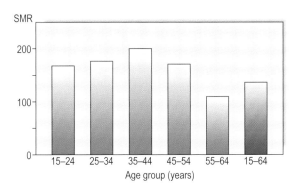

Fig. 2 **Standardised Mortality Ratio 1971–1981** among men seeking work in 1971, by age at death. (Moser et al 1984.)

STOP THINK A most important debate regarding the explanation of the findings relating to unemployment and mortality has been waged between Eyer (1977) and Brenner (1983). Brenner claims that a 1% increase in unemployment can account for a 2% increase in death rates after a lapse of 3 years. For Eyer the delay is much smaller and he believes, contrary to Brenner, that the sources of social stress which occur with an economic boom are responsible for the increase in the death rate. What do you think?

Mechanisms

Recent research has been able to capitalise on the volume of work carried out in the 1980s and gives more attention to the mechanisms which cause ill health. In order to understand the relationships between unemployment and ill health and mortality, four mechanisms are important:

- the role of relative poverty
- social isolation and the role of self-esteem
- health-related behaviour
- the effect that a spell of unemployment has on subsequent employment patterns.

Psychological health is seen to be affected by financial problems which increase the frequency of stressful life events. Mental health is also affected by decreasing social activity and participation, and diminishing social support. Although alternative social networks may eventually be formed, these may involve groups who have withdrawn from the norms and values of mainstream society. They may thus be more likely to indulge in health-damaging behaviours. In terms of physical health the 'stress pathway', involving physiological changes (for example raised cholesterol and lowered immunity), is believed to be the main mechanism. The importance of relative rather than just absolute disadvantage has also been highlighted in the recent literature (see pp. 44–45, 48–49).

Case study
The Johnsons — The loss of a job

David: *'The relief feeling was very short, it only lasted a month. I can't sit about, you see. I was really shaken when my first job went sour, then the psychological effects came in, because I thought the job would be easy to get. It may have been my attitude, my elevated ego, thinking that I was better than anybody else.*

I think the family started disintegrating then. I started to drink too much, getting into vicious tempers, I was easily angry and upset and I used to snap at the children all the time. I started having these deep depressions, and nobody could help me. Then I started to withdraw. I would take a bottle of wine and finish it within the hour. Then I would sleep. I would do nothing constructive around the house. Just sit around, with no energy, I didn't want to go out of the doorstep. Nobody could talk to me and I had nothing to talk about. I wasn't sociable. Then I tried to pull myself together for the girls coming back from school. It wasn't my character at all.'

(From Fagin & Little 1984)

Unemployment and health

- There is a growing consensus that unemployment has detrimental effects on people's health.
- The major pathways to illness include unemployment as a 'stressful life event'.
- Psychological studies of the unemployed have discovered three stages through which the unemployed person passes: an initial stage characterised by denial, an intermediate stage of active distress, and a final stage of fatalism.
- All cross-sectional studies show the employed to be in better health than the unemployed. Longitudinal studies strongly suggest that the contrast is caused by unemployment rather than by selection within the labour market.
- The main causes of mortality among the unemployed are malignant neoplasms (particularly lung cancer), and accidents, poisonings and violence (particularly suicide).
- Relative poverty, social isolation and the lack of self-esteem, and damaging health-related behaviours are the major factors associated with the production of ill effects among the unemployed.

WAR, CONFLICT AND DISASTER

As a result of war or disaster, people may lose not only their lives, but their close relatives, belongings and also the jobs or other roles they occupied in the community. Sometimes communities are completely destroyed, and their members are forced to become refugees. These different forms of loss are referred to as losses of identity. The identities we possess, as worker, family member or group member, provide us with roles which shape our activities and give meaning to our lives. If these are destroyed, the sense of who and what we are is severely threatened.

CAN WAR OR DISASTER IMPROVE PSYCHOLOGICAL WELL-BEING?

There are several difficulties in assessing the impacts of war and disaster and these may lead to misleading conclusions about the extent of distress experienced by populations (see Table 1). For example it is important to distinguish between a fall in psychiatric admissions which might be due to closure of hospitals and a fall which is a genuine result of reduced levels of depression in the community. Nonetheless, it is possible for mental health to improve during times of war. One reason for this is that wars usually require people to think of themselves as part of a group, working together against a common enemy, rather than as individuals. If the group is doing well, this may give people a sense of well-being, just as watching one's own country win the World Cup can lead to feelings of happiness. Also, when the group part of our identity is in the forefront of our mind, our personal problems are at least temporarily forgotten. A second source of well-being during war may arise from the acquisition of new roles and identities. During war, many accepted rules and practices are put aside, allowing some people greater freedom and choice in life. For example, during the Second World War, married women were entitled to paid work for the first time and were permitted to work in occupations from which they had previously been excluded.

> **STOP THINK** What reasons can you suggest to explain why mental health casualties might be unrecognised or untreated during or following war or disasters?

Case study
Disaster at Buffalo Creek

A major disaster which occurred at Buffalo Creek, in the United States, provides a graphic example of the effects of loss of community. A dam collapsed at the top of a valley, flooding many small mining villages and marooning families in different parts of the valley, in unfamiliar groupings. Two years after the disaster, 80% of the villagers were still experiencing the symptoms of post traumatic stress disorder. Prior to the disaster, the villagers had lived in tightly knit communities, where friendships were of long standing and much time and energy was invested in community activities. When the disaster occurred, people found that they no longer had a community in which to invest their energies and had profound difficulties in creating new social relationships or finding new goals to pursue. For these people, whose identity was centred around their sense of belonging to a recognisable village, the disaster literally took away their knowledge of who they were and their sense of purpose in life (Erikson 1976).

Table 1 **Difficulties in measuring the psychological effects of war, conflict and disaster**

Baseline measures	Measures of people's psychological adjustment before they experienced a traumatic event are rarely available so it is difficult to assess changes
Self-report biases	During conflict, war or disaster people may be too preoccupied with practical concerns to take part in research studies Rescue workers, such as police, firemen, doctors, nurses and members of the armed forces may fear dismissal or ridicule if they disclose emotional difficulties
Service provision	Although official figures, for example of psychiatric admissions before war-time, may appear to provide useful comparison statistics it is important to remember that psychiatric admissions depend on the number of beds available. During WW2 psychiatric hospitals were used as general medical hospitals to receive wounded military personnel Figures on the number of people seeking counselling after a disaster will be influenced by the level of provision of counselling services, not just by level of need

COPING WITH THREAT

Stress reactions depend to a large extent upon the ways in which people perceive events (see pp. 52–53). One factor which is very important in determining whether we experience threat and how we cope with it, is the extent to which we believe we can control it. Disasters are, by their very nature, events over which individuals have little control. During war-time, people have very little warning of violent attacks and minimal ability to control their effects. In these circumstances, people have to develop coping strategies to deal with unpredictable threats. One way people do this is by becoming accepting or fatalistic about the possibility of threat. If they do this, they may be able to reduce their sense of anxiety, but are unlikely to take precautionary action to protect themselves. Another coping strategy is to deny the existence or severity of the threat. A study of people living with the threat of violence in Northern Ireland (Cairns and Wilson 1984) investigated the possibility that denial was used as a means of maintaining psychological well-being. People living in two different towns, one where there had been a lot of violence and one where there had been very little violence, were asked to complete a questionnaire which measured mild psychiatric disturbance. They were also asked to say how much violence they felt there was in the area where they lived. The results showed that people living in the high violence town who acknowledged that there was a lot of violence going on reported more psychiatric symptoms than people who denied or avoided thinking about the level of violence (Fig. 1).

POST-TRAUMATIC STRESS DISORDER

Although at present post-traumatic stress disorder (PTSD) is not an official psychiatric diagnosis according to the International Classification of Disease used in Britain, it is an official diagnostic category in the American Diagnostic and Statistical Manual and it is widely used to assess the casualties of war and disaster all over the world.

Case study
Living with conflict in Northern Ireland

The following extracts are from interviews conducted with students living in Northern Ireland in 1987. The extracts reveal how they viewed the conflict around them and managed it in their everyday lives.

- *'We don't let it affect us. We just go where we want and take a chance. A few years back we wouldn't go outside the immediate area but now we just go anywhere and hope we don't get into any trouble. That's part of the way my attitude's changed ... I was found guilty of something I didn't do [rioting], it could easily happen again, so I don't really have any control over what might happen. What the hell, if you get done you get done, if you don't you don't ... As soon as I finish here I'm just going to start looking for a job somewhere else.'*
- *'I stay in a lot ... I absorb myself in TV, videos, fantasise about different places. ... Most of the time I do have a barrier up but I know it's there. I don't block it out completely. The reason I don't block it out completely is that I know what's happened to my mates. I want to know it's there. If I blocked it out completely and then something happens like getting your door busted in or something like that I'd just go to pieces ... I can't afford to do that because I want a future for myself. I can only do that if I keep a grip on myself.'*
- *'All my family are in the security forces. My fiancé as well. You can't go places. You can't go to pubs or discos. You always have to check the car, you always have to look behind you and look out the window before you go anywhere ... You have to smile ... I do get very frustrated about it but I can't do anything about it ... I think of the security forces as my group. Wives and girlfriends or whatever. I identify with that. Everyone supports the next one, it's sort of like a clan. We arrange parties and discos. The only thing is they have to be arranged inside the police barracks. I don't have too many friends outside of the security forces group. It makes you feel more secure.'*

Re-read the extracts of young people in Northern Ireland talking about the ways they manage to live with the conflict. What types of coping strategies do the students describe? What factors do you think might influence the type of coping strategy a particular person uses to reduce stress?

A person can be said to have PTSD if he or she experiences the following symptoms:

- a history of a recognisable traumatic event
- re-experiencing the trauma in recurrent dreams, in intrusive waking recollections of the event or by suddenly feeling or acting as if the traumatic event were occurring again
- reduced involvement in and responsiveness to the external world, characterised by diminished interest in previously salient activities; feelings of detachment from others and diminished emotional reactions.

In addition, the person may experience some of these symptoms:

- a marked startle response, disturbed sleep, survival guilt, impaired concentration or memory, avoidance of activities that bring the trauma to mind and increased symptoms in connection with events similar to the trauma.

Of these symptoms, vivid re-experiencing is the most characteristic. PTSD can affect trained soldiers, rescue workers and health professionals as well as civilians caught up in war or disasters. Just over a third of police officers who helped evacuate people from the Bradford football stadium fire disaster experienced PTSD. In a study of Israeli troops following the Lebanon war, 10% of men who did not experience a stress reaction during the war itself were found to be experiencing PTSD 3 years later. PTSD often appears to begin some time after a traumatic event has occurred. This may suggest that people initially are able to block out the events they experience, perhaps because circumstances often demand it, but when the crisis has passed the emotional impact becomes apparent.

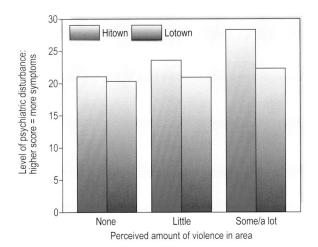

Fig. 1 **Effects of level of violence and perceptions of violence on psychiatric disturbance in two Northern Irish towns.** (Adapted from Cairns and Wilson 1984.)

War, conflict and disaster

- Wars and disasters lead not only to loss of life, personal injury and damage to property, but to changes in the roles people occupy in their communities. These changes can have profound effects on the sense of self and lead to changes in psychological health.
- Post-traumatic stress disorder is increasingly being recognised as a specific reaction to severe traumatic events, requiring specialist treatment. It affects rescue workers and health professionals as well as civilians.
- In order to understand the extent to which people experience anxiety about the threats created by war or disaster, it is necessary to examine the ways they perceive and cope with it. The extent to which people feel they can control threat is an important determinant of the coping strategy they adopt.

WHAT IS PREVENTION?

THE GOALS OF PREVENTION

The goals of prevention are to preserve and promote good health in society by preventing disease and minimising its consequences. It is useful to distinguish between three types of prevention, usually referred to as primary, secondary and tertiary prevention. The distinction between these three types of prevention is that each has a different goal. Have a look at Table 1 showing the goals of prevention before you read on.

PRIMARY PREVENTION: THE PREVENTION OF DISEASE INCIDENCE

The incidence of disease is measured in terms of the number of new cases of disease occurring in society, usually during a specified time period such as 1 year. Primary prevention can be undertaken whenever the cause of disease has been identified.

Perhaps the best known form of medical intervention in primary prevention is the development of mass immunisation. Over the years, immunisation has been introduced against poliomyelitis, tuberculosis, measles and many other diseases. However, since it usually takes several years of medical research before a virus is identified and a vaccine developed, the impact of immunisation on disease incidence is sometimes very small. Poliomyelitis immunisation is probably one of the few medical interventions to have had a demonstrable primary prevention effect in the last century (Fig. 1).

Health education (e.g. advice to use condoms during sex) and public health measures which help people avoid contact with viruses and bacteria may be particularly valuable early interventions.

The major causes of death in developed countries today are diseases of the circulatory system and neoplasms (see p. 42). These diseases have been linked to particular behaviours, such as smoking cigarettes. Figure 2 shows that smokers' life expectancy during the last century

has increased only half as much as that of non-smokers, a remarkable finding given the improvements in nutrition and sanitation which have occurred during the same period. In developed countries, therefore, primary prevention efforts have been particularly concerned with health education regarding personal behaviours (see pp. 70–71).

SECONDARY PREVENTION: THE PREVENTION OF DISEASE PREVALENCE

Prevalence is defined as the number of people who have a particular disease at any one time. Clearly, if diseases are left untreated and new cases are occurring all the time, the prevalence of a disease will increase. Although doctors are continually involved in secondary prevention, from time to time campaigns are mounted to increase the likelihood of doctors detecting particular diseases. For example, skin cancer may go unrecognised by patients and doctors unless specific efforts are made to identify it during consultations. Some forms of secondary prevention, such as screening for relatively rare diseases such as cervical cancer, require the participation of practically all

women in society if those with the disease are to be detected and the screening programme is to prove cost-effective. Efforts to provide education to persuade people to take part may therefore be seen by some as efforts to compel people to participate in secondary prevention programmes, and doctors delivering these services need to be aware of the anxieties people have about screening tests (see pp. 66–67).

TERTIARY PREVENTION: THE PREVENTION OF ADVERSE CONSEQUENCES OF DISEASE OR GENETICALLY CAUSED IMPAIRMENT

As a result of increased life expectancy and a reduction in the birth rate, there is increasing concern for the care of people who survive treatment of, for example, heart disease, cancer or stroke. This means ensuring that patients experience the best possible health for the longest possible period of time following diagnosis. Tertiary prevention is concerned with a wider range of health indices than either primary or secondary prevention. For instance, tertiary preventive interventions might have as their goals the reduction of disability and promotion of

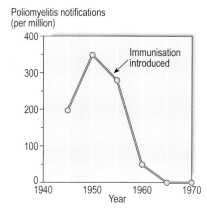

Fig. 1 **Poliomyelitis notifications before and after introduction of immunisation: England and Wales.** (Adapted from McKeown 1979.)

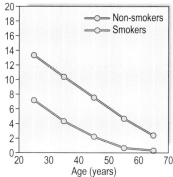

Fig. 2 **Increase in expectation of life of men 1838–1970.** (Adapted from McKeown 1979.)

Table 1 **Goals of prevention**

Type of prevention	Distal goal	Proximal goal	Behavioural goal
Primary prevention	Prevent new cases of disease		
	Prevent new cases of AIDS	Prevent infection with HIV	Use of condoms during sexual intercourse
Secondary prevention	Reduce number of people with disease at a given time		
	Reduce cases of cervical cancer	Identify cervical cancer early and treat effectively	Uptake of test to detect cancer and pre-cancer Uptake of treatment
Tertiary prevention	Minimise consequences of disease or impairment		
	Minimise disability in children with cerebral palsy	Identify disability	Uptake and maintenance of skills training

psychological well-being. Exercise and rehabilitation programmes may be provided in medical settings and during follow-up care to enable stroke survivors to walk and acquire control over a range of movements (see pp. 116–117).

Chronic conditions which are genetically acquired or acquired during childhood or early adulthood are also a focus of tertiary prevention. These conditions cannot be cured but much can be done to minimise the extent to which they result in disability or distress. A person with asthma can exercise control over his or her condition by using medication effectively and practising behavioural strategies to avoid attacks.

BEHAVIOURAL CHANGE IN PREVENTION: LEVELS OF INTERVENTION

The success of prevention depends to a great extent upon the ability of the health care system and health care professionals to deliver preventive interventions to people who believe themselves to be in good health, and on the extent to which people take up interventions and are motivated and able to comply with behavioural recommendations. However, in order to bring about behavioural change it is important to acknowledge the cultural and social influences which govern behaviour (see pp. 72–73).

Strategies to change behaviour occur at many different levels (see Table 2).

Action by governments is important in facilitating health-related behavioural change, among both doctors and patients. For instance in 1990 the British government changed the General Practitioner contract in order to encourage greater participation in preventive health care. One target for change was in primary and secondary prevention of heart disease. General Practitioners were offered financial inducements to encourage them to screen patients with respect to their diet, smoking habits, exercise and blood cholesterol levels and to offer appropriate treatments or behavioural change clinics to help people to modify their life-style. Governments may also seek to prevent heart disease by imposing taxes on cigarettes to limit their consumption or passing legislation which ensures that the fat content of food is clearly marked on labels so that people are able to make informed choices about their diet.

A second level of change concerns attempts to modify the social environment or commonly held views about health and health-related behaviours. Clearly, people will be unable to change their diet if they have limited access to fruit and vegetables in local shops or works canteens. Community and organisational level interventions can do a great deal to assist individual behavioural change. People are very much influenced in their behaviour by what they see or believe others do, and particularly by what they think will be approved or disapproved

of by others (see pp. 54–55). Screening for heart disease risk, for example, depends upon changing people's views about the appropriateness of consulting the health care system when they are in good health.

At an individual level, health care professionals are directly involved in communicating to patients what preventive strategies they might use and advising them on how to implement these strategies. Doctors' advice to patients can be very effective in motivating people to change. However, many preventive behaviours require people to acquire new skills and confidence in their ability to control or promote their own health. It is on the development and delivery of effective behaviour change strategies that much of primary and tertiary prevention depends (see pp. 70–71).

DILEMMAS AND PROBLEMS IN PREVENTION

For many years, prevention has been seen to be the province of a speciality of medicine known as Public Health Medicine. A shift towards prevention requires that all health professionals acquire new skills in the effective communication of health education messages and behaviour change strategies.

Some forms of prevention rely upon the participation of everyone in society in order to make them cost-effective. For example, infectious disease control depends to a large extent on what is known in epidemiology as herd immunity. These considerations may have led some to question how we distinguish between education, persuasion and compulsion. Other forms of prevention which are now becoming available rely on the detection of fetal abnormalities. The introduction of genetic screening has raised concerns about the ethics of parental choice and society's view of those with genetic disorders (see also pp. 68–69).

Table 2 **Levels of intervention to achieve behavioural change: fat in the diet**

Level of intervention	Example of intervention	Behavioural changes
Governmental/societal	Legislation requiring manufacturers to specify the fat content of products on packaging	Agricultural policies to restrict animal fattening Research investment to develop low-fat food products Department of Health incentives to doctors to undertake prevention
Social/environmental	Mass media health education	Provision of low-fat choices in schools/worksite canteens
Individual	Screening by doctors to assess risk and provide motivation and healthy eating advice	Rehabilitation programmes by nurses and doctors to promote diet change, e.g. following heart attacks Food and cookery demonstrations and workshops in community centres School health education to provide motivation and skills

STOP THINK
- How might you go about making a case for spending money on prevention?
- What ethical issues are associated with preventive programmes to (a) immunise all children (b) screen all women for cervical cancer (c) ban worksite smoking (d) conduct genetic tests for fetal abnormalities?
- What skills do doctors require in order to practise preventive medicine effectively?

What is prevention?
- Primary prevention refers to the prevention of disease incidence.
- Secondary prevention refers to the prevention of disease prevalence.
- Tertiary prevention refers to the prevention of disease impact.
- Preventive efforts occur at many levels; the governmental or societal policy level, the social or environmental level and the individual level.

MEDICAL SCREENING

Medical screening is potentially very valuable as part of preventive medicine. In those who screen positively there is the possibility of early diagnosis or early identification of risk with the resulting benefits of early medical intervention. Those who screen negatively are likely to benefit from reassurance. However, the usefulness of medical screening may be limited if the uptake rate is low or if no benefits are obtained by patients found to be positive on screening. In addition, there may be disadvantages to patients if the techniques simply serve to increase their anxiety.

Procedures have been developed for screening patients for disease (e.g. phenylketonuria, breast cancer), for precursors of disease (e.g. cervical cytology, HIV test) or for risk factors for disease (e.g. smoking, poor diet, hypertension). For screening to be useful, it must be possible to take some action such as changing life-style or taking medication to reduce the impact or risk of disease.

The potential to develop new screening procedures has been greatly increased by the identification of risk factors for disease such as cardiovascular disease. It will increase as a result of the Human Genome Mapping project as it becomes possible to screen for genetic defects or for carrier status.

SCREENING: PROCESS AND RESULTS

Usually those found to be positive will go on to have further tests which will determine whether the first result was a true or false positive. Since no screening test is perfect, there will always be a number of

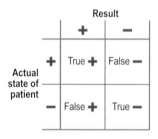

Fig. 1 **Four possible outcomes of a screening test.**

false positives and false negatives and the number will depend on the sensitivity and specificity of the test. The four possible outcomes of screening are shown in Figure 1.

Patients found to be positive in the definitive test may then go on to medical treatment or further monitoring, or they may be advised to make changes in their life-style.

UPTAKE OF SCREENING

No test achieves 100% uptake by the relevant population. Doctors may fail to recommend the test and patients may not accept it if offered. While the reasons for patients declining a test have been investigated in some detail, recent research suggests that doctors may not offer a test even when it would be appropriate, perhaps when the doctor thinks the test is ineffective or believes the patients would not take the appropriate actions (e.g. change diet, adopt safer sex procedures), or simply forgets to offer the test.

Those offered a test may refuse to take it because it is incompatible with their health beliefs (see pp. 54–55), for instance, they may not think they are susceptible to the condition being tested. For example, women were more likely to have amniocentesis if they thought they were likely to have a Down's baby; and uptake was related to *perceived* risk, but not to *actual* risk as indicated by the maternal age. Lack of information may also reduce the rate of uptake. Additionally, patients may make a rational decision not to have a test, for example when a pregnant woman declines tests on her fetus because she would not consider termination of pregnancy.

ADVERSE EFFECTS FOR THOSE TESTED

Patients show high levels of anxiety when being screened and awaiting results. Informing the patient that the test is negative lowers anxiety more effectively than telling them to assume the result was normal if they hear nothing more. However, even communicating a negative result can have adverse effects. A *true negative* result can be harmful if the individual overgeneralises the reassurance; pregnant women screened negative for spina bifida and Down's syndrome frequently believe the tests showed that their babies would be normal. A *false negative* result can be harmful if it prevents the patient from receiving appropriate treatment or advice on life-style; a false negative HIV test might result in the patient putting others at risk by sexual transmission and remove the motivation to adopt safer sexual practices.

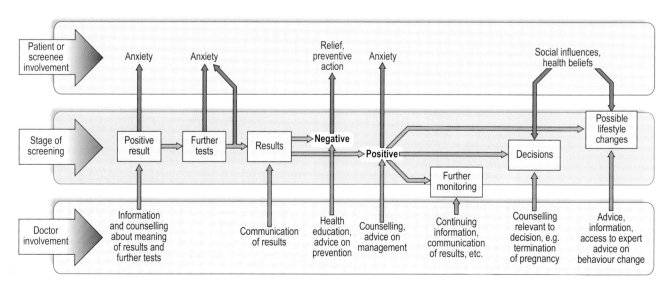

Fig. 2 **Schematic outline of medical screening and the social and behavioural factors involved — the process following a positive result.**

Patients testing positive

Following a positive screening test result, there are further stages of tests, results and medical management. Each of these involves further social and behavioural processes, as shown in Figure 2.

False positives

When the initial test result is positive or ambiguous but is followed by a clear negative result, i.e. the patient has received an initial false positive or invalid result, patients may continue to be anxious long after being told the negative result.

True positives

If the result is a true positive, patients' reactions will tend to vary with the implications of the results, depending on the seriousness of the condition and the available preventive or curative medical treatment. Nevertheless, there may be unexpected reactions. For example, individuals found to be positive for genetic disease such as Huntington's chorea or polyposis have reported feeling relieved, perhaps because their uncertainty was reduced.

When screening identifies people at risk of disease, there may be adverse effects of labelling the individual and it has been found that they may respond *as if they are ill* rather than just at risk (see pp. 120–121). Studies of people shown on screening to have hypertension have found that they subsequently show higher levels of distress, report more symptoms, take more time off work, and participate less in social activities. The level of distress is affected by the way in which the diagnosis is communicated. For example, those informed that they were hypertensive and given leaflets describing hypertension as 'the silent killer' were more anxious months later than those fully informed that it was a risk factor and reassured about management (Rudd et al 1986).

IMPLICATIONS OF A POSITIVE RESULT

For some test results, such as Huntington's chorea, the result carries no specific implications for action in a clinical context, although the recipient may choose to make relevant plans for the future. For other tests such as genetic tests with a probabilistic rather than certain result, there may be continued uncertainty

and further clinical monitoring will be required. For yet others, such as hypertension, appropriate medical management may reduce the likelihood or severity of the condition.

Other positive results may require the recipient to make critical decisions (such as whether to terminate a pregnancy) or to consider changes in behaviour and life-style (such as reducing fat intake or practising safer sex). While there is ample evidence that many people will make these changes successfully, a substantial number of people will attempt to change and fail. The overall success of the screening programme may be limited by failures to change behaviours in those screening positive.

 Consider one area of medical screening such as in pregnancy, for genetic disease, or for cardiovascular risk factors. Follow the flow charts in Figure 2 and consider what adverse effects might arise at each stage. How might doctors minimise these adverse effects?

THE ROLE OF DOCTORS

Doctors may play key roles at every stage (see Fig. 2 and list below). The results of screening, both in terms of successful detection and management of clinical conditions and in terms of the potential adverse effects for those tested, depend on the doctors' behaviours.

The role of doctors in screening includes:

- inviting the individual for screening: motivating the individual to attend without raising unnecessary fears
- counselling about screening: indicating the potential benefits while outlining the limitations; enabling the individual to reach an informed decision
- giving health education: before screening, e.g. for serum cholesterol or HIV; after positive screening, e.g. for risk factors for cardiovascular disease
- communicating results which may be complex: providing enough information to enable patients to understand; achieving a balance between raising unnecessary anxiety and giving inappropriate reassurance
- advising on decisions following positive results: giving information to enable informed choice and consent
- clinical management: varies depending on the type of screening
- assisting individuals to make necessary life-style changes: e.g. smoking, diet, exercise, medication, safer sex, repeated screening or monitoring.

Case study

Mrs Green had been alarmed to be recalled for further tests after blood tests suggested something might be wrong with her baby. She had taken a long time to conceive and this was a much wanted child. Although she thought the pregnancy might already show, she felt she could not tell her friends at work until she got the result of the amniocentesis and could be sure the baby was all right. After the amniocentesis, the obstetrician said there was nothing to worry about as the test result was normal. However, Mrs Green continued to be concerned — why had the original test been positive? Surely that indicated something was wrong, after all 'There's no smoke without fire' — if one test was positive and one was normal, how could the doctors be sure which one was right? Her continuing anxiety led her to be on the lookout for signs that things were going wrong. She worried over every little sensation in her body.

When the baby was born she was reassured that he looked like a normal baby boy, but wondered if there had been a more subtle abnormality which had made that first test positive and which would show itself over time.

Medical screening

- For any screening test, a substantial number of those offered the test do not accept — a result of poor information, social influences or, in some cases, good rational decisions.
- Screening may have adverse effects, especially raised anxiety, which may persist even when the result is normal.
- The way in which results are communicated can affect the impact of the results on the individual.
- Those being screened require information and counselling.
- For some tests, those being screened may need health education and advice on behaviour and life-style change.
- People do not always succeed in making life-style changes without further professional assistance.

THE SOCIAL IMPLICATIONS OF THE NEW GENETICS

Developments in molecular genetics have major implications for society and individuals, doctors and patients. The knowledge and techniques which have arisen from the development of recombinant DNA are likely to affect profoundly how we think about and deal with health, risks to health, disease and illness. The search for genetic components to a range of diseases, behaviours and traits is well underway.

The new genetics touches the social, cultural, ethical and personal realms as well as the biological, and has implications for some of the fundamental principles which guide research and clinical practice — confidentiality, autonomy, informed consent and individual choice (see pp. 154–155). The new genetics promises great improvements in health and increased control and choice for individuals, especially in relation to reproduction. Many scientists, clinicians and others take the social and ethical implications seriously and contribute to the important debate about how this knowledge may be used (Nuffield Council on Bioethics 1993). Genetic testing and screening are areas where the impact on both individuals and society has to be considered, and where clinicians and other health care professionals have a crucial role.

GENETIC TESTING

The genes for many single gene disorders have been identified, and genetic components in common multifactorial conditions are now being researched. Testing for a range of genetic diseases (e.g. for late onset dominant conditions or for carrier status for single gene recessive disorders) is now available in many industrialised countries. Experience gained in the introduction of existing genetic testing programmes provides a good illustration of the social, cultural and ethical issues involved, and may help shape the application of scientific developments in the future.

Predictive testing: Huntington's disease

Huntington's disease is an autosomal dominant condition. All those who inherit the gene will develop the disorder; it is of late adult onset, fatal and untreatable. Definitive testing is now available which can identify those who will develop the disease. At first glance, the provision of predictive testing within families known to be at risk of Huntington's disease may seem to be desirable, not least because an individual who has been identified as inheriting the gene may wish to control their own reproduction. It can be anticipated that any testing brings with it specific concerns about the rights of individuals to know or not know their genetic status, the rights of other family members to information and the psychological impact of a positive result. However, the experience of introducing predictive testing for Huntington's disease has thrown up other pertinent issues, and few individuals have actually come forward for testing. Those who have fall into three different groups:

- those who want to be tested in order to plan their lives or avoid passing the gene on to children
- those who wanted to obtain an early diagnosis (they were already suspecting symptoms)
- those who wanted to establish that they were free from the disease (they were passing the age when they would be likely to develop symptoms).

Several reasons have been identified to explain why people have not come forward for testing. Firstly, a positive test result would have implications for their existing children, some of

Case study

Susan is 32 years old and has two young daughters. Her mother died from breast cancer at the age of 46 and her grandmother when she was 50. She thinks other female relatives may have had breast cancer, but she is not really sure. Although Susan knew that breast cancer was 'in the family', she had not really given it much thought and certainly viewed herself as a healthy person. However, when she read in the papers that a gene had been identified (BRCA1) for some familial breast cancers and that the test was available to those at risk, she began to think whether this could explain her family history and what the consequences of that would mean. Would she want to be tested? What if she carried the gene? When would she tell her daughters or other family members? What might be done to her — would she have to have both her breasts removed or would she just have regular check-ups? After worrying about all these things for several weeks, she decided to see her GP. Since her GP could not answer many of Susan's questions, she referred her to a clinical geneticist.

whom may have inherited the disorder. Secondly, there is no effective treatment for the disease, so testing may not bring any medical benefits. Thirdly, some people were worried about the loss of health insurance. Lastly, some felt that the completion of their own childbearing removed any reason to have the test. It has also been found that both positive and negative results can cause distress to individuals and their families. Those found to be free of the disease may experience survivor guilt. The certainty provided through testing is not always welcomed. Families have lived with uncertainty in terms of the risk status of its members, and this uncertainty forms a crucial part of identity and experience (Richards, 1993). The experience of introducing testing for Huntington's disease suggests that the information is not always desired by those at risk, and that an individual's right to refuse to be tested must be preserved. Some of these dilemmas are present in the case history.

Carrier testing for recessive disorders: beta-thalassaemia

Beta-thalassaemia is an inherited blood disorder. If both parents are carriers of the trait, there is a one in four chance of passing the disease on to their child, while carriers themselves remain free from the disease. The disease can be fatal without proper treatment, and this treatment is complex. Knowledge of carrier status makes possible greater reproductive choice, particularly the use of prenatal diagnosis and the abortion of affected foetuses where this is personally and culturally acceptable. In Cyprus, where the trait is common, the Orthodox church insists that people are aware of their carrier status for beta-thalassaemia when they marry. Where both partners are carriers, the couple then use prenatal diagnosis and abortion to avoid the birth of an affected child. Abortion is accepted on these grounds, but not on others. This programme has virtually eliminated the births of children with beta-thalassaemia in Cyprus. Where the abortion of affected foetuses is personally or culturally unacceptable, testing is unlikely to be taken up by people.

Other factors may also come into play. For example, screening for sickle cell trait in the USA demonstrated that stigma can be attached to carrier status which led to further discrimination of black people (see pp. 48–49). Additionally, where people do not perceive themselves to be at risk, because they have little direct knowledge of the disease being detected through carrier testing, uptake has been low, for example with testing for cystic fibrosis carrier status in parts of the UK (Marteau and Anionwu 1996).

Population screening for susceptibility to disease

Most diseases are multifactorial in aetiology, involving the interaction of many genes with each other and with the environment. Research may lead to tests to identify genetic susceptibility to a range of common diseases in individuals. This could be beneficial where treatment or lifestyle modification improves health outcome. However, this possibility also raises problems and concerns (Clarke 1995). Firstly, screening whole populations in order to identify individuals with genetic susceptibility to common diseases is commercially attractive to those corporations developing tests and treatments. Such interests may precipitate the introduction of population screening, without good regulation or control. Secondly, population screening may lead to a view that genes determine health, and that individuals must respond with lifestyle modification if they are at risk. Thirdly, like other forms of screening, those not considered at high risk may view themselves as invulnerable to disease, while those at high risk may not necessarily be helped, especially if lifestyle modification is difficult or treatment options limited. The geneticisation of disease may lead to a neglect of other causes of illhealth and other solutions, such as social and environmental interventions: 'Geneticisation exaggerates personal responsibility for health, denigrates the collective solutions to health problems that may be the only hope for those with few resources, and favours corporate profits over the collective and equitable provision of health care around the world' (Clarke 1995).

LIMITS TO THE USE OF GENETIC TECHNOLOGY AND GENETIC EXPLANATIONS FOR DISEASE

Genetic testing for disease or susceptibility to disease raises a range of concerns both for the individual who may come forward for testing, the doctor and for society as a whole. Two general issues are relevant to the application of knowledge gained from research into the genetic components of diseases, traits and indeed behaviours: eugenics and individual choice.

Eugenics

Concerns about eugenic control of populations are sometimes raised. The identification of genes implicated in disease can quickly lead to the availability of tests, such as those for Huntington's disease and beta-thalassaemia outlined above. Where such testing aims to provide people with the information to make informed decisions (e.g. greater choice in relation to reproduction in order not to pass on the disease to their children), this can mean aborting affected foetuses. The elimination of disease in this way may add to the stigma and discrimination currently experienced by disabled people in our society, and may affect the resources available for their care. Concerns also relate to the potential increase in the number of tests available and therefore the range of diseases which may be deemed serious enough for interventions of this kind.

Individual choice

Many of the concerns expressed about eugenics can be checked by the emphasis on individual choice present in democratic societies, where the rights of individuals to choose whether to be tested and whether to abort affected foetuses are considered paramount. There should be no coercion to make a particular decision. While the preservation of individual choice is important, it is also crucial to recognise that decisions are not made in a social vacuum. There are many constraints on individuals which can make one choice more favoured than another. There may be subtle rather than overt pressures to conform to what is expected to be the obvious or right decision, or people may not have sufficient information with which to make informed decisions. Where there are inequalities and discrimination and concerns about the costs of care, the extent of choice available to individuals is culturally and socially restrained. Figure 1 provides examples of how some people perceive this to be the case, drawing on research based on focus group interviews with the lay public.

PRACTICAL APPLICATION

Those involved in health care should be aware of the effects on individual patients and on society more generally. Within consultations, it will be important to discuss social and ethical issues with patients, and consider the context within which decisions are made. It is also important for doctors to work towards ensuring that the possible negative outcomes of genetics (e.g. increased discrimination, stigma and inequality) are minimised. This can be achieved through self-regulation, through engaging in open and public discussion, and through actively promoting regulation and control of those institutions whose functioning is likely to be directly influenced by genetic research and application — insurance, employment and health care provision.

- Will research into the genetic basis of disease lead to geneticisation, where other causes are ignored?
- How can we avoid stigma and discrimination which those with genetic disease may face?
- What sort of information will help informed decision-making for patients?

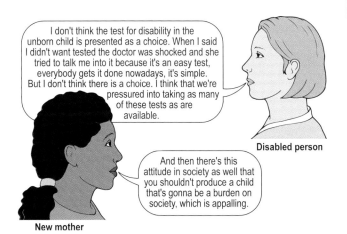

I don't think the test for disability in the unborn child is presented as a choice. When I said I didn't want tested the doctor was shocked and she tried to talk me into it because it's an easy test, everybody gets it done nowadays, it's simple. But I don't think there is a choice. I think that we're pressured into taking as many of these tests as are available.

Disabled person

And then there's this attitude in society as well that you shouldn't produce a child that's gonna be a burden on society, which is appalling.

New mother

Fig. 1 **Two examples of cultural social restraints on individual choice in genetic testing.** (Source: Amos et al 1998).

The social implications of the new genetics

- Research into the genetic basis for disease can quickly lead to applications in clinical practice.
- Genetic testing raises important social and ethical issues for individuals, doctors and society.
- Decisions taken by patients and doctors should be understood within their social, cultural and economic context.

CHANGING INDIVIDUAL BEHAVIOUR

LIFE-STYLE AND HEALTH

Lifestyle and health behaviour factors contribute significantly to ill-health, disease and death. As a result health professionals are becoming increasingly aware of people's ability to contribute to their own health choices and are seeking to influence their intentions and supporting them to change their health behaviour. Adopting specific *health-enhancing* (e.g. exercise) and *health-promoting* (e.g. health screening) behaviours and changing *health-damaging* (e.g. smoking) behaviours are ways in which people realise their potential to enhance their physical well-being.

Health professionals have the task of promoting the idea of individual choice and empowering individuals to overcome barriers to implementing and maintaining their good intentions to improve their health.

WHAT FACTORS INFLUENCE INDIVIDUALS IN THEIR HEALTH CHOICES?

When people are engaging in a health behaviour then it is assumed that they are in some way doing something to protect, promote or maintain their health so as to avoid ill health and prevent disease. Many people mistakenly think that in order to reach a planned health-related target, e.g. stop/reduce smoking or increase exercise, then all that is required is willpower. But this does not enable us to explain or understand the processes involved.

Individual differences in attitudes towards a particular behaviour often stem from:

- different beliefs about vulnerability to illness
- perceived threat of disease
- perceived benefits
- costs of engaging in healthy behaviour
- the ability to perform a health action
- personal and important others' attitudes towards target behaviour
- perceived control over one's own behaviour
- or belief that one's health is controlled by others or by chance.

These variables represent some of the reasons why certain people intend to engage in healthy behaviours or disengage from unhealthy ones, while others do not.

In more recent years this gap between intention and behaviour has been narrowing with the introduction of explanations such as the transtheoretical model (Prochaska and Diclemente 1983) and the health action process model (Schwarzer 1992). According to Schwarzer (1992) the probability that people will engage in healthy behaviours is dependent on several foresights they may have:

- that a life situation is dangerous (smoking and lack of exercise may trigger diseases)
- that behavioural change will reduce the threat
- that one is sufficiently competent to adopt the positive behaviour or to quit the negative behaviour.

CHANGING BELIEFS AND ATTITUDES — METHODS OF PERSUASION

Conflict and persuasion are goals of behaviour change methods, and are prerequisites for intentional change. Therefore one role for health professionals is to find methods of providing people with information in a way that effectively initiates and supports them in their behaviour change. This will involve identifying people's beliefs and developing strategies to persuade them to adopt a healthier life-style.

One model of persuasion is the Elaboration Likelihood Model (Petty and Cacioppo 1986). This theory provides a framework for understanding how people's attitudes can be positively influenced in a convincing way. Two routes of persuasion are distinguished: the *central*, which identifies persuasion as operating through factual arguments relevant to the issue at hand, and *peripheral*, where rousing people's mood is the medium for persuasion (Fig. 1). Much of the research in this area has concluded that attitude change is more enduring, defiant and prognostic in terms of behaviour change when initiated by the central as opposed to the peripheral route.

Health messages (e.g. government television campaigns about AIDS in the early 90s), have been used as a medium for persuading and changing people's knowledge and attitudes towards specific behaviours, but have not been proven to successfully change actual behaviour. One reason is that while knowledge is

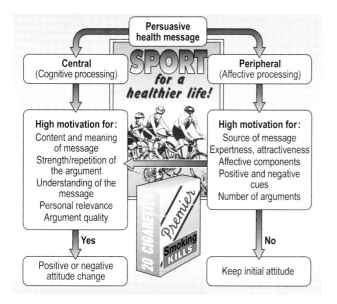

Fig. 1 **A simplified model of the central and peripheral routes to persuasion.** (Adapted from Petty and Cacioppo 1986.)

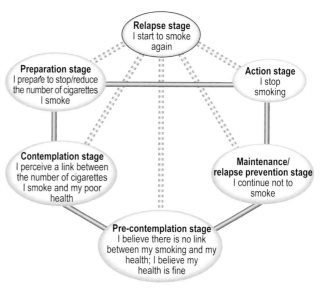

Fig. 2 **Transtheoretical model as it relates to stopping smoking.**

certainly necessary for behaviour change, it is not sufficient on its own to induce actual change. Adopting a new behaviour involves more elaborate cognitive, social, behavioural and self-regulatory skills. Stopping smoking may require the ability to identify situations where smoking is less under personal control (a cognitive skill), to assert the desire not to smoke when socialising with peers (a social skill), and to adhere to a previously made decision not to smoke (a self-regulatory skill). If people do not possess the necessary skills to maintain a new health behaviour, then they are are not likely to begin to make a change in their behaviour, let alone keep it going once change has been successfully initiated.

Dissonance theory (Festinger 1957) provides another way of understanding attitude change. Health professionals often want to induce *cognitive dissonance* as a method of motivating individuals to change current unhealthy behaviours and/or adopt healthier ones.

For example, 40-year-old Mr Maguire attends his local general practitioner reporting that over the past few months he has been experiencing shortness of breath and a productive cough with green and sometimes blood-stained phlegm. The doctor points out smoking 60 cigarettes a day may be contributing to his symptoms and requests that he cut down. According to cognitive dissonance theory Mr Maguire can respond in two ways: (1) having not previously made a connection between his smoking and his symptoms he feels very uncomfortable about

the amount he smokes and decides that he will make an effort to cut down over the coming weeks; or (2) having not previously made a connection between his smoking and his symptoms, momentarily he feels uncomfortable about the amount he smokes, but decides that he has always been healthy, rarely visits the doctor anyway, and that his symptoms are caused by the recent cold weather and not his smoking. In both responses a state of consonance has been achieved.

INFLUENCING BEHAVIOUR CHANGE THROUGH INTENTIONS

Raising awareness of the need to alter one's behaviour is often just the first stage in the process leading to specific behaviour change and maintenance of that change over time.

Prochaska and Diclemente (1983) introduced the idea of encouraging people to maintain changes in their behaviour in their stages of change model. They propose that up to six separate stages can be identified relating to behaviour change in individuals. These are precontemplation, contemplation, (preparation), action, maintenance, and relapse (Fig. 2). In one early study, the transtheoretical model was applied to 872 subjects who were independently attempting to alter their smoking habits. This was a cross-sectional study in which data on the stage of change and smoking status of the subjects was collected at an initial assessment. They found that people attempting to change their smoking habits fell into the categories as described by the transtheoretical model of change (with the exception of preparation which is a stage introduced in later studies), with each stage using different change processes.

Once a person's stage of change has been assessed relative to a particular health behaviour, the person can be guided towards a specific behaviour change. In the precontemplation phase, the focus is on providing information and feedback so that an awareness of the problem behaviour is increased. People at this stage often do not have any intention of changing their life-style practices. In the contemplation stage people may be considering change but key beliefs need to alter before behaviour change can occur (one role of persuasion and conflict). In the action stage the focus may be on intention strength, goal setting and the removal of negative prompts. However, when people make a change in the way they behave, this does not guarantee that the change will be maintained. In the maintenance stage, reinforcement and shaping may be critical to turning a small behavioural change into a consistent and more substantial change in life-style.

Case study
Patient-directed behaviour change and smoking cessation

Bella suffers from chronic back pain, tension headaches and hypertension. She has been a smoker for the past 20 years, smoking between 20 and 30 cigarettes a day during this time. She recently went to her GP as she was feeling generally unwell and complaining of dizziness. Her GP checked her blood pressure, which was 120/180, and immediately advised Bella to stop smoking completely.

Bella became very motivated to make the effort as she values her health a lot and does not want to develop any more problems. She is now very worried about the effect that her smoking is having on her blood pressure.

Bella has tried to give up cigarettes numerous times before but she has failed. She has tended to go for an all or nothing approach, cutting out all cigarettes at once. She admits that she enjoys smoking so much as it helps her to relax and eases her back pain at the same time. She realises that it is difficult for her to give cigarettes up even though she really wants to for health reasons. She feels encouraged to stop but is at a loss to understand why she cannot as she feels so determined and motivated. She does not know how to get started and has decided to go back to her GP for more advice.

STOP THINK A 26-year-old male patient with a 10-year history of insulin dependent diabetes mellitus attends for results of a recent fasting blood sugar. His result is a blood sugar of 28 mmols. You are aware of his history of excessive drinking. What advice do you give? Increase insulin, reduce drinking, refer patient for counselling for his alcohol problem or offer advice about how he can better manage his diabetes?

Changing individual behaviour

- Changing health behaviour involves supporting individuals to adopt *health-enhancing* and *health-protecting* behaviours and to reduce *health-damaging* behaviours.
- Key correlates of health behaviour are rooted in people's beliefs and attitudes about their health. To change health behaviour successfully, these cognitions need to be identified.
- Health messages are a common mode of encouraging people to change their health behaviour. They can be delivered by central (factual arguments) or peripheral (affective) routes, as described by the Elaboration Likelihood Model.
- Cognitive dissonance can change people's attitudes towards health by providing individuals with information which conflicts with their current health practices. A state of consonance may be reached without the intended behaviour change taking place.
- Six stages of behaviour change have been identified: precontemplation, contemplation, preparation, action, maintenance and relapse.

THE SOCIAL CONTEXT OF BEHAVIOURAL CHANGE

Few people would dispute that the enjoyment of good health is a worthy goal for individuals and for states/governments to pursue. In the UK, government health education bodies now promote healthy and discourage unhealthy behaviour. The emphasis on the individual's responsibility to make good health choices is evident in the messages which these health education authorities promulgate. We could sum up this idea in the recent slogan: 'Be all you can be'. However, individuals operate within a social context and we need to take this into account when considering behaviour change.

This spread looks at two ways in which behaviour change can be seen in a social context. First, the social context in which individuals come to alter their behaviour; second, the role society and the state play in influencing citizens' health behaviour.

THE SOCIAL CONTEXT OF INDIVIDUAL BEHAVIOUR CHANGE

There is clear evidence that behaviour such as smoking, eating large quantities of animal fats and failing to exercise is detrimental to health. Lay people are aware of this evidence (health warnings are printed on the sides of cigarette cartons, for instance) and it seems only 'common sense' that people will make rational decisions to change their behaviour on the basis of information of this kind. So why do people often fail to do so?

You have seen that the health belief model (see p. 54) and the theory of planned behaviour (see pp. 70–71) endorse the assumption that the individual will weigh up the evidence, the costs and benefits of particular behaviour and come to a rational *choice*. These conceptions have much in common with a research tradition that attempts to understand the process of persuasion, i.e. how attitudes can be altered. Attitudes were targeted for change, not behaviour, as it was assumed that attitudes cause behaviour in a fairly unproblematic way. Early health education messages therefore assumed that information, once disseminated, would be sufficient to alter beliefs and hence behaviour: they were wrong!

Interestingly, advertising companies had long recognised that the most successful of campaigns will usually be effective in altering the consumption habits of only a small percentage of the targeted audience. Initial health education promotions probably had too high expectations of behaviour change, and importantly (unlike advertising campaigns designed to, say, switch the consumer's allegiance to another brand of soap powder), they were often aimed at altering behaviour which was *pleasurable*, such as smoking, and therefore of considerable consequence to people. Further, in some cultural contexts, hazardous behaviour may be valued and engaged in precisely because of the associated risk: e.g. a type of cigarette marketed under the brand name 'Death Cigarettes' has sold successfully (Bunton and Burrows 1995).

Investigating 'unhealthy' behaviour

One study which illustrated the importance of taking the social context of a behaviour such as smoking into account was that by Hilary Graham (1984). Graham argued that caring for children and managing the financial and organisational burdens of domestic life may be so arduous that behaviour such as smoking can be conceptualised as a coping strategy. One of her respondents, for instance, said:

> After lunch, I'll clear away and wash up and put the telly on for Stevie [her son]. I'll have a sit down on the sofa, with a cigarette … It's lovely, it's the one time in the day I really enjoy and I know Stevie won't disturb me. I couldn't stop, I just couldn't. It keeps me calm. It's me [sic] one relaxation is smoking.

Here, smoking fills a critical role for the carer in that it actually *enables* her to be an effective mother and domestic worker. Graham has termed this phenomenon 'the responsibility of irresponsible behaviour' (see pp. 50–51).

Studies like this give us some indication of how behavioural change is constrained by social circumstances and hint at some of the reasons behind social class differences in health behaviour (and outcomes), e.g. why working class mothers (with fewer material resources) may find it harder to give up smoking than middle class mothers (see pp. 46–47). It would be difficult

---

Case study

Mrs Berry, a 29-year-old mother of three young children, visited her GP, Dr Hall, complaining of excessive tiredness. After examining her, Dr Hall prescribed a vitamin supplement and told her that she should be more responsible about eating regular healthy meals. He handed Mrs Berry a leaflet entitled: 'Cooking sensibly can be fun!'.

Several months later, Mrs Berry attended her medical practice again with her youngest child, who had a persistent cold. Dr Stephens, who dealt with the child's problem, noticed that Mrs Berry was looking unwell, and enquired after her health. In the supportive atmosphere of Dr Stephen's surgery Mrs Berry revealed that she was worried about the whole family's health in that, although she tried hard to provide nourishing food, it was difficult to do so given their relatively low household income. Fresh fruit, vegetables, cheese, meat and so on tended to be expensive so she rarely bought these items.

It became clear that the Berrys' food budget consisted of whatever money was left after the 'inflexible' items in the family budget such as rent and electricity were paid every week. If heating costs happened to be high, there was relatively little left for food.

Dr Stephens was aware that as a result of a recent road traffic accident, and of general anxiety over the local levels of childhood asthma, local parents were actively seeking the establishment of a protected play area. Dr Stephens asked Mrs Berry, who had not heard of the scheme, whether she would be interested in expanding the project into other health-related areas, such as diet.

Mrs Berry subsequently joined the group and took the main responsibility for developing and organising the thriving food co-operative which it now runs for the benefit of the local community.

indeed to get an idea of the sheer *complexity* of the role played by smoking in this woman's life from an investigation solely of psychological factors such as her attitudes and beliefs towards giving up the habit.

 Financial constraints mean that treatment priorities in the area in which you work are being reviewed. You have heard the suggestion that high cost cardiac surgery should in future be denied to middle-aged, heavy smokers. Do you believe such an idea should be entertained?

THE SOCIAL CONTEXT OF MASS BEHAVIOUR CHANGE

Mass education campaigns directed at people's attitudes may have limited success in changing behaviour. In certain situations the state can target the behaviour itself by introducing sanctions. Just as we might privately decide to deny ourselves a chocolate bar if we fail to complete an assignment on time, so the state may bring in external incentives in the form of legal penalties if we do not conform to a particular rule.

The introduction of car seat-belt legislation is a good example of this strategy: after failing to persuade people to wear seat-belts, the Swedish government passed legislation making it compulsory for front-seat passengers in private cars to do so. Seat-belt use increased from 30 to 85% (Fhanér and Hane 1979).

Many people would probably agree that it would be unacceptable for the state to legislate directly to forbid habits such as smoking or drinking — except perhaps in public places. In these cases, persuasive health promotion campaigns aimed at our views and beliefs are the alternative.

Be all you can be?

Let us consider the basic tenet of the UK government's current health message, in which we are seen as having responsibility for our health and the freedom to choose a healthy life-style.

There are some problems with this conception. We may not be *able* to choose healthy options — for instance if the state organises a dental service on a fee for treatment basis, we may not be able to afford oral health no matter how strongly we value it. Poverty appears to have its own dynamic — the Alameda County study in California (Berkman and Breslow 1983) showed that after taking into account the influence of all known behavioural risk factors there were still substantial differences in morbidity and mortality between high and low income families. Life-style and behavioural factors are not the only influences on our health: the material and environmental conditions we live in can play a significant role and are an important explanation of health inequalities (Whitehead 1988, 1995). Poor people are more likely to live close to factories and major roads which generate air-borne pollution and hence encourage respiratory problems, which may be exacerbated by mould spores arising from damp, under-heated housing (see pp. 56–57).

Addressing these sorts of issues must be the responsibility of governments and industry, and the potential financial costs are enormous. Clearly the state has conflicting responsibilities and interests. While wishing to promote the health of its citizens, it also needs to support industrial development to generate wealth but in doing so produces the pollution and dangerous work conditions which help to make some of us ill. As sceptical social analysts we notice that while the state-endorsed message, 'look after your own health', is a liberal sentiment in that it allows individuals control over their lives, it also serves to *deflect attention* from the role of material and environmental factors in illness. It can therefore be seen as a politically expedient message. One sociologist (Prior 1995) has likened the use of such individualistic (behavioural) explanations of ill health to explaining variations in the homicide rate in Northern Ireland in terms of personal shortcomings such as failing to fit bomb alarms or failing to belt one's flak jacket. The ignoring of cultural/political factors in explaining homicide in Ulster, or ill health in general, is equally absurd.

In addition, the government receives vast revenues from the sale of tobacco and alcohol, and it is perhaps not surprising that it has for so long resisted demands to ban tobacco advertising at sports events. The 'look after your own health' ideal has of course also supported a burgeoning health industry; we are enjoined to purchase every conceivable 'health' product from yogurts to leotards! The overall context in which we play out our behaviour is thus determined ultimately by political considerations, and therefore can only be influenced by collective action.

The role of health professionals

As a body, health professionals are repositories of knowledge about the lives of lay people and can operate as powerful pressure groups which can influence local government (for example by supporting community self-help groups) or national government (for example by recommending a reduction in the amount of alcohol which drivers may legally consume).

Of course, trying to influence another person's behaviour raises ethical and moral questions: if a person fails to take responsibility for their health should they be denied certain treatments? Should governments only have the power to attempt to change behaviour by informational means (the condom campaign in relation to HIV and AIDS is an example) or, as in the case of water fluoridation, should they be able to introduce sweeping changes to our lives for our own good?

The social context of behavioural change

- The social context of behavioural change can refer to the background to an individual's efforts to stop a deleterious (or start a beneficial) behaviour or to the overall societal influences upon how we behave and how we think about behaviour.
- Individuals' behaviour is embedded within complex social circumstances and is not always best understood by accessing the beliefs and attitudes associated with it.
- Attempts to effect mass behaviour change are often more successful if behaviour itself is targeted (e.g. legal sanctions for failure to conform are introduced) as opposed to trying to persuade people to change their behaviour through informational means.
- The idea that individuals can exercise choice over their health status, while partially true, can nevertheless act in a politically convenient way to deflect attention from environmental/material explanations of inequalities in health.
- Trying to influence behaviour always has ethical and moral implications.

HEALTH PROMOTION IN MEDICAL PRACTICE

WHAT ARE THE OBJECTIVES OF HEALTH PROMOTION?

The World Health Organisation defines health both as the absence of disease and as a positive sense of well-being. Thus the objectives of health promotion are

- to prevent disease (see pp. 64–65)
- to promote health in the sense of well-being.

In practice the two are related. For example, the management of chronic pain (see pp. 132–133) can involve the patient maintaining as full and positive a life as possible — maximum well-being despite the intractable pain, which in turn leads to reduction of the pain symptoms.

These two objectives could cover almost the whole of medicine, but health promotion is normally most concerned with diseases which have a substantial life-style component in their aetiology or with the way patients cope with their condition (Table 1).

Tones and Tilford (1994) have suggested three philosophies of health promotion: social engineering, individual prevention and individual empowerment.

Social engineering

Social engineering assumes that ill health is caused by social phenomena such as poverty, poor living conditions, lack of education, inappropriate cultural norms and inadequate health care. Objectives should be to improve living standards, change norms and improve health care access. Social engineering can be effective: for example, in Southern India for cultural reasons birth control is often not used, but increasing women's literacy also makes them more likely to adopt and encourage birth control. Unfortunately, mass social engineering is often expensive and it can also be criticised for imposing change without consultation. For example, some people are opposed to the fluoridation of water, despite the dental benefits.

Individual prevention

This school of thought believes that health is caused by the behaviour and conditions of individuals and can therefore be changed by changing the individuals' health behaviours. Methods of changing behaviour include education, advertising, specific physical interventions, such as seat belts, and special medical treatment and screening. This approach fits with much medical thinking, which tends to be oriented towards treating individual patients. Much current health promotion is of this kind, the most common form probably being the provision of leaflets informing patients about life-style factors such as exercise, diet, drug abuse, smoking, alcohol, or the management of their particular disease. Unfortunately individualistic prevention involving education alone is rarely effective. Specific material interventions, such as seat belt laws, or the reduction of salt intake by making salt cellar holes smaller, can succeed, but they infringe people's autonomy. Also, there can be an element of patient-blaming in individual health promotion. This may be inappropriate because in most diseases addressed by health promotion, such as cardiovascular disease, the patient's behaviour is only one causal factor among many (see pp. 50–51).

Individual empowerment

Individual empowerment involves giving people the means to take responsibility for their health and to change their social conditions. Empowerment can be effective, but people may choose not to make health their priority. There is a tension in medicine concerning which decisions about health the patient has a right to make. Most doctors would agree that patients are free to choose their own diet, but few would allow a patient to decide which anaesthetic they would prefer. The difference is in the level of knowledge and expertise involved in making the decision and in the risks involved. Much health promotion claims to be empowering, while strongly encouraging people to make the 'correct' health decision. What does one do, for example, with someone who chooses to smoke and risk dying early? Many doctors find it difficult to respect such a decision.

THE PRACTICE OF HEALTH PROMOTION

Doctors can provide patients with information via leaflets (Fig. 1), other written sources, computer systems and other media, or serve to facilitate social change, for example by pressing for improved housing conditions. But doctors probably do most health promotion via personal contact.

Doctors are highly respected and can promote health by example. Being seen

Table 1 **Main current areas for health promotion**

Smoking
Diet and weight
Contraception and HIV prevention
Blood pressure monitoring
Screening for cancers
Alcohol and substance abuse
Responsible medication use
Child care
Exercise

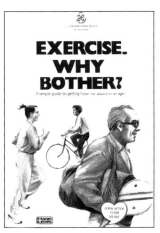
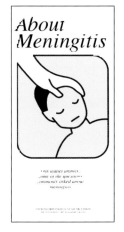
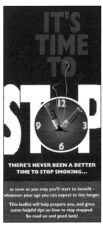
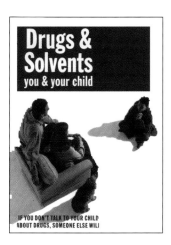

Fig. 1 **A selection of health promotion leaflets found in a GP's surgery.**

to cycle to work, or not to smoke, can affect their patients' behaviour.

The doctor's attitude and approach to patients can also promote health. A paternalistic pill-pusher is liable to develop patients who believe in quick medical repairs for their ailments, rather than prevention. A doctor with better communication skills may listen to patients and discuss how they should deal with their health problems. This may help inform and empower patients on health issues (see pp. 86–87, 92–93).

Many consultations provide scope for *opportunistic health promotion,* where the doctor promotes health in a consultation concerning something else. Two examples: a patient with a head injury from falling may also have an alcohol problem and the doctor should take the opportunity to enquire about this; a patient over 40 attending their GP these days is likely to have their blood pressure monitored, whatever their problem.

A related way of promoting health is to take detailed histories of health behaviours and social circumstances. Such histories allow doctors to notice unhealthy behaviours and behaviour changes, then praise or warn as appropriate. Until recently, health behaviours were rarely recorded. Even a polite warning from a doctor has some impact on patient behaviour (minimal intervention: see below).

Accurate histories also allow patient behaviours to be followed up on subsequent visits.

Doctors also provide specific facilities, programmes and clinics for different health behaviours. It is often appropriate to offer patients available aids for behaviour change. These range from simply monitoring change, for example by weighing the patient on each visit, to prescriptions, for instance for nicotine gum or patches for heavily dependent smokers, to advisory leaflets. Many health centres now also have access to dieticians, specialist nurses and psychologists to help with a range of health behaviours.

Minimal intervention

If doctors systematically ask all patients about their smoking or drinking and simply suggest to the smokers that they stop, or the drinkers that they cut down, without providing further intervention, then about 10% of patients successfully comply. This is low, but success rates for any attempt to change health behaviours are only about 20%, and such minimal intervention is quick and cheap.

Fear messages

It is commonly believed that the best way to change people's behaviour is to warn them of the frightening consequences of their behaviour. The doctor's role would

be to spell out to patients the risks of coronary heart disease, cancers, AIDS and other diseases. Fear can be a powerful motive for changing behaviour, but it can easily 'misfire' because fear generally leads people to avoid the situation where they became afraid.

- They may avoid the doctor or lie about their behaviour, rather than change their behaviour.
- They may explain away the dangers, to reduce cognitive dissonance (see pp. 70–71). This may include their rejecting the doctor as a credible source of information on the topic.
- Not everyone is afraid of the same things, and some fear messages may be irrelevant.
- Patients can be motivated to change, but be unable to change. Fear messages may simply add anxiety and guilt to their problems, reducing their ability to cope and making change less likely.

Generally, the people most impressed by fear messages are those least at risk. For them, the message reinforces their current beliefs. For this reason, messages which downplay fear may even offend the public. For example, messages which are realistic about the dangers of drug abuse are often accused of going 'soft' on drugs.

Case study

Andrea is a married woman aged 48. She is severely obese, with high normal blood pressure. She is moderately active, given her obesity. Andrea attended because she wanted help to lose weight. In what follows the GP expresses concern about her smoking, but does not risk alienating the patient by pushing the issue.

GP: *'So you take about five or six drinks a week. That's well within the safe limits and I don't think it will be having much effect on your weight. Do you smoke?'*

Andrea: (Laughs) *'Yeah, I've always got something in my mouth.'*

GP: *'How many a day?'*

Andrea: *'About 40.'*

GP: *'That's quite a lot. Have you ever thought of quitting?'*

Andrea: *'One thing at a time, doctor. I don't need to put on more weight.'*

GP: *'Actually, your smoking is worse for your health than your weight problem. I would like to see you try and stop.'*

Andrea: *'I'd rather get this fat off first.'*

GP: *'OK. Would you like to make an appointment with our dietician? I'll talk to you about smoking again in a few months.'*

- What is the difference between health education and health promotion?
- When might giving patients leaflets about their condition not affect their behaviour?
- What steps might a doctor take to ensure that leaflets were effective?
- Health information is sometimes seen by patients as patronising and unrealistic. Why might this be so?

Health promotion in medical practice

- The objectives of health promotion are to prevent disease and promote health.
- Objectives can be achieved by social engineering, individual prevention, empowerment.

The doctor can promote health by:
- information provision
- facilitating social change
- setting an example
- communicating effectively with patients
- including health behaviours in history-taking
- recommending healthy behaviours
- providing support for behaviour change.

ILLEGAL DRUGS

Illegal drug use amongst young people is quite common (see Fig. 1). Most users use cannabis and occasionally other drugs. Aside from breaking the law, they rarely come to harm. Such use does not lead inevitably to addiction or other drugs, such as heroin. However, use of most drugs — even cannabis — can occasionally cause acute harm through overdose, accidents while intoxicated, fatal adverse reactions (notably to ecstasy or solvents), severe psychological distress or psychosis. Casualty departments often treat such patients. A minority use drugs excessively and problematically. They are the most likely to seek medical help for drug problems and also need general health services (see Table 1).

DEFINING DRUG PROBLEMS

Drug misuse is a medico-legal term: *use of a drug other than for its intended or lawful purpose*. For controlled ('illegal') drugs, this generally means any use without prescription.

Drug abuse is a psycho-medical term: *use of a drug in dangerous or harmful ways*. There is dispute about whether all misuse constitutes 'abuse' or whether occasional, recreational use of drugs can be harmless. An example of a rarely harmful pattern may be the use of cannabis, amphetamines, LSD and ecstasy in conjunction with the dance scene.

Drug addiction is a psycho-medical term: *use of a drug in a highly frequent and obsessive manner, with withdrawal symptoms when use ceases*. Addiction is supposed to be caused by neurochemical adaptation to repeated drug use. However, much addictive behaviour is difficult to explain fully by neurochemical means and 'addiction' is now being supplanted by the two more general concepts, drug dependence and problem drug use.

Drug dependence: *use of a drug in a dysfunctional and self-harming manner, which is difficult to stop*. Dependence has no single defining feature, but typically a dependent user will spend considerable time and money taking drugs, obtain money by criminal means, have difficulties with family and friends,

repeatedly try and fail to stop and show substantial distress when stopping. Also common are wider psychological problems including depression, delinquent or anti-social behaviour and substantial disturbances such as having been abused as children.

Problem drug use: *any use of a drug which causes users, or those around them, problems*. Some problems are worsened by society's approach. For example, some of the damage caused by heroin is due to its being illegal and hence contaminated and expensive. Not all problem drug users are in any sense dependent. For example, someone's drug problem can be that they keep getting into debt with loan sharks to buy cannabis. Obviously such a person needs treatment other than detoxification, or a prescription, and may need more counselling about life-style than about drugs.

Table 1 **Situations where drug users may require special treatment**

Situation	Special problems
Obstetrics	Maintenance or reduction of prescribing and counselling may be required to minimise harm to mother and fetus
Surgery	May show high tolerance to anaesthetics and sedatives
May be HIV positive
General practice	Can be disruptive and deceptive. May require specialised support services
Internal medicine	May fake pain to obtain painkillers. May continue to use drugs which interact with their prescribed medicines
Infectious diseases	HIV, hepatitis
Casualty	Overdose, injuries through accidents while intoxicated, violence related to the drugs trade

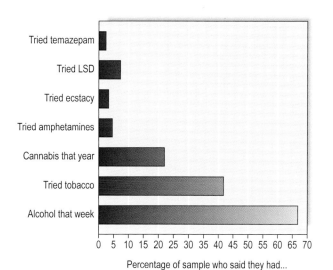

Fig. 1 **Drug use in 1990 by 908 Glaswegians aged 18–19.** Cocaine and heroin use were both below 1%. (Data from West and Sweeting 1992.)

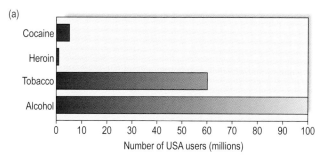

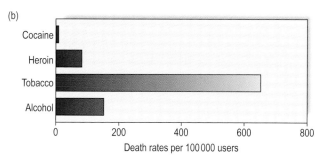

Fig. 2 **Estimated number of users (a) and death rates from drug use in the USA (b).** (Source: Ostrowski 1989, p. 47.)

DRUG DEPENDENCE AND PROBLEM DRUG USE

Most drug-dependent and problematic users use a wide variety of drugs. As many as 10% drug injectors become dependent or have problems, but even injection is not inevitably problematic. Drugs injected include heroin, buprenorphine, benzodiazepines including temazepam and diazepam, amphetamines and cocaine. Smoking heroin or smoking crack cocaine are also likely to lead to problems. Finally, some people prescribed oral benzodiazepines become dependent. Drug users who avoid the preceding drugs and practices are relatively unlikely to develop problems requiring medical attention. To put the problem in perspective, less than 1% of the population is dependent on controlled drugs, and the problems caused by alcohol and tobacco are far more widespread. Figure 2 shows estimates of American death rates; equivalent figures are not available for the UK. There are no known fatalities from cannabis use and fatalities from hallucinogens (other than ecstasy) and amphetamines are very rare.

TREATMENT

Treating drug dependence is difficult and it can take a decade before a drug-dependent person stops, during which time they may have repeated involvement with health and other services. They will usually have tried to stop or moderate their use several times, by several methods, relapsing each time. In the meantime, they should be provided with the information and means to minimise the harm their drug use causes. This also benefits users who are not dependent (see Table 2).

No single treatment works best for dependence but treatment which includes cognitive type therapy that addresses motivational and thought patterns tends to come out best in controlled trials.

Do doctors push drugs? Some doctors see prescribing methadone as selling addicts drugs to keep them quiet and feel that this is immoral. Others feel that the practical benefits of methadone outweigh the moral issue. Another issue is the prescription of minor tranquillisers to make anxious, stressed or emotional patients feel better. Where is the line between taking a drug to feel better and taking a drug for fun? Should doctors encourage people to use drugs to feel better?

Table 2 **Harm minimisation strategies for drug injectors.** (Adapted from Department of Health 1991 Drug Misuse and Dependence)

Education	Hazards of injecting (especially equipment-sharing)
	Safer sex
	Getting sterile equipment and condoms
	Cleaning equipment
	Avoiding overdose
	First aid
Direct action	Hepatitis B immunisation
	Provision of sterile injecting equipment and condoms
	HIV testing (with counselling)
	Substitution of oral methadone

Case study

Mike is a 23-year-old drug injector with a history of criminal convictions and drug abuse going back to age 16. Two years previously he had been discharged from a residential detoxification programme for using drugs. He told the GP that he was now highly motivated by having a steady partner and a newly-born daughter, but cannot give up heroin. The GP prescribed methadone and established a good relationship with Mike. With the prescription his general health improved and his previously hostile approach to NHS staff decreased. He was also referred for dental treatment because of numerous caries due to neglect and a sugary diet, the pain of these previously being concealed by high doses of drugs. Unfortunately, 6 months later Mike was arrested for burglary. He denied involvement and the GP testified in writing on his behalf, but as a persistent offender he was nonetheless convicted and sentenced to 2 years. In prison his maintenance regime was replaced by a rapid reduction of methadone dose. Mike was unable to manage and began to inject again occasionally, sharing a syringe. As a result he contracted hepatitis C. On release he was determined to stop injecting. However, his GP was now reluctant to prescribe methadone as Mike had not used opiates regularly in prison. This, and a serious quarrel with his partner, led Mike to resume heavy drug use and crime for some months. He returned to the GP requiring treatment for a large abscess (see Fig. 3). He is now back on methadone, requires regular monitoring for liver damage from hepatitis C and has re-established a relationship with his family, although he no longer lives with his daughter's mother.

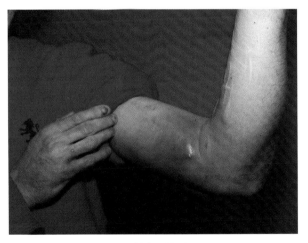

Fig. 3 **Damage to arm by use of injectable drugs.**

Illegal drugs

- Illegal drug use is quite common.
- Much illegal drug use is not a medical problem, but most drugs do cause occasional acute problems, even deaths.
- Drug dependence is quite rare.
- The dependent drug user may take a long time and repeated attempts to stop. Prior to stopping he or she may benefit from help with:
  — harm reduction, including substitute prescribing such as methadone for heroin
  — general medical care
  — life problems as well as drug dependence

ALCOHOL PROBLEMS

Alcohol is the most widely-used recreational drug in the western world. While many users come to no harm, its use can cause medical, psychological and social problems.

THE MEDICALISATION OF ALCOHOL PROBLEMS

In the 18th and 19th centuries alcohol was generally regarded as a wholesome foodstuff. Excessive drinking was seen as a vice rather than a medical problem, although the main medical effects of alcohol had already been noted. For example, in Britain there was particular concern about the working classes abusing gin, and drinking levels were much higher than today. Between about 1850 and the late 1950s alcoholism came to be considered a disease caused by some biological reaction to alcohol. This reaction was supposed to be permanent, so the only palliative treatment for alcoholism was permanent abstinence. Still widely believed, this idea is faulty:

- Many problem drinkers come to harm from drinking but are not alcoholics.
- Even dependent drinkers have some control over their drinking. Some, not all, people with severe alcohol problems can moderate their drinking to problem-free levels, often without help.

Alcoholics Anonymous emphasises abstinence (see below), as do some professional treatments. Other treatments include monitored detoxification for severely dependent drinkers, counselling to enable the patient find methods of coping other than drinking, or therapeutic communities where patients stay off alcohol and undertake group therapy. Given the choice, some patients opt for abstinence and some for moderating their drinking. Occasional relapses to heavy drinking are common, even for those trying to abstain, and patients are taught to expect and cope with this. Controlled follow-up studies suggest that approximately 80% of people treated for alcohol dependence by any method have relapsed within 2 years. Alleged better rates tend to be due to bias (for example treatment programmes which only admit people who have virtually stopped drinking already) or poorly controlled research.

The 12-steps approach

Alcoholics Anonymous consists of groups of recovering alcoholics who provide mutual support and aim at complete abstinence from alcohol. The philosophy is the famous 12-steps approach, which requires that the alcoholic surrender to a higher power (or God), admit their wrongs and try to rectify them (see pp. 136–137). This requires some spiritual feeling, accepting abstinence as a goal, and usually works better for those who were heavily dependent. AA has less to offer people who are not dependent. Doctors often suggest AA as a supplement to treatment. There are also professional residential programmes which offer a 12-steps approach.

DRINKING PROBLEMS

Even quite moderate drinking increases morbidity (Table 1) and mortality (see pp. 76–77). This has led to the BMA recommended safe limits shown in Figure 1. Many people, especially young men, drink above these limits (Fig. 2).

At the legal limit for driving (UK: 80 mg alcohol in 100 ml blood), reactions are slowed by about 20% and thought is impaired. People who are drunk may generally behave in risky, anti-social or foolish ways without adequately considering their actions. This causes some of alcohol's pleasurable effects — people are more likely to dance, flirt, or converse. Unfortunately, drunkenness also contributes to quarrels, violence, disorder, suicide, fires, and other accidents. Over 40% of serious traffic accidents involve alcohol, as do at least 27% of violent casualties. It is quite easy to overdose on alcohol, which can kill through respiratory depression.

CONTROLLING THE NATION'S CONSUMPTION

Increasing the price of alcohol by taxation reduces national consumption, which in turn reduces alcohol-related problems.

Table 1 **Alcohol, disease and possible benefits**

Liver disease	Fatty degeneration, fibrosis, acute alcoholic inflammation, cirrhosis
Cardiovascular disease	Hypertension Heavy drinking increases stroke risk and coronary heart disease
Cancer	Oesophageal cancer, possibly stomach cancer
Neurological disease	Korsakoff's syndrome, alcoholism
Beneficial effects?	1–2 units per day may reduce the risks of CHD Red wine lowers cholesterol levels Small occasional dose of alcohol may serve as a sedative or tranquilliser

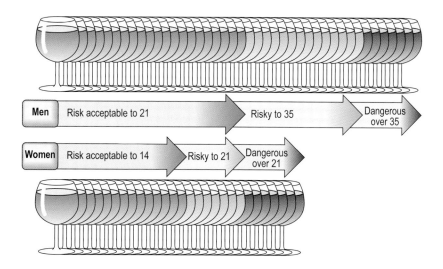

Fig. 1 **Recommended limits on alcohol consumption per week.** A unit = approximately 1 glass wine, 1 pub measure of spirits, half a pint normal strength beer or two-thirds of a bottle strong lager. (Source: BMA, 1995.)

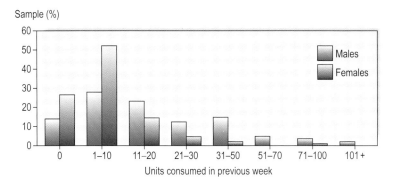

Sample (%)

Units consumed in previous week

Fig. 2 **The self-reported previous week's alcohol consumption of a sample of 433 19-year-olds in Lothian.** (Adapted from Plant, Peck & Samuel 1985.)

STOP THINK Some medical students and doctors drink excessively. Could you, or your colleagues, benefit from cutting down? How might you go about this? Doctors often drink as part of medical school culture, to 'cope' with stress and to relax, although drinking can end up worsening the stress and their work can be affected by drinking or hangovers. What other methods of coping might be more constructive? Would any changes to your school's culture help?

Case study
Minimal intervention with a heavy drinker

Ralph is 35 and a travelling salesman. He presented with frequent abdominal pains, which he attributed to stress. From examination and tests there was no evidence of physical abnormality and non-specific gastritis was diagnosed. When Ralph attended the GP again to discuss the test results the GP asked him to go through the previous seven days and list all the alcohol he had consumed (a retrospective drinking diary). Ralph was drinking over 50 units of alcohol a week — about 2 pints (4 units) or equivalent at lunchtime and a further 2 in the evening to relax.

GP: *'You don't drink that much a day, but it's steady. Now the recommended safe limit for men is 21 units a week — that's about ten and a half pints of beer a week.'*

Ralph: *'Is that all? How much did I get through last week then?'*

GP: *'A bit too much, 58 units. I think that your stomach pains are made worse by your drinking. I'd like you to stop for a week or so and see what happens to your pain.'*

Ralph: *'I can't give up drinking! It goes with the job. A lot of my clients wouldn't stand for it if I didn't have a couple with them.'*

GP: *'I'm not suggesting you give up for ever, just for a week to see what happens, then maybe try and cut down a bit. Try not to drink every day, or have some soft drinks sometimes, or low alcohol beer.'*

Ralph: *'That's going to be hard, but I guess I have to, don't I, doctor, if it's affecting my stomach and that?'*

GP: *'Yes. Come back and see after you've stopped for your week. If you want to know more about cutting down then there's a good book, 'Let's Drink to your Health'.'*

Ralph now has the advice of the doctor as a motive for cutting down and can also use his health as an excuse when he feels social pressure to drink.

Another approach is to attempt to change the ways people drink, by:

- Education about safe levels and risks. This may have helped change society's attitude to drunk-driving.
- Continued control over where, when and by whom alcohol may be consumed, with licensing laws. For example, increased under-age drinking may require a reduction in tolerance of violations of existing law.
- Manipulation of the physical and social settings where drinking problems are common. For example, the banning of alcohol and increased provision of seating at football grounds to prevent disorder.

A major barrier to such changes is a widespread indifference to, and minimisation of, alcohol problems. The health professional's role is in part to raise the problems' profile, by routinely taking alcohol histories and treating alcohol use as a priority health care issue.

THE ROLE OF MEDICINE

- To counter the drinks industry's promotion of its products.
- To press for better controls on the sale and pricing of alcohol.
- To routinely ask patients about their drinking and relate this to illness and disease.
- To advise patients of safe drinking levels and suggest that they adopt these levels.
- To monitor patients drinking and praise and encourage them when they improve their drinking.
- To be aware of the contribution which alcohol can make to illness and injury in general practice and hospital specialities.
- To serve as a role model by drinking moderately, within safe limits.
- To be aware of and refer to local specialised alcohol treatment services.

Alcohol problems
- Alcohol causes many problems.
- Some people require treatment for dependence.
- Others require advice to moderate their drinking.
- Alcohol use should be a routine part of history-taking.

MEDICINE AND SMOKING POLICY

Cigarette smoking causes cancer, cardiovascular diseases, and other disease. A quarter of all smokers will die of a smoking-related disease. About one third of teenagers who try at least three cigarettes will go on to be lifetime smokers, which suggests cigarettes are more addictive than heroin or cocaine. Many smokers find it difficult to stop and only about 10% of quitters succeed. Nicotine patches, gum or nasal spray (still being evaluated) help a little, but it is better to prevent new smokers.

Smokers tend to start as young teenagers. Health education about the risks of smoking has limited effects on this group because they see health damage 20 years on as irrelevant to them and believe that they can easily give up. While informing everyone about the risks of smoking is important, other means of preventing smoking are also necessary.

THE TOBACCO INDUSTRY

The industry is large and powerful and devotes considerable resources to defending and promoting its product. It does this in several ways:

- by playing down the health effects of smoking (Fig. 1)
- by devising means of advertising cigarettes which get around advertising controls
- by associating cigarette brands with positive activities through funding sport, music and other cultural events
- by targeting new markets, such as the Third World, to replace decreased sales
- by maximum 'product penetration'; in the UK there is probably no other item which is retailed at so many outlets, including supermarkets, corner shops, off licences, pubs, restaurants and petrol stations, and any of these shops bear prominent advertising for tobacco brands
- by lobbying governments, over which it exerts influence because it is a large industry, which can provide inducements to politicians and substantial tax revenue obtained from cigarettes
- by presenting controls on smoking as an issue of individual freedom, although most smokers regret starting and wish that they could stop
- by legal and media attack on prominent anti-smoking lobbyists, including the British Medical Association.

PRACTICAL STEPS TO PREVENT TOBACCO USE

Enforcement of current age limits

Smoking by under-16s is rarely taken seriously, but most lifetime smokers start by 16. Shops should not sell to the under-16s and this should be enforced.

Control of smoking in public and workplace

This reduces the social acceptability of smoking and can lower tobacco consumption, especially by less dependent smokers (see Case study).

Raising prices

Increasing price makes a small number of smokers give up, but the effect is temporary. However, it also reduces the number of young people who begin smoking.

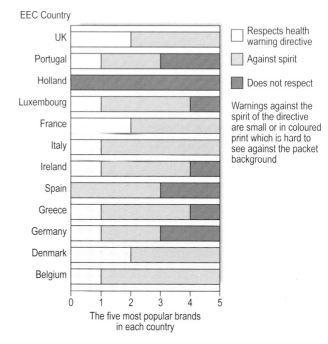

Fig. 1 **Health warnings on cigarette packets: the top five cigarette brands' compliance with the EEC directive** (European Bureau for Action on Smoking Prevention, Brussels.)

Case study
A smoking policy in the workplace

Greater Glasgow Health Board negotiated the following with the union for its headquarters:

i)   No smoking anywhere in the building except in designated smoking areas and for the exceptions given in v) below.
ii) Provision of designated smoking areas for use at meal and coffee breaks.
iii) Provision of health education material for staff.
iv) Provision of therapeutic resources and counselling services to help staff within the workplace. This was offered as a group led by clinical psychologists.
v)   Recognition that certain individuals would have difficulties coming to terms with the new arrangements — in such cases efforts were made to accommodate staff in separate areas or single rooms (i.e. with other smokers or by themselves).

Particular effort was expended in getting the most visible staff, such as receptionists and lift attendants, to adhere to the policy. After a year only 18% of staff disapproved of the policy and over 50% positively approved of it as 'setting an example' and for a cleaner, smoke-free work environment.

This policy is fairly typical of workplace smoking policies, which are probably more important as methods of changing attitudes and expressing disapproval than as methods of stopping people smoking. GGHB has since banned smoking in all its hospitals, hospital grounds and other premises.

(From Lock et al 1985)

Control of sales outlets

Some countries restrict where tobacco can be sold. Wide availability makes it easy for under-age youth to buy tobacco, normalises tobacco products and tempts ex-smokers to relapse.

Banning advertising

The industry argue that advertisments are aimed at adult smokers, to encourage them to change brand and NOT at youth to encourage them to smoke. They also argue that banning advertising does not influence rates of smoking. However, the content of many advertisements and sponsorships (e.g. sport) might seem attractive to youth as well as adults. Young teenagers are aware of tobacco advertising and can name tobacco brands, which suggests that advertising may influence the decision to smoke. Banning advertising has a modest effect on national smoking rates and also reinforces society's committed opposition to smoking.

Health education

Most smokers and youth contemplating smoking are aware of the health risks. Education needs to mantain this awareness and to address fatalism. Both youth and socially-disadvantaged groups tend to view future health effects of smoking as irrelevant

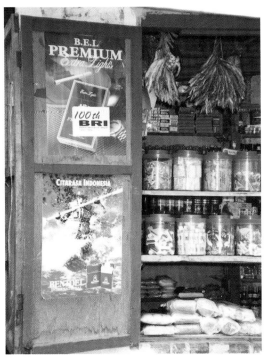

Fig. 2 **Around the world the tobacco industry is eager to associate its product with positive imagery as shown in these cigarette advertisements in Indonesia.**

STOP THINK Smoking is a good example of many modern health problems where a purely biological individual model of disease is insufficient and a biopsychosocial approach is required. Other such issues include diet, drug and alcohol problems, pollution, poverty and accidents. To tackle smoking, the range of necessary interventions have included surgical, pharmacological, behavioural, social, economic and political measures. Smoking also illustrates that medical science does not function independently of social forces. What roles can medicine play in tackling smoking?

to their current concerns. For youth, emphasis on lack of fitness or unattractiveness may be more relevant. Empowering youth to accept responsibility for their health is also important.

Minimal intervention by GPs

If GPs consistently enquire about whether their patients smoke and simply suggest to all smokers that they stop for their health, then about 10% do stop, which is good success for such a cheap intervention. In subsequent consultations it may help to ask in a non-judgemental fashion if they have quit, cut down, or have stayed quit and to praise any success. Minimimal intervention also supplements general health education.

STRATEGIES FOR A SMOKE-FREE EUROPE

The First European conference on tobacco policy, 1988, resolved on the following strategies:

1. Recognise and maintain people's right to choose a smoke-free life.
2. Establish in law the right to smoke-free common environments.
3. Outlaw the advertising and promotion of tobacco products and sponsorship by the tobacco industry.
4. Inform every member of the community of the danger of tobacco use and the magnitude of the pandemic.
5. Assure the wide availability of help for tobacco users who want to stop.
6. Impose a levy of at least 1% of tobacco tax revenue to fund specific tobacco control and health promotion activities.
7. Institute progressive financial disincentives.
8. Prohibit new methods of nicotine delivery (except as smoking cessation aids) and block future industry marketing strategies.
9. Monitor the pandemic and assess the effects of countermeasures.
10. Build alliances between all sections of the community that want to promote good health.

SMOKING AND THE DEVELOPING WORLD

The prevalence of smoking is falling in most of Western Europe and North America, although some places, such as Scotland, still have a high prevalence. There is also still concern about the number of young people, particularly women, who continue to smoke. Unfortunately, rates of cigarette smoking are rising in many developing countries in Africa, Asia and the former Eastern Bloc. In these countries smoking and its promotion are not always highly regulated or taxed, and current poverty is a more pressing concern for many than future health. Cigarettes are also often associated with an affluent, glamorous 'western' lifestyle (Fig. 2). Globally, smoking will continue to be a major health problem well into the next century.

Medicine and smoking policy

- Treating the individual patient is not enough.
- The tobacco industry vigorously defends its product.
- Prevention requires enforcing current laws, banning smoking in public, banning advertising, raising prices and controlling sales.
- Doctors should consistently tell patients to stop smoking, or not to start.

EATING AND ITS EFFECTS ON BEHAVIOUR AND ON HEALTH

The diet in both the USA and Western Europe has shown a consistent trend this century towards increased consumption of sugar, animal fats and proteins and reduced consumption of fibre. People are in general eating fewer vegetables, fresh fruit and cereals and consuming more meat and sugar in the form of soft drinks and processed foods. Diet has been related to increased incidence of atherosclerosis, hypertension, and cancer. But such epidemiological studies are not easy to interpret, and it is unclear whether some associations such as high fat/low fibre diets and increased cancer prevalence are confounded by increased longevity associated with better nutrition.

UK epidemiological studies suggest that over 70% of adults have blood cholesterol levels in excess of a target level of 6.5 mmol/litre, and that fat consumption should be reduced to less than 35% of the total energy intake. Before advocating dietary change on such a massive scale, we need to understand more about the potential influences of diet on behaviour. For example, studies of the behavioural effects of the carbohydrate/ protein composition of the diet have identified a range of effects on biochemistry, mood and food intake. Single meal studies suggest that dietary fat influences mood and arousal, with low fat content promoting feelings of vigour. Conversely there is evidence from animal studies that low fat diets may have negative emotional consequences. Changing food habits is not an easy task and reflects the diverse influences on what determines our likes and dislikes from the start.

LEARNING ABOUT FOOD PREFERENCES

Humans are omnivores and our food preferences are largely the result of learning in which the experiences of early childhood are especially powerful. Neonates show an innate liking for sweet tastes and a similar aversion for bitter tastes. Between about $1\frac{1}{2}$ and $2\frac{1}{2}$ years of age, children are relatively neophobic about food, i.e. they tend to reject new foods offered to them and they may restrict their food choices to a very limited range. Mothers often worry about the adequacy of their child's diet and this is a frequent topic of enquiry to GPs and health visitors.

Unfortunately many parental practices designed to encourage food consumption in these pre-school years can have completely the opposite effect. Research has shown that using common reward strategies such as 'if you eat all your X, then you can have some Y', serve only to increase the child's liking of Y and further increase the dislike of X. Although consumption of green vegetables is unlikely to be increased by offering them as a reward for consuming chocolate ice-cream, the chances of successful acceptance of a novel food at this age will be increased by offering the new food as a reward. Another powerful influence on children's eating is their peer group — children sitting at a nursery lunch table will switch their food preferences in accordance with others in the group; and role models such as super-heroes are used in advertising food products because of their strong effects on liking.

Psychologists have demonstrated an important and unique form of learning restricted to taste and which is responsible for often very long-lasting food aversions. In this long-delay learning, we could, say, eat a distinctive flavoured Chinese meal, and then for entirely unrelated reasons several hours later, develop a fever and become nauseous and vomit. Subsequently a pronounced aversion to the distinctive taste of Chinese food will result. In classical conditioning (see p. 20), however, the conditioned stimulus (sound of bell) must precede the unconditioned stimulus (sight of food) by a few seconds for the conditioning to be successful (salivate to sound of bell). What is special and unique about this form of taste aversion learning is that the association occurs across such a long period of time and is only possible with novel or unusual tastes (we do not for example form an aversion to the restaurant itself or to any other distinctive cues associated with the meal). Yet the learning is not open to cognitive persuasion: for instance, we would not be able to overcome such aversions even if it could be convincingly demonstrated that the nausea and vomiting were not caused by eating the meal. This form of learning is then very distinct from a food allergy (you eat strawberries and subsequently develop a facial rash); here you must avoid eating strawberries but you continue to like their taste and the idea of eating them. Temporary food aversions often develop in cancer patients when they first experience chemotherapy treatment that produces nausea.

CULTURAL INFLUENCES AND EATING DISORDERS

Anorexia nervosa

In the Western world, this century has seen the rise of a number of eating disorders particularly characteristic of young women. Anorexia nervosa has been recognised since the seventeenth century and it is a salutary thought that in 1990 'it may be more dangerous and life threatening to be a fashion model, a PE student, at a ballet school, a single-sex girls' school … than to be a coal miner, a stunt man or working on a North Sea oil rig'. This reflects the very high levels of mortality in people with anorexia compared with other psychiatric conditions.

The defining characteristics of anorexia (an unfortunate name, as loss of appetite is rare) are a refusal to maintain body weight over a minimal normal weight for age and height; an intense fear of gaining weight or becoming fat; a distorted body image; and in girls, the presence of amenorrhoea. The disorder is more common among sisters and mothers of sufferers than among the general population, and some believe this is good evidence for a possible genetic basis to the illness. People with anorexia are a very difficult group to treat successfully because they steadfastly deny or minimise the severity of their illness and are uninterested in and often resistant to therapy. The

---

Case history

I stepped on the machine, only to find that, fully clothed as I was, I weighed five stone ten pounds — or, naked, as I reckoned, five stone eight. My first reaction was one of overwhelming relief, but it was followed at once by a feeling of bewilderment. How could I have got it so wrong? Instead of having gained two stone, as I had feared and imagined, I had lost almost half a stone. I didn't feel five stone ten or eight: I felt much larger: I felt fat. And yet the weighing machine — the only one I could trust — couldn't lie. I must be thin.

(From an autobiographical account of anorexia nervosa, MacLeod 1981, p.116.)

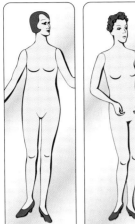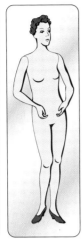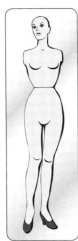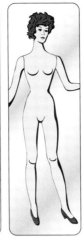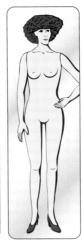

Fig. 1 **Changes in the appearance of fashion mannequins from 1920s to the present day reflect changing ideals for women's bodies.** It is calculated that the body fat depots on contemporary mannequins would be insufficient to permit normal menstruation. (Adapted from Rintala M, Mustajoki P 1992 Do mannequins menstruate? BMJ 305: 1575–6)

body fat/lean mass ratio would not support reproductive capacity. Fashion models of anorexic proportions assume the status of superstars. Little girls from an early age play with 'Barbie' dolls with similar proportions, and report dieting at younger and younger ages (Fig. 1).

Patients with eating disorders see weight as being extremely important, equate their personal value with the weight of their bodies, and devote much of their time and energy to weight regulation. Measurement of these concerns has traditionally relied on self report questionnaires such as the Eating Attitudes Test (EAT) and Body Shape Questionnaire (BSQ), which have been able to pinpoint those aspects of shape and eating which are of particular concern for an individual.

comments which people with anorexia make about food and their own bodies often seem curiously inappropriate. They may insist they are terribly overweight when clearly very slim, or maintain they have just eaten an enormous meal which in fact consisted of three grapes and a lettuce leaf.

Bulimia nervosa

An even more prevalent condition, and one which is rapidly changing in its presenting symptoms, is bulimia nervosa, first described by Russell in 1979. It has been estimated that upwards of 4–5% of female students in the UK have a history of bulimia. Unlike the anorexic patient, bulimic patients usually have a normal body weight, but are subject to repeated episodes of bingeing followed by immediate self-induced vomiting. A typical binge occurs in the evening, averages 4 800 calories, is usually sweet or salty carbohydrate foods, and is conducted in secret. Whereas anorexia seems more

prevalent in middle-class families, bulimia is less restricted to a particular socio-economic grouping.

People with bulimia exhibit great concern about their weight and make repeated attempts to control it by dieting, vomiting, or the use of drugs. Treatment outcome is more satisfactory than with anorexia, perhaps because patients usually refer themselves for treatment, with a form of cognitive therapy being particularly successful.

Dysfunctional attitudes to weight and shape play a central role in the psychopathology of anorexia and bulimia nervosa. They have been described as examples of an 'ethnic disorder', meaning they arise as a direct product of the unique pressures within a particular culture (Gordon 1990) — in this case the ever-present urge to be slim and attractive put across in women's magazines. Measurements of the size of mannequins in successive decades this century show how after 1960 calculations of the likely

EXPERIMENTAL STUDIES OF DIETING

A very useful model with which to consider bulimia is that of counter-regulation, developed by Peter Herman and Janet Polivy in conjunction with their measure of dietary restraint. The latter is a simple instrument for determining an individual's tendency to show concern about body weight and to restrict body weight through dieting.

Laboratory experiments show that restrained eaters (those who score highly on the dietary restraint scale), respond to increasingly large pre-loads by exhibiting more eating subsequently, whereas unrestrained eaters decrease the amount eaten as function of size of preload. This behaviour, which is opposite to what one might predict if eating was entirely under physiological control, is referred to as counter-regulation. This model suggests that dieting causes bingeing rather than vice versa, and that the relentless media pressure on young girls to maintain a slim figure pushes the vulnerable restrained eater into a pattern of bingeing and purging resulting in bulimia.

STOP THINK
• What do you think the implications of long-delay learning might be for the treatment of cancer with chemotherapy?
• The prevalence of eating disorders in our society has been attributed to 'cultural pressures'. What steps could be taken in schools to counter some of these pressures?
• Why do we find it so difficult to follow nutritional advice on adopting a more low-fat, high-fibre diet, and yet can change our food habits overnight in response to a food scare such as salmonella?

Eating and its effects on behaviour and on health

● Different kinds of learning play important roles in the acquisition of food preferences.
● Parental practices designed to encourage eating particular foods are often counter-productive.
● The increase in eating disorders is a result of cultural pressures.
● Dieting causes bingeing rather than vice versa.

DECIDING TO CONSULT

This spread examines the factors that help to explain why some people with symptoms choose to consult a doctor and why others delay. Understanding why people do or do not consult is important because some doctors feel frustrated and angry about 'inappropriate or trivial' consultations, and some patients feel frustrated and angry about doctors whom they perceive as uninterested in their problems. Both sets of feelings influence subsequent consulting behaviour, medical treatment, adherence and health. Delay may seriously affect a patient's risk of disease progression and the development of complications.

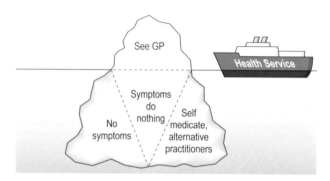

Fig. 1 **The symptom iceberg.**

THE SYMPTOM ICEBERG

Over a 2-week period about 75% of the population will experience one or more symptoms of ill health. About one third of these people will do nothing about their symptoms. About one third will self-medicate or seek the advice of an alternative practitioner (see pp. 96–97), and about one third will consult their general practitioner (Fig. 1).

Hannay (1979) has shown that the proportion of people with significant medical symptoms who do not consult a doctor is higher than the proportion of people with minor medical symptoms who do consult a doctor (26% and 11% respectively).

> **STOP THINK**
> A GP in Scotland (Usherwood 1991) produced a booklet to help parents decide when to seek professional advice for children with symptoms. The overall effect of the booklet was a small reduction (28%) in day-time home visits for booklet symptoms but a large increase (173%) in out-of-hours, night-time consultations.
>
> Why do you think the booklet had this effect on consultation behaviour?

DIFFERENCES IN SYMPTOM PERCEPTION

Three features of symptoms are important for people's perceptions of their seriousness: the intensity or severity of the symptom, the familiarity of the symptom and the duration and frequency of the symptom. For example, a severe headache may cause a person who has rarely had a headache to go to the doctor, whereas a person who has experienced migraine for some years is unlikely to consult. This person may consult, however, if the symptoms are unusual in some way or if the headache persists for longer than usual or recurs more frequently than usual (see pp. 110–111). Patients' anxieties as to the potential seriousness of symptoms may be strongly associated with their perceptions of severity.

Figure 2 contrasts the health concerns of a sample of consulters with symptoms of dyspepsia and a sample of non-consulters with similar symptoms and shows that consulters were significantly more likely to be worried that their symptoms indicated a serious or fatal condition, particularly heart disease or cancer. People with a family history of stomach cancer were also more likely to consult.

Many patients 'temporise': they wait and see if the symptoms go away in time and only decide to consult if they do not. Hannay has shown that people are most likely to consult a doctor with symptoms which they perceive as 'social' (50% of people

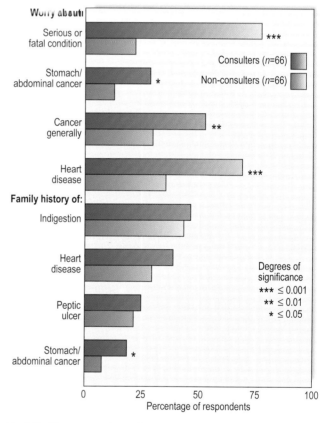

Fig. 2 **Health concerns of consulters and non-consulters.** (From Lydeard S, Jones R 1989 Journal of the Royal College of General Practitioners 39: 495–498)

with social symptoms took them to a doctor), considerably more than those with symptoms perceived as physical (34%), and least likely to consult when symptoms are perceived as mental (17%). He suggests that this may relate to people's reluctance to admit to mental health problems or to reveal their more personal problems because of a fear of 'giving themselves away'. Hence the importance of trust developing between patient and doctor.

DIFFERENTIAL EVALUATION

People weigh up for themselves what the relative costs and benefits will be of going (and of not going) to the doctor or other health practitioner. People often decide that other things in their lives are more important than dealing with symptoms of ill health; indeed doctors themselves are classic examples of people who battle on at work because they perceive themselves as indispensable.

People also weigh up what they think the doctor will think of them and what the doctor or other health worker can actually do for them and their symptoms. Research with people with breathing difficulties has shown that people who perceive their symptoms to be serious may delay going to see their doctor if they believe that they will not be able to communicate the seriousness to the doctor.

It is also common for people to consult their doctor with symptoms that appear minor to the doctor but the decision to consult reflects *anxiety* that things might be serious, and they are consulting in order to seek *reassurance* that things are in fact all right.

ACCESS

Figure 3 shows that people experiencing symptoms are less likely to visit their doctor if they live farther away from the

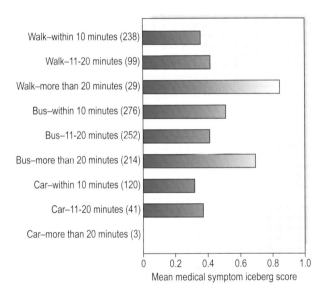

Fig. 3 **Travel to health centre, and the medical symptom iceberg.** Bus includes the 1% of subjects who travelled by train, and car includes taxi. (Reproduced with permission from Hannay 1979.)

Case study

A qualitative study of mothers' accounts of how they recognised and dealt with children's illness reported that 'not wanting to bother the doctor' and 'not wasting his time' were dominant themes for mothers when they were deciding whether or not to consult:

R62: *'Sometimes you think, well, is it worth bothering him, but so far, what they've had, if it hasn't cleared up within a couple of days I sort of try to make an appointment to see the doctor or call him in … I know there must be people that 'phone up just for anything and they've got to be sure that you need a doctor.'*

R47: *'I got to a stage that I wouldn't go to him because I felt like he was … here she comes again just purely wasting his time …'*

Adapted from: Cunningham-Burley & Maclean (1991)

surgery. Studies of the use of Accident and Emergency services have shown that the relative distance from the GP's surgery and the A&E department is a key factor in deciding which to consult: the closest being the most favoured.

Access to child care arrangements or the provision of a sitting service for a dependent relative, the availability of a telephone to make an appointment, the availability of a suitable appointment slot, and the approachability and friendliness of the doctor and the practice staff are also important factors affecting accessibility.

INFLUENCE OF FAMILY AND FRIENDS

According to some studies, up to 50% of symptoms are taken to a doctor on the advice of family or friends. It appears that family are more likely than friends to recommend a visit to the doctor, possibly because they have the responsibility for caring for the individual.

Research with pregnant women has found that social class V women with extensive and strong lay support and advice, sometimes referred to as people's lay referral network, are less likely to attend hospital ante-natal classes compared with women from social classes I and II with less lay support. It has been suggested that both the relative number of lay advisers and the degree of congruence in culture between the woman and the doctor will affect the woman's decision whether or not to consult.

People who move to a new area away from their friends and family have been found to make more visits to a doctor in their first year after moving. This raised consultation rate may reflect not only the absence of social support but also the increased risk of ill health arising from the stress of moving house.

TRIGGERS

Several studies have shown that it is not always the experience of symptoms that brings a person to see the doctor. A symptom or an anxiety may have been present for some time but something else in the person's life 'triggers' the person to consult: a relative may become concerned about a continuing problem and suggest a visit to the doctor; a change at work or in one's personal life may make the symptom more noticeable or incapacitating than before. For example, research suggests that unemployment increases consultation rates not only as a result of people becoming less well, but also by increasing people's awareness of their existing health problems, problems which had previously been put to one side in favour of involvement in their work.

Deciding to consult

- The decision to consult a doctor is a complex interplay of physical, psychological and social factors.
- Many people go with relatively minor symptoms because they are anxious that something serious may be indicated.
- There is often a mismatch between what doctors and patients perceive as appropriate reason for consulting.
- The perception of what the doctor can do for them and how they will treat them is a significant factor in a person's decision to consult.
- A change in a person's social setting or relationships may trigger a consultation even when there has been no change in the symptoms.

SEEING THE DOCTOR

Every day in the UK about 1 million people consult their general practitioner. They attend with very different problems and are seen by doctors with very different styles. This spread examines how the process and outcome of care may depend as much upon the relationship between patient and doctor, as upon the patient's problem.

TYPES OF DOCTOR–PATIENT RELATIONSHIP

Four models of the doctor–patient relationship have been proposed.

Paternalistic

The 'paternalistic' relationship has, until recently, been the most commonly observed type of relationship, and is relatively disease-focused. The doctor, a medical expert, makes a systematic enquiry, with the patient answering relatively specific and closed questions, carries out appropriate tests and reaches a diagnosis or a range of possible diagnoses. The doctor then decides on the appropriate treatment, which the patient is expected to follow without question.

More recently, studies of doctor–patient relationships have suggested that patients are also 'experts' but in different aspects of the relationship, and that there are areas of potential disagreement or conflict, particularly as patients become more knowledgable and critical of their care. They may have rather different expectations, and different knowledge and beliefs.

Mutual

The 'mutual' relationship is now becoming more common, partly as a result of greater patient knowledge particularly about chronic disease, and partly because of a general cultural shift not to be passive followers of authority. It is characterised by a willingness on the part of the doctor to recognise that patients' beliefs and knowledge are important to understanding the patients' health, illness and illness behaviour.

Consumerist

The 'consumerist' relationship is relatively uncommon in Britain but is becoming more common as a result of the extension of private health insurance, the introduction of patient charters, and the increasing emphasis on extending patient choice. It is characterised by patients 'shopping around' for their preferred care, and is accompanied (as exemplified

Table 1 **Patient reports after GP consultations**

	Short consultations (n = 585–721)	Long consultations (n = 579–722)
GP gave you the feeling your opinions were important	89%	95%
GP gave you a chance to say what was on your mind	67%	83%
GP helped reduce your worries	54%	68%
GP explained things fully	84%	91%
Patient more able to cope with life	23%	32%
Better able to understand illness/problems	41%	57%
More able to cope with illness/problems	38%	53%
More able to help self	5%	46%
More confident about health	39%	47%
More able to keep healthy	34%	46%

(Source: Howie et al 1991 BJGP 41: 48–54)

in the USA) by relatively high levels of investigation, treatment and litigation.

Default

The fourth model, sometimes categorised as 'default', is characterised by relatively low levels of engagement between doctor and patient. It is perhaps best observed in situations where the doctor can find nothing organically wrong to explain the patient's symptoms, or where patients are unable, or unwilling, to accept continuing responsibility for their own health and health behaviour. There are very particular problems associated with the way doctors respond to such situations, and there is a considerable risk that patients will become trapped in a cycle of over-investigation and treatment with nobody taking responsibility for addressing any underlying issues.

PATIENT-CENTRED CONSULTATION

There has been some debate about whether the paternalistic or the mutual relationship is the more appropriate but there is now growing agreement that, wherever possible and within the constraints of the urgency for medical intervention, patient involvement is most productive. Although there is some evidence that patients with specific physical problems prefer doctors to be relatively directive and disease-focused (Savage and Armstrong 1990), other research

(Howie et al 1991, 1992) has shown that patients are more likely to be satisfied and to feel more able to cope with ill health when doctors are more patient-centred, take longer with patients (Table 1) and identify and deal with more psycho-social issues. In such settings, they are less likely to give the patient a prescription (Howie et al 1992).

The 'patient-centred' consultation still involves taking a systematic note of the patient's presenting and underlying problems but it differs from the more traditional paternalistic relationship by integrating it with an enquiry into the patient's ideas, knowledge, beliefs, expectations and feelings (see pp. 38–39, 54–55). In their study of doctor–patient relationships, Tuckett et al (1985) showed that consultations were most likely to break down and patients were most likely to be dissatisfied and non-compliant when doctors failed to elicit and respond empathetically to patients' beliefs and expectations. Of course, patients will sometimes hold unrealistic or inappropriate expectations. In such cases it is important that the doctor and patient are clear what the patient's expectations and beliefs are, and that the doctor explains in a manner that does not make the patient feel stupid or defensive, why the belief or expectation is inappropriate. In some cases this will involve negotiation. Some of the strategies that patients and doctors use to control consultations are

STOP THINK

The development of an 'internal market' in the UK has given general practitioners the dual roles of providers of health care and purchasers of care. At the same time, the Patients' Charter has emphasised the development of patient choice. In what ways would you predict that these two developments will affect the relationship between doctors and patients?

How, as a future doctor, do you feel about this?

What evidence can you find for your views?

Table 2 **Negotiation strategies**

Patients	Doctors
Disclose	Physical setting of room
Suggest	Language
Demand	— technical/non technical
Leading question	— open/closed questions
Non-verbal behaviour	— tone of voice
Hesitation/silence	Clarifying/functional uncertainty
Delaying tactics:	Listening/interrupting
'While I'm here …'	Picking up/ignoring cues
See a different doctor	Non-verbal behaviour
	Interest/uninterest
	Calm/haste
	Prescription

Table 3 **Tasks and skills of clinical consultations**

Tasks	Important skills and behaviours
Opening the interview	1. Make eye contact, greet patient by name and shake hands 2. Invite patient to sit, and indicate where 3. Make eye contact and introduce self (name and title/position) 4. Explain purpose of interview and indicate time available 5. If necessary, explain reason for note taking and check it is acceptable
Eliciting the patient's problems	1. Use open questions to encourage patient to talk 2. Listen carefully and keep interruptions to a minimum 3. Facilitate verbally (e.g. 'Go on') and non-verbally (e.g. head nods) 4. Carefully observe patient's NVC while he/she talks 5. Reflect important points or feelings 6. Clarify details or ambiguities using closed questions if necessary 7. Elicit patient's ideas about cause or diagnosis 8. Summarise understanding of patient's problems and confirm accuracy 9. Check whether patient wishes to add anything or ask any questions
Examination and investigation	1. Describe procedure and what patient should expect to experience 2. Elicit any concerns or confusion 3. Observe patient's reactions during examination and clarify if appropriate
Discussing test results, diagnosis and treatment	1. Indicate what information you are going to give 2. Summarise patient's problems and confirm accuracy 3. Provide clear, structured, comprehensible explanation 4. Observe patient's reactions for signs of confusion or emotional response 5. Clarify patient's thoughts and feelings about information given 6. If appropriate, negotiate agreed management plan 7. Summarise main points of discussion 8. Check whether patient has any questions or concerns
Closing the interview	1. Indicate verbally and by NVC that interview is coming to an end 2. Ask patient if there is anything else they wish to say or ask 3. Confirm follow-up plans where appropriate 4. Offer a friendly goodbye

(Source: G. Deans, personal communication)

summarised in Table 2. Working-class people may sometimes express themselves rather directly, which doctors may interpret as a demand for a particular test or treatment. On occasion, no resolution may be found and both patient and doctor are likely to feel dissatisfied with the consultation.

It is also important to remember that a single consultation between a patient and a doctor does not occur in isolation, particularly in general practice. A 5- or 10-minute consultation may be but one of a series of consultations during which patient and doctor may negotiate the diagnostic and treatment possibilities, and the implications for the patient's general well-being.

Lack of time may frequently constrain a doctor from being as person-centred as he or she would like and put pressure on the doctor to be disease-focused, and on the patient not to bring up their anxieties. Patients often feel intimidated by doctors and are reluctant to ask questions or mention anxieties. Given that people frequently have anxieties that relatively minor symptoms may indicate something more serious, and given their reluctance to present with mental health problems (see pp. 84–85), it should not be surprising that they often feel unable to mention their worries lest the doctor think that they are either wasting their time with trivia or that they are 'stupid'.

Campbell and Elton (1994) and Howie (1992) have shown that general practitioners tend to develop a style of working which is relatively consistent and inflexible, a finding confirmed in a study of how Canadian surgeons break bad news (see pp. 94–95). However, it is possible for students and doctors to be taught how to improve their communication and patient-centred skills (see pp. 92–93). Table 3 summarises the main tasks and skills associated with clinical consulting.

Case study
Time and guilt

All patients, except the two with consultations under 5 minutes (patients 88 and 101), complained of shortage of time. Although most patients said that they were not rushed and could have asked more, this was the major reason given for not asking questions.

'… you're thinking of the person behind you so you don't want to keep him waiting too long and I wasn't sick, so I'm forgetting the things I want to ask him …' (Patient 73)

The doctor's time was seen as short and valuable. Patients felt that they themselves actively limited the length of their consultation. Most patients felt guilty while consulting, for two reasons — wasting the doctor's time and taking more than their fair share:

'You always feel you want to cut corners if you can and get it over as quick as possible so he's not too late finishing because he works so many hours.' (Patient 51)

'The only reason I feel guilty is for taking up other people's time … I feel personally that, you know, let's hurry up because he's got other people waiting especially sometimes when you go in there and there's four or five people behind you …' (Patient 73)

(Cromarty 1996 BJGP 46: 525–528)

Seeing the doctor

- Doctors and patients have different knowledge, beliefs, wants and expectations, and consultations often involve negotiation.
- The process and outcome of care differs not just between patients but between doctors and especially in doctor style.
- Patient-centred doctors are more likely than disease-centred doctors to identify patients' psycho-social problems, and to deal with their anxieties.
- Patients are often reluctant to voice their ideas and anxieties in case they are thought of as inappropriate, stupid or time-wasting.

PLACEBO

A remedy without any direct action on a disease, given to keep the patient happy, or to persuade the prescriber that he is doing something positive and useful, or both.

Penguin Medical Encyclopaedia

The placebo effect is important to understand because it lies outside the usual scientific analysis of medicine yet it has a great effect on the treatment of patients. Placebos are used and abused but often little understood.

THE EMERGENCE OF PLACEBO EFFECTS

Until comparatively recently, there could be no neat distinction between drugs whose mode of action for a specific disorder was known and understood, and any other drug (see Fig. 1). Effective herbal remedies were given, and are still given all over the world, without the physiological response being known. With the development of scientific medicine, people then began to identify active ingredients and to become more suspicious of drugs whose action was not understood. This introduced the notion that there were drugs which would treat a particular condition by a particular route and other substances that might be placebos.

However, the evidence for the efficacy of placebos is impressive, both in everyday clinical practice and in experimental conditions. Placebos have been shown to bring about clinical improvement in many branches of medicine: surgery, the treatment of cancer, dentistry, psychiatry, paediatrics and numerous others. They can produce the phenomena observed with other drugs:

- side-effects
- habituation (a tendency to increase the dose over time)
- withdrawal symptoms
- dependency (an inability to stop taking them without psychiatric help)
- inverse relationship between severity of symptom and efficacy of placebo.

In order to demonstrate the efficacy of any new treatment now, clinical trials include a placebo for comparison so that such effects can be separated from the effects of the experimental compound. These are often 'double blind' trials, i.e. neither the patient nor the member of staff who gives it knows which is the experimental drug and which is the placebo. This ensures that nothing can influence a patient's expectations about the drug and therefore the response.

TYPES OF PLACEBO

- *Pure placebo*: thought to contain no active ingredient, for example a sugar pill.
- *Impure placebo*: contains an active ingredient, but one which is not known to have any effect on the condition being treated, e.g. a Vitamin C tablet being given for headache.
- *Placebo procedure*: a procedure, for instance taking blood pressure, which is not known to produce any clinical change.

In practice, where placebos are used they are likely to be the 'impure' ones, substances which have some beneficial effect but may not be known to help the patient's particular condition.

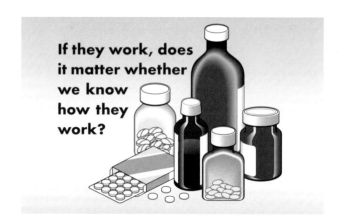

Fig 1 Drugs and mode of action.

WHAT MAKES SOMEONE SUSCEPTIBLE TO A PLACEBO?

There are no personal characteristics — age, race, gender, intelligence or personality — that will predict whether or not a patient will respond to a placebo. *Circumstances and presentation* are more influential. It has long been observed that perception of pain depends on the situation: people injured in combat appear to tolerate pain better than those with similar injuries in hospital. In war, an injury means evacuation to safety and thus brings great relief: this is not the same in civilian life. With placebos, experiments have demonstrated a number of factors that produce a response, for instance:

- The physical appearance of the placebo, whether this is a pill or a procedure, can amplify a treatment; for example, green tranquillisers reduce anxiety more than yellow or red ones (Shapira et al 1970).
- The reputation of the setting helps, e.g. a university research unit will enhance treatment more than a backstreet clinic.
- The patient's perception of staff attitudes affects response — for example, where doctors are judged as more interested and enthusiastic, the results are more positive.

HOW DO THEY WORK?

There are various possibilities:

Social influence Doctors are perceived as people in authority and therefore their direction and expectations are followed. If the doctor says the treatment will help, the patient obediently gets better.

Role expectation The doctor's role is to organise treatment, and the patient's role is to get better, so he or she plays that role.

Classical conditioning For a patient, past experiences of taking drugs led to improvement, so the administration of a new drug is more likely to produce the same response, i.e. an improvement, simply because the patient has been conditioned (see pp. 20–21).

Operant conditioning The doctor rewards the patient who shows any sign of improvement with smiles, praise and encouragement, thus increasing the probability that the patient will continue to report improvement (see pp. 20–21).

Cognitive influence The patient has firm beliefs about medical treatment, such as 'Modern medicine is based on scientific evidence, therefore this drug will be effective.'; 'My doctor is qualified, trustworthy and therefore competent, so this procedure is bound to work'.

Such beliefs then influence mood and behaviour so that the patient gets better. Of course, the opposite would also be true: if the patient believes modern medicine to be useless, he or she would be less likely to respond.

Any or all of these processes may be involved in an observed placebo response. Whichever theory you follow, there is some evidence that such psychological processes produce physiological changes, as shown in the case study.

 Many people in prison are vulnerable and have in the past been dependent on drugs or alcohol. They feel the need to continue to take something 'to help with nerves'. Part of this dependence is psychological rather than chemical and they frequently come to the medical officer asking for medication.

Should a medical officer prescribe a placebo in this case, 'to keep the patient happy, or to persuade the prescriber that he is doing something positive or useful, or both'?

Case study

Levine and colleagues hypothesised that placebo effects which relieve pain are mediated by endorphin release. If that were the case, then naloxone (an opiate antagonist) would block them. They gave medication to patients after surgery in a double blind trial (Fig. 2). The patients had all had wisdom teeth removed. Group 1 were given morphine, Group 2 had naloxone and Group 3 got a placebo. Of those initially given a placebo (Group 3), half were given another placebo an hour later (Group 3a), and half were given naloxone an hour later (Group 3b). Our interest lies in these two groups of patients. When they were initially given the placebo, 39% reported a significant decrease in pain, but if they were in Group 3b that were later given naloxone, the pain increased again. For those who had not responded to the placebo, the naloxone made no difference. So it appeared that some patients obtained significant pain relief from a placebo, but this was reversed by an opiate antagonist. The experimenters concluded that endorphin release must have occurred with the placebo.

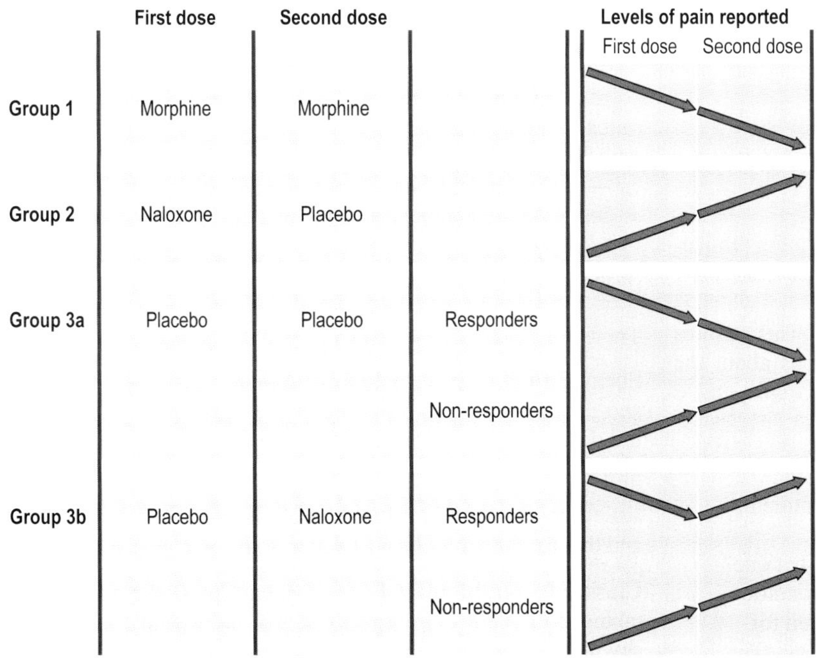

WHAT ARE DOCTORS' ATTITUDES TO PLACEBOS?

Many doctors have strong feelings about the use of placebos in medicine: some are positive, but many are negative, perhaps because the placebo effect is similar to faith-healing, when many doctors prefer to see medicine as a science. Views can range widely:

- The placebo effect is akin to witchcraft and some gullible people are susceptible, but it is outwith the remit of medicine.
- Placebo effects are a nuisance that interfere with the understanding and practice of medicine.
- Placebo effects are powerful, but to use placebos in practice is a betrayal of trust between doctor and patient.
- Placebo effects are powerful and should be usefully incorporated to enhance treatment.

Placebo

- Placebo effects have been demonstrated in many branches of medicine.
- They show various phenomena associated with established drugs.
- Placebo effects ought to be controlled in experimental trials of medical procedures.
- There are no established personal characteristics that will predict a response to placebo.
- Effects are influenced by context: culture, expectations and beliefs.
- There are ethical issues involved in the clinical use of placebos.

	First dose	Second dose		Levels of pain reported	
				First dose	Second dose
Group 1	Morphine	Morphine			
Group 2	Naloxone	Placebo			
Group 3a	Placebo	Placebo	Responders		
			Non-responders		
Group 3b	Placebo	Naloxone	Responders		
			Non-responders		

Fig. 2 **Levels of pain reported in double blind trial, naloxone/placebo.** (Reproduced with permission from Levine J D, Gordon N L, Fields H L 1978 The mechanisms of placebo analgesia. Lancet: 654–657.)

PATIENT ADHERENCE

WHAT IS ADHERENCE?

Adherence refers to following the advice of health care professionals. It includes:

- preventive health behaviours (e.g. reducing alcohol consumption)
- keeping medical appointments (e.g. keeping a follow-up appointment requested)
- self-care actions (e.g. caring for a wound after surgery)
- taking medication as directed (e.g. in relation to dose and timing).

Non-adherence is usually defined as a failure to follow advice which will lead to health damage or a decrease in the effectiveness of a medication regimen.

Most medical interventions rely on patient adherence. For example, correct diagnosis and prescription can only affect patients' health if they pick up their prescriptions and take their medication. A shared understanding of the patient's health problem and the suggested action is likely to promote adherence (Ley 1997).

MEASURING ADHERENCE

Patients' own reports, pill counts and analysis of blood or urine samples can be used to measure adherence. These different measures have been shown to provide very similar results but patients consistently overestimate their adherence in relation to non-report measures (Ley 1997).

HOW GOOD IS PATIENT ADHERENCE?

About 40–45% of patients are consistently found to be non-adherent (Ley 1997). This suggests that:

- almost half of all prescribed medication has a reduced health impact
- doctors may only be effective with 55–60% of their patients
- patients are becoming ill unnecessarily due to non-adherence.

It is estimated that 10–25% of hospital admissions are due to non-adherence.

When do patients follow advice?

Reviews of adherence research have identified a number of interconnected factors influencing adherence. These are illustrated in Figure 1. Adherence is most likely when patients understand what they are being asked to do and why. Patients must also remember what they are told if they are to act on it later. Satisfaction with the doctor and the consultation also makes adherence more likely.

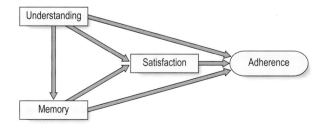

Fig. 1 **Key determinants of patient adherence.** (Adapted with permission from Ley 1997.)

How can doctors increase adherence?

Patients are more likely to feel satisfied and to understand advice when the doctor finds out what the patient thinks is wrong and discusses this. The doctor should seek to reach an agreement with the patient about what is wrong and what should be done about it (see pp. 86–87). The importance of such co-operation has been underlined by a recent proposal that adherence be replaced by the concept of concordance. Mullen (1997) has emphasised the need for joint and negotiated decision making about treatment and suggested that initial prescriptions should be regarded not only as trials of the effectiveness of treatment but also as tests of the feasibility of the regimen for each particular patient.

PROMOTING PATIENT SATISFACTION

If a patient feels her doctor is not very interested in her problem or has not understood it properly this will undermine confidence in the doctor's advice. For example, in a well-known study of paediatric consultations Korsch et al (1968) found that mothers who were very satisfied with their doctor's warmth, concern and communication were three times more likely to adhere than dissatisfied mothers.

Satisfaction depends upon the patient's perception of the doctor's sensitivity, concern, respect and competence. Reducing waiting time, taking time to greet the patient in a courteous manner and engaging in friendly introductory exchanges are all likely to increase satisfaction. Asking open-ended questions which cannot be answered 'yes' or 'no' and allowing the patient time to express his or her worries is also likely to make the patient feel satisfied with the consultation.

INCREASING PATIENT COMPREHENSION

Using simple words to describe the body or treatments and encouraging the patient to express his or her understanding is essential to ensuring that the patient understands.

Clear communication also depends upon knowing what others already know and what they expect from us. The doctor's task may be a little like giving directions. Deciding upon the most effective directions involves establishing some common understanding of local geography. Similarly, the doctor may need to assess the patient's health knowledge, beliefs and expectations before deciding how to explain the problem and treatment. Assessing the *health beliefs* (see pp. 54–55) specified by the health belief model and clarifying any misunderstandings regarding, for example, symptom severity, treatment effectiveness or side effects may motivate the patient to follow an agreed treatment plan.

Finding out how motivated the patient is and what others may think of their illness or of the suggested treatment may also help identify problems that could lead to poor adherence. Encouraging and supporting patients to take action to improve their health is likely to be worthwhile because unless the patient follows advice, the consultation may have no impact on their health.

Changing health beliefs to increase adherence

Jones et al (1987) showed how the health belief model could be used to increase adherence amongst patients attending an accident and emergency unit with asthma symptoms. Patients' health beliefs were assessed and they received information relating to their *susceptibility* to asthma complications, the *seriousness* of such complications and the *benefits* of visiting their GP to obtain treatment and avoid complications. 91% of this group made a follow-up appointment with their doctor compared to 43% in a control group who had not received the educational intervention. More importantly 75% kept these appointments compared to 10% in the control group.

STOP THINK A patient taking anti-hypertension medication returns for a routine check-up. You find that his blood pressure is high. What do you do? Increase the dose, change the medication, refer the patient for further tests or talk to the patient about the medication and any problems which may be involved in taking it?

HELPING THE PATIENT TO REMEMBER

Telling someone what you are about to tell them makes it more likely they will remember because this assists with the process of encoding in memory. This labelling of information is called 'explicit categorisation'. For example, a doctor might say, 'I'm going to tell you what is wrong with you' or 'I'm going to tell you when to take your tablets,' before conveying these important pieces of information. Instructions may also be remembered more easily if the doctor stresses that they are important and repeats them.

Specific advice, for example 'Cut the number of cigarettes you smoke by half' or 'Make an appointment for two weeks time', is easier to remember than general suggestions such as 'Cut down the amount you smoke,' or 'come in again soon'.

Simple advice and regimens are easier to understand and remember. Therefore, where possible, doctors should negotiate regimens which suit the patients' routines. For example, the progestogen-only pill may not be an appropriate contraceptive for a woman who thinks she is unlikely to remember to take it at the same time every day.

Finally, encouraging patients to take notes in consultations and providing printed information can ensure that patients have accurate information when they come to check later. Using techniques like these has been shown to improve the amount of information remembered by patients in general practice.

Helping patients remember in general practice

Ley et al (1976) assessed the amount of information which the patients of four GPs remembered. The researchers then developed a brief manual for the doctors which explained how they could simplify information, use explicit categorisation and repetition and give specific rather than general advice (see pp. 26–27). The amount of information their patients remembered after they had read the manual was then assessed. The results suggest that the doctors' adoption of these memory-enhancing communication techniques increased the amount their patients remembered (Table 1).

Table 1 **Percentage of information remembered by patients**

	Before	After
Doctor A	52	61
Doctor B	56	70
Doctor C	57	73
Doctor D	59	80

From Ley 1976

Case study
A change in treatment?

Janice was using an inhaled bronchodilator to control her asthma symptoms. She wrote a short letter to her GP asking for the usual repeat prescription and was asked to make an appointment because she had already had five previous repeat prescriptions. Janice was disappointed because work was hectic and she had little time to spare.

She arrived at the surgery on time but had to wait 40 minutes before being called. Her doctor took a few minutes to finish some notes while she waited in his room. When she explained that she needed a new prescription for her inhalers he announced that he wanted her to try a new approach using inhaled steroids. She was to take two puffs each morning and evening and to use a peak flow meter every morning. She would also be able to use her previous inhaler when she needed it. This all seemed a bit of an inconvenience to Janice who was worried about missing her driving lesson in fifteen minutes' time. However, it seemed clear and she left without asking any questions.

She was able to take the steroid inhaler and use the peak flow meter. For the next few days she recorded morning and evening readings on her grid but she forgot how many measures she was supposed to take for each reading. She decided one was probably enough. She could not remember whether her doctor had told her what lung capacity to expect and so could not decide whether she was doing well or badly. She was also unsure how she was supposed to take her usual inhaler. She remembered that her doctor had said he would expect her to use it less and she thought it might be bad for her to take the steroid inhaler without reducing her usual drug dose. She began resisting using her bronchodilator and her asthma got worse over the next few days.

Then she watched a television programme about the side-effects of steroids on body-builders. She began to worry about how her steroid inhaler might affect her and why her doctor thought she should use it. Combined with her concern about what her doctor said about oral thrush, this was enough to discourage Janice. She reverted to her usual treatment which had worked well for many years. Three months later Janice needed another prescription and went back to see another member of the practice.

Patient adherence

- 40–45% of patients are non-adherent and between 10% and 25% of hospital admissions may be due to non-adherence.
- Adherence is more likely when patients understand and remember what they have been told.
- Adherence is also more likely when patients feel satisfied with the consultation.
- Doctors can increase understanding by simplifying information and taking account of patients' knowledge and beliefs.
- Doctors can increase patients' recall by using explicit categorisation, stressing and repeating instructions and giving specific advice.
- Doctors can increase satisfaction by being friendly and considerate.

COMMUNICATION SKILLS

Medical science has provided increasingly sophisticated diagnostic and treatment techniques. However, there is no point in being expert in those techniques if you cannot enable your patients to understand how they may be helped by them. The consultation therefore remains central to effective medical practice because it largely determines the quality of the doctor–patient relationship. Research has shown that if doctors' communication skills are poor there is increased risk of :

- failing to identify the patient's main problem
- inaccurate diagnosis, inappropriate investigations (Stewart et al 1979)
- poor adherence with treatment (Ley & Llewelyn 1995)
- patient dissatisfaction and complaints (Richards 1990)
- patients choosing litigation if an error is made (Shapiro et al 1989).

It is therefore important for doctors to understand the kinds of factors and skills which affect communication and to use this awareness to improve their communication with patients.

FACTORS AFFECTING DOCTOR–PATIENT COMMUNICATION

These can be considered under four broad headings.

1. Physical setting

The environment within which a doctor interviews a patient is important.

- **Seating**. It is helpful if a doctor sits at an angle of about 45° to the patient. A patient is likely to feel more uncomfortable if the doctor sits directly facing them, sits behind a desk, or stands when the patient is sitting or lying down.
- **Privacy**. Unless patients believe they won't be overheard they are unlikely to talk freely.
- **Noise and interruptions**. Intrusions which disturb the patient's (or doctor's) concentration can make a consultation less effective.

2. Non-verbal behaviour

Non-verbal communication (NVC) refers to behaviour, other than speech, which influences social interaction. NVC is not normally under conscious control and can at times contradict what is said. Awareness of the significance of NVC, their own and patients', can enhance doctors' clinical interviewing. Among the most important aspects of NVC are:

- **Proximity**. Sitting a comfortable distance from a patient assists communication. Being too distant makes the doctor seem aloof, while being too close may feel overly threatening.
- **Posture**. Sitting upright but relaxed, with arms and legs uncrossed and leaning slightly toward the patient, conveys attentiveness. Leaning back, slouching or sitting with chin resting on hand suggests boredom or lack of interest.
- **Eye contact**. This is the most powerful NVC for initiating, maintaining and ending communication. The doctor's gaze should be in the direction of the patient without staring. This allows the patient to make eye contact as wished. Avoiding eye contact for long periods inhibits communication.

- **Facial expression**. Facial expressions often give away how a person is really feeling. Doctors can be alert to patients' expressions showing emotions like fear, embarrassment or confusion, and can by their own facial expressions show interest, compassion and concern for the patient. However, if the doctor's expression reflects disgust, anger, or disbelief the relationship with the patient may be damaged.
- **Head nods**. Head nods convey understanding and encouragement to say more. However, vigorous nodding may be interpreted as impatience. Similarly, nodding when a patient expresses a strong opinion may inadvertently imply the doctor's agreement.
- **Touch**. Within medical relationships touch can be *facilitative* (e.g. in helping to establish a friendly relationship with the patient by shaking hands on meeting), *functional* (e.g. to carry out physical examinations) or *therapeutic* (e.g. touching a distressed patient on the hand, arm or shoulder to console). However, not all patients find the latter comforting so its appropriateness must be judged for each individual.
- **Paralinguistic features**. This refers to aspects of verbal messages which serve to modulate their meaning. Variations in vocal attributes such as tone, pitch and volume can determine whether the same words, e.g. 'You took all the tablets', are expressed as a statement of fact, surprise, or as a question.
- **Silence**. Silences may occur when a patient is taking time to decide how to answer a question, trying to recall a detail or is experiencing a difficult emotion. It is important not to 'fill' this silence immediately with another question but instead to allow the patient time to respond. If the patient begins to appear very uncomfortable with the silence, use of a reflection, e.g. 'You seem upset', can often lead to a clarification of thoughts or feelings.

Used skilfully, non-verbal behaviours offer a doctor powerful tools with which to encourage a patient to talk, and to demonstrate interest in, understanding of and empathy with the patient's predicament.

 Patients often complain that doctors do not ask about their feelings or emotional responses to illness. But some doctors argue that their job is just to treat disease, not deal with how people cope with it.

What's your opinion on this view of medical practice?

3. Verbal communication

To practise medicine well, doctors need to be able to obtain details of patients' problems accurately, explain diagnoses clearly and discuss treatment options sensitively. It is therefore also important that they can use language effectively to achieve these goals. Different aspects of verbal clinical communication can be identified.

Questioning

There are different types and functions of questions but two broad categories can be distinguished:

- **Closed / narrow questions**. These are so called because they tend to limit the patient to one- or two-word answers. Closed questions are useful for obtaining or clarifying details. Examples include questions which invite:

  – an item of detail — When did the pain start?
  – choice of alternatives — Is it sharp or dull pain?
  – yes/no response — Is the pain still there?

- **Open / broad questions**. These questions allow patients more discretion in replying and are good for eliciting beliefs, opinions or feelings. Open questions are also useful early on in an interview for encouraging a patient to describe fully their problems, for instance:

– what's been troubling you?
– what do you think is wrong with you?
– how do you feel about the operation?

Blended skilfully, questions of these two types will allow you to explore, and confirm understanding of, a patient's difficulties. It is also important to avoid asking more than one question at once, and to avoid leading questions.

Reflecting

Reflection is an important verbal skill for encouraging a patient to talk and for demonstrating active listening. Thus if a patient says, 'I can't believe it's cancer', a doctor might reflect back:

– using the patient's words — you can't believe it
– an interpretation of those words — It's too much to take in
– or, an impression of the patient's feelings — You feel shocked.

Summarising

A summary draws together the significant aspects of what has been said. Doctors may summarise their understanding of the patient's symptoms or the key points of treatment. This provides an opportunity for clarifying misinterpretations on the part of the doctor or patient.

Explaining

The ability to deliver lucid, coherent explanations is critical to providing patients with an understanding of their illness, diagnosis, investigations or treatment. An explanation should be presented in a way that takes account of the patient's needs and is easily understood. When giving an explanation it helps to:

- use a series of logical points
- avoid or explain any jargon
- repeat and emphasise key points
- use examples and diagrams
- give specific rather than vague advice
- ask for feedback on understanding.

4. Psycho-social context

This refers to characteristics of doctors or patients which may affect how they relate to each other. Such attributes include personal values, attitudes and beliefs which may reflect the influences of family, socio-economic, religious or ethnic background. These factors may have particular significance when issues with ethical or moral overtones arise, e.g. sexual matters, drug taking, AIDS. Organisational context is also very important, with short appointment times providing little opportunity for patient-centred consultations (see pp. 86–87).

Case study

Consider the following different responses of a Consultant to a patient. In what way do they differ and what factors might account for the difference?

Peter was a 26-year-old Physiology PhD student with a recent history of passing blood following mild exercise. At a busy out-patient clinic he had just undergone an IVP to X-ray his kidneys and was called to see the Consultant, Mr Brown.

Mr Brown (looking at X-ray on screen): *Well, Peter, I can find nothing wrong with your kidneys. I think you have a touch of long-march haematuria which sometimes happens to people who exercise a lot.*
Peter (in a hesitating voice): *Oh? I ... I've read a bit about that condition and I don't think it fits with what happens to me.*

Response 1

Mr Brown (turning to stare at Peter with an expression of disbelief and annoyance): *Oh, you don't! (pause) Well young man, in that case you've just talked yourself into a cystoscopy! We'll send you an appointment for a few weeks' time. (Walks off briskly.)*
Peter (looking very anxious) *Oh dear. Thanks.*

Response 2

Mr Brown (turning with an expression of surprise but interest): *What makes you say that, Peter?*
Peter: *Well, the blood I pass is bright red and in this condition I believe it's usually a dark brown colour.*
Mr Brown: *I see! That's possibly significant. (pause) Well, we could do a cystoscopy to have a look in your bladder. That would mean giving you a general anaesthetic and passing a fine optic fibre up through your penis. How would you feel about us doing that?*
Peter (looking apprehensive): *Well ... OK, if you think it will help find out what's wrong with me.*

Peter underwent cystoscopy and was found to have calculi which had been causing inflammation in the lining of his bladder.

Communication skills

- Good doctor–patient communication is central to the effective practice of medicine.
- Poor communication increases the risk of inaccurate diagnosis, patient dissatisfaction and non-adherence with treatment.
- Four factors which influence the effectiveness of doctor–patient communication are:
  – physical setting
  – non-verbal communication
  – verbal communication
  – psycho-social context.
- Effective clinical communication requires the ability to use the relevant skills flexibly in response to the needs of different patients.

BREAKING BAD NEWS

WHAT IS BAD NEWS?

One of the most difficult jobs a doctor has is that of breaking bad news to a patient or a relative. Bad news has been defined as 'any news that drastically and negatively alters the person's view of her or his future' (Buckman 1994). Bad news may be giving a terminal or life-changing prognosis, e.g. metastatic cancer or multiple sclerosis, but it could also be news of sudden loss, e.g. telling a young wife that her husband has died after a massive heart attack or parents that their teenage son has been killed in a motorbike accident.

WHY IS IT DIFFICULT?

There are several reasons why breaking bad news is an especially difficult task for doctors, irrespective of their age, speciality or professional experience. These may be personal (related to their own personality or past experience), social (to do with society's attitudes), professional (influenced by role or peer values), or legal/political (Buckman 1994). Some of these are listed in Table 1. In addition, it may be made more difficult if family members want to protect the person from bad news and distress. Under these circumstances, the doctor may be asked to collude with the relatives in order to withhold the truth from the person. This situation often puts strain on a previously healthy relationship and can lead to feelings of mistrust and isolation on the part of the patient. Nowadays, most doctors believe that people should be made aware of their diagnosis and prognosis if they wish, and will tell the person if asked directly. In situations of collusion the doctor should find out the reasons for the relative's wish. If it appears that not telling is causing problems, the doctor should try to negotiate permission from the relative to tell the person (Faulkner et al 1994).

Several studies have found that doctors find the breaking of bad news so stressful that they adopt a variety of strategies to make the task easier for themselves. The use of these strategies in turn can affect the amount of information doctors give to patients, i.e. their policy of disclosure (Fig. 1).

Although the doctor may be able to do little to minimise the physical outcome of the bad news, the way a doctor breaks news of this kind can affect later adjustment and coping. There are several ways in which a doctor can manage this situation to make it easier for those receiving the news.

MANAGING THE INTERVIEW FOR THE PATIENT'S SAKE

Check the person's physical ability to take in news

Before attempting to give any information of this kind it is important to make sure that the patient or relative is physically able to understand (Faulkner et al 1994). In the case of a serious diagnosis such as untreatable cancer, the patients may already be experiencing symptoms which are preventing them from thinking clearly, such as confusion due to hypercalcaemia or drug-induced drowsiness. It is necessary therefore to treat any condition which will prevent the person from comprehending the news, before attempting to impart it.

Check own appearance and readiness

The way doctors present themselves at the consultation can also help patients to accept the news more easily. Making sure that you appear comfortable, relaxed and are not rushing will portray to patients that you have the time to spend with them and feel at ease with the task. Appearing in a blood-stained coat and looking tense and harassed will only serve to heighten patients' stress.

Setting the scene

The context of where the news will be broken is as important as how it is broken. The most appropriate place will be a quiet side room on the ward to ensure the person's privacy and concentration. People will absorb the news better if they feel as relaxed and comfortable as possible. Most doctors find it helpful to be accompanied to the interview by another member of staff, e.g. a nurse, social worker or chaplain, as well as allowing the person to be joined by a relative or friend. The presence of other people can often help to clarify information which was given by the doctor after the interview, as well as providing emotional support when the news is broken. The news being given may be shocking or devastating for the recipient. For these reasons it should never be given during the doctor's round from the bottom of the bed or in the middle of the ward corridor where other patients, visitors and staff can see and overhear.

Table 1 **Difficulties involved in breaking bad news**

Personal	Fear of own illness/death Fear of expressing own emotions, e.g. crying Recent bereavement Identification with own experience (for example victim may be same age) Embarrassment/distress/discomfort
Social	Removal of death from home to institution makes death unacceptable and taboo Sickness stigmatised
Professional	Lack of experience or training Fear of eliciting a difficult response, e.g. anger Fear of being blamed by person or superiors Failure to provide cure Fear of causing pain/emotional damage Fear of destroying hope
Political	Fear of litigation

Source: Buckman 1994

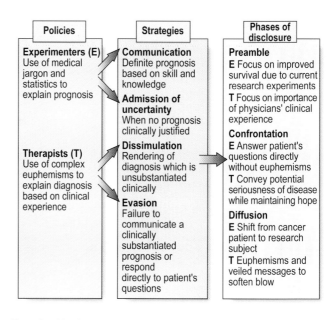

Fig. 1 **Breaking bad news: phases of disclosure, strategies and policies in Canadian study.** (Source: Taylor 1988.)

Case study

John is a 34-year-old man who is engaged to be married next year. For the past 2 years he has periodically experienced pins and needles in his arms and legs. Although his fiancée and family urged him to go to the doctor he had shrugged the symptoms off. In the last few weeks however an episode of blurred vision and a temporary loss of power in his right leg precipitated his referral to a neurologist by his General Practitioner. A series of tests confirmed a diagnosis of multiple sclerosis. Unfortunately, the neurologist was unable to give the news himself because a prior commitment to present a paper at a conference meant that he had to be absent from the ward for a few days. He therefore asked his house officer to break the bad news in his place. This worried the house officer because he had never had to do this before. To minimise his anxiety, he decided he would do it while taking blood from John as this would give them both something to concentrate on. On hearing the news, John was devastated. He began to weep uncontrollably and then became angry with the house officer and demanded to see the consultant. Not knowing how to respond to this reaction, the house officer fled to find the ward sister.

STOP THINK Imagine you were the house officer in this situation. How would you have broken the news to John? What factors might have caused John to react the way he did? If you were the ward sister, what would you do to help John now?

BREAKING BAD NEWS — THE CONSULTATION

The process of breaking bad news can be described as a series of stages to be worked through by the doctor and the recipient (Buckman 1994; Faulkner et al 1994).

Stage 1. It is essential before breaking the news to find out what the person already knows and understands about his illness. This will inform the doctor of the degree of insight and provide a baseline on which to build. Sometimes the person will indicate that he already suspects that something is seriously wrong. This may be especially true of people who have been experiencing difficult symptoms or have known a relative or friend who has had the same illness.

Stage 2. Before continuing, the doctor should find out what the person wants to know about his/her illness. This can be done by asking the person directly, and should leave the doctor in no doubt about how much information to give. For example, some people will require only to know about their treatment without wishing to speak about their diagnosis or prognosis.

Stage 3. If the person wants to know more, the news should be broken frankly and clearly. To begin with, some information should be given by the doctor to warn the person that the news is not good. For example, 'The results of the tests are more serious than we thought'.

Stage 4. Allow time for news to sink in.

Stage 5. Listen and respond to how the person reacts. You can keep giving information as long as the person is asking for it and understands what is being said.

Stage 6. Plan treatment or next course of action with the patient or relatives (for example with bereaved relatives it may be to view the body). It is vital that the doctor arranges to see the patient at a follow-up interview in order to help clarify any misunderstandings or anxieties the person may have about the news.

Some doctors now provide an audio-tape of the interview which the person can play back in the privacy of his/her own home or to other relatives or friends who were not at the interview. Other doctors give written information to back up what they have said.

NO NEWS IS BAD NEWS

An important part of communicating news to patients is conveying the results of tests. It can be difficult to reassure patients who have been anticipating bad news that the news is good. Studies show that patients who are experiencing symptoms but have negative test results may remain anxious long after the consultation and continue to experience the same symptoms, often leading them to consult again. Reasons for this anxiety may be a misunderstanding of what the doctor has said or disbelief (McDonald et al 1996). In these circumstances doubt may be fuelled by conflicting evidence from an individual's personal circumstances — for example, knowing someone with the same symptoms who has died or who has had a false negative result. In these circumstances direct discussion of the patient's concerns is advocated rather than referring the patient on for further tests (McDonald et al 1996).

SUDDEN BAD NEWS

In cases of trauma, the task of breaking bad news may be even more difficult because of the suddenness and unexpectedness of the death, illness or accident. In addition there will usually have been no time to establish a relationship with the person beforehand or warn him/her that the news is serious. Often the situation is complicated by the fact that the victim may be young, the next of kin may be difficult to establish or contact and it may be less easy to control the context in a busy Accident and Emergency department or intensive care unit (McLauchlan 1990). In these situations the police may be a useful source of help in contacting and supporting relatives.

REACTION TO BAD NEWS

The way a person reacts to bad news will vary widely. Its impact will depend on the difference between what the person hopes for and the medical reality (Buckman 1994). Reactions may be dictated by the person's past experiences, personality, coping strategies or the impact of the news on the individual. They may be unrelated to the type or stage of the disease. For these reasons reactions may vary from calm or resigned acceptance to acute distress, anger, shock or denial.

Breaking bad news

- Ensure the person is physically able to take in the news.
- Find a quiet room where the news can be broken in privacy and undisturbed.
- Allow the person to be accompanied by a friend/relative/staff member of their choice.
- Check what the person already knows and understands and requires to know further.
- Give warning to alert the person that the news is serious.
- Continue giving information if the person is understanding and responding positively to it.
- Monitor the person's reaction and respond.
- Plan next course of action with the person and always arrange follow-up.

SELF-CARE AND ALTERNATIVE TREATMENT

People experiencing physical discomfort or emotional distress do not always turn to a doctor for advice and treatment. In all societies there is a range of ways in which people either help themselves or seek help from others. Kleinman (1985) has suggested that health care systems are composed of different sectors or arenas — the popular sector, the folk sector and the professional sector — although they may partly overlap with each other (Fig. 1). In Western industrialised societies, the professional sector is predominantly bio-medicine. However, doctors certainly do not see all the illness and disease that occurs in a community. Indeed, they only see what has been called the tip of the iceberg of both symptoms and disease (see pp. 84–85). This means that there is a considerable amount of unmet need in the community, where people may be experiencing health problems which would respond to medical treatment. However, it also means that many people are dealing with a range of both self-limiting and chronic illness themselves, by using self-care or alternative treatments. We can begin to understand this by examining the popular and folk sectors in more detail.

THE POPULAR SECTOR

The popular sector is where ill health is first recognised and defined. It is also where much ill health is treated; and where various health maintenance activities take place (for example ensuring healthy diets, taking vitamin supplements). It includes all the therapeutic options which people use without consulting either medical or folk/alternative practitioners. Three components of the popular sector are important: the lay referral system, self-care and self-help.

The lay referral system

Most people discuss their symptoms with someone else, whether this is a member of their family or a friend. Indeed, some people in the community have an important place in these lay networks — those with experience of an illness; those with experience of raising children; and those who are or were health professionals. This system of lay referral may influence health and illness behaviour. For example, if the network or subculture is incongruent with doctors, in terms of beliefs and situation, there may be a low rate of uptake of services (Freidson 1975).

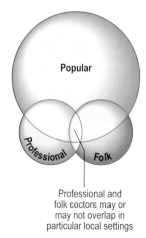

Fig. 1 **Three sectors of health care.** (Redrawn from Kleinman 1985 and Scambler 1997.)

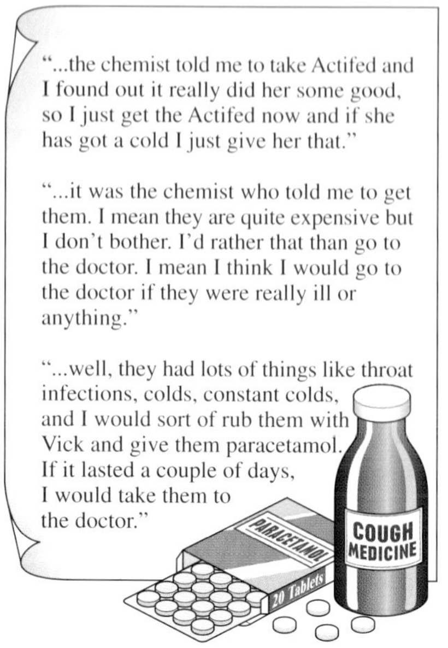

Professional and folk sectors may or may not overlap in particular local settings

Self-care

Self-care, and specifically self-medication, is a large and important part of the popular sector of health care. This can include both over-the-counter medicines and home remedies. For example, research carried out in Scotland on mothers and young children (Cunningham-Burley and Irvine 1987) found that these were the most common responses to children's symptoms. In this study, mothers were asked to complete health diaries and participate in an in-depth interview: 42 women completed health diaries, and the results show that the mothers closely monitor their children, and often notice changes which may indicate illness. Something was noticed on 49% of all recorded days. On 65% of these days the mothers took some kind of action in dealing with their children's symptoms, yet they made contact with a health care professional on only 11% of these days. The main ways in which mothers cared for the symptoms were through home nursing and home remedies (some of which activities may have been previously recommended by doctors) and providing over-the-counter remedies, particularly analgesics and cough medicines. Using the pharmacist was an important part of the lay referral system and self-care activities amongst this group, as these extracts show from interviews with mothers of young children (Fig. 2).

How people deal with illness themselves will depend on their beliefs, attitudes, resources and access to formal health care. In this same study, the mothers thought that you could 'catch an illness early', thus obviating the need to go to the doctor for an antibiotic. They

"...the chemist told me to take Actifed and I found out it really did her some good, so I just get the Actifed now and if she has got a cold I just give her that."

"...it was the chemist who told me to get them. I mean they are quite expensive but I don't bother. I'd rather that than go to the doctor. I mean I think I would go to the doctor if they were really ill or anything."

"...well, they had lots of things like throat infections, colds, constant colds, and I would sort of rub them with Vick and give them paracetamol. If it lasted a couple of days, I would take them to the doctor."

Fig. 2 **The chemist and self-care: mother's view.** (Cunningham-Burley and Irvine, 1987; Cunningham-Burley et al 1983-85.)

also knew from their own experience that many illnesses were self-limiting — they would thus try something first, and only go to a doctor if symptoms did not clear up. They also did not want to bother their doctors when they could attempt to treat the child themselves.

Self-help

A third component of the popular sector is self-help (see also pp. 136–137). Self-help groups in relation to health have grown in recent years, often providing an alternative to formal medical care. They are important both for the individual members of the group, but also at a more collective level, where they may lobby for a change in attitudes or in the provision of health care. Some groups emphasise the former and are 'inner-focused', and some the latter and are 'outer-focused' (Katz and Bender 1976). There are different reasons why self-help groups have developed to be an important part of the popular sector of health care. Firstly, existing services sometimes fail to meet the needs of people with a particular condition; secondly, self-help groups provide a panacea to the isolation many feel when experiencing a chronic illness. Self-help groups have several characteristics which give mutual support and help. Members have a common experience of the problem, and there is no distinction made between helper and helped. Reciprocity is an important part

Case study

Kelleher (1994) investigated self-help groups for people with diabetes. These are a recent development in the UK, and reflect grass root activities and recognition of need. They are affiliated to the British Diabetic Association, which is a large national organisation, but are small locally-run groups. They meet to discuss problems around managing diabetes. This provides an important forum for people to express their worries, to learn from others about how they manage, and to admit to temptation. Members begin to feel less guilty about how they manage their condition as part of their everyday lives, and become more confident.

of self-help, and the sharing of problems. Groups may provide important information to members, and may help people overcome stigma or feelings of being different.

THE FOLK SECTOR

The folk sector refers to all types of traditional, alternative or complementary healers or practitioners which exist in different societies. This sector is large in non-Western societies, and is increasingly recognised as an important element which needs to be integrated into any biomedical health care system. The folk sector is also of growing importance in the developed world. Historically, before the development of Western medical science, the traditional sector was paramount. The reasons behind its resurgence are various. There has been a decline in faith in scientific medicine; a realisation that there is a range of conditions which medicine cannot cure; and as people become more active consumers, they are better able to exert choice in the care they seek. However, many people use

alternative treatments in parallel to, rather than instead of, professional medicine. Sharma (1990) conducted research on 30 people who used alternative medicine in England. She identified 4 main types of usage (Fig. 3).

The sector encompasses a range of formal and informal types of practice and practitioners. Some receive formal training, and have professional bodies similar to medicine. Others are more informal. For these reasons it is difficult to estimate the numbers of practitioners in any one country. However, in the UK, research carried out in 1981 recorded that there were over 11 000 therapists belonging to a professional body in the UK (Threshold Survey; Fulder, Munro 1982). The largest group is osteopathy, then acupuncture. Yet the folk sector contains a vast range of therapies, from homoeopathy to therapeutic massage. Estimates suggest that up to one in four people in Britain use some kind of alternative practitioner.

Alternative medicine tends to view the patient holistically: it treats the patient's symptoms as part of a total health profile, and does not see these in isolation from

the whole person. Alternative practitioners spend more time with their patients — a first consultation usually lasts about 1 hour.

 Some general practitioners are integrating specific complementary medicine skills like homoeopathy and acupuncture into their daily practice. Others are very sceptical. Why do you think this is happening? Would you consider doing so, and why/why not?

PRACTICAL APPLICATION

Recognition of the vast amount of health care which takes place in the popular sector is important both for doctors working in the community and for those planning health care services. When self-care represents appropriate treatment, doctors should respect this expertise when someone does eventually consult them. Reassurance that the initial response to symptoms is appropriate is one way of doing this; and education about other options helps to develop a patient's own resources for care. It is also important for doctors to recognise the value of self-help, to be aware of groups in the area, and to alert patients to them. This may be particularly important for people living with a chronic illness, although other problems and conditions are also relevant. Many patients will now be using alternative practitioners as well as, or instead of, doctors. It is important to recognise why patients may find this beneficial, and work with, rather than in opposition to, this sector of health care.

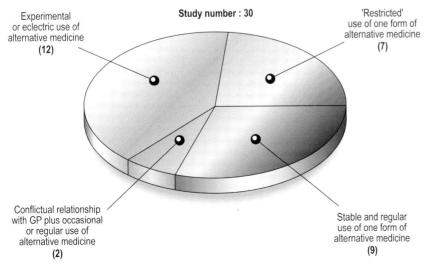

Fig. 3 **Types of usage of alternative medicine.** (After Sharma 1990)

Self-care and alternative treatment

- Most illness does not come to the attention of doctors but is dealt with by people themselves through self-care within the popular sector of health care.
- Self-help is a growing area of health care, based on mutual aid and support.
- Alternative medicine is becoming a more significant component of the health care system.

THE EXPERIENCE OF HOSPITALS

More and more people go to hospital at some point in their lives (see Fig. 1) but hospitals are changing from places where one goes to die, to places for acute conditions and specialist care. In the past there was a greater risk of dying in hospital, so it is not surprising that for many old people hospitals are places with negative associations. Modern hospitals may appear quite different, and offer cafes and shops to serve patients, visitors and staff.

Nearly all first births in the UK take place in maternity hospitals. This means that about 90% of women will experience a stay in hospital, and nearly everyone will have known a relative who has stayed in hospital. Elderly people are more likely to be admitted than younger people, although efforts are made to care for them in the community (see pp. 14–15, 146–147). However, less time is spent as inpatients and there are more day cases and earlier discharge into the community. Hospitals also play a part in maintaining health, and many people go to hospitals for check-ups or rehabilitation programmes.

THE EXPERIENCE OF BEING A PATIENT

When someone is admitted to hospital, even if only for a day or overnight stay, then they enter the role of a *hospital patient* (see pp. 102–103). Goffman (1968) suggested that the person becomes invisible, leaving only the illness visible. Doctors and nurses may talk about the patients as if they were not present (see Fig. 2). Being a patient also carries certain expectations. They must move parts of their body on command, respond to probes in parts of their anatomy with declarations of pain and answer questions about the name of the current Prime Minister.

Patients may also resent their loss of freedom. They may wear night clothes throughout the day, and be dependent on others for basic functions. They may have little or no choice about the timing of meals or visits. Lights will go off at a set time and they may be forbidden to get out of bed, or not allowed to stay in bed. They lose their familiar social roles at work and at home.

Not all patients are perceived in the same way by medical and nursing staff. The patients who obey instructions, make no demands, do not ask questions, and never complain may be labelled as 'good patients'. 'Good patients' are appreciated by staff and may be easier to manage, but their health may actually suffer. Taylor (1986) points out that 'good patients' may not ask for information and may not report important clinical symptoms. The hospital environment may actually encourage patients to become helpless. The more that patients feel they cannot control the environment around them the more they will feel helpless.

The patients who ask questions, demand attention and complain may be labelled as 'bad patients'. 'Bad patients' who are not seriously ill may be perceived as difficult patients. However, they may be angry and demanding because they are anxious. These patients may assert their sense of control and independence by breaking the rules. Being a 'bad patient' could be good for health, although not if they are poor at coping with stress. If more questions are asked, more information will be given, and if symptoms are reported, they may help the diagnosis and treatment.

CONTROL

The feeling of losing control is unpleasant. Taylor (1986) divides control into behaviour control, cognitive control, decision control and information control.

- **Behaviour control** involves being able to influence procedures in some way. Allowing a patient to control the progress of a painful procedure such as an enema can reduce anxiety. If anxiety before an unpleasant event can be reduced the unpleasant event will be more tolerable.
- **Cognitive control** is used in cognitive therapy and is very effective. In cognitive control the idea is to think about something neutral or irrelevant (distraction technique) or to concentrate on the positive aspects of the procedure. In childbirth the pain of contractions can be borne by learning to apply distraction techniques such as recalling a tune or a poem.
- **Decision control** — if a patient can choose when to have an unpleasant procedure, e.g. an injection, then they will experience less discomfort.
- **Information control** — it is often assumed that the more information the patient receives the better, but this is not so for everyone. Information may be reassuring because it may reduce fear of the unknown and enable people to adopt coping strategies.

STRESSFUL ASPECTS OF HOSPITALS

Medical students may quickly get used to hospitals, but patients and relatives may find them stressful for a number of reasons.

Privacy

This will be determined to some extent by the architecture of the hospital or clinic. In a single-bedded ward patients have more control over their own activities, but if they are not seriously ill a multiple-bedded ward can be a friendly place.

The ward environment

Patients and visitors may find noise, smells and elaborate instruments stressful.

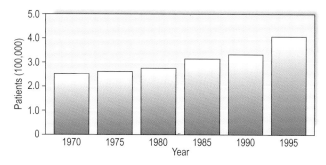

Fig. 1 **Hospital inpatients in Scotland 1970–1995.** (Source: ISD 1996.)

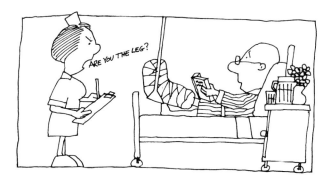

Fig. 2 **The person may become invisible on admission, and be identified only by the condition.**

The professional role

Uniforms and name badges help to maintain role relationships and tell the patients who people are. Uniforms can also be a barrier and are not always worn by staff in psychiatric wards. Nurses, junior doctors and medical students have different social identities and roles. Each social role has role-related rights such as being allowed to inflict pain, to administer drugs, or to ask intimate questions. Each role also has obligations to be respectful, to be caring and to preserve confidentiality.

 In what ways may a hospital's teaching and research interests conflict with the interests of patients? What could be done to reduce this conflict?

SURGERY

Many patients get very anxious before operations (see pp. 100–101). Johnston (1980) suggested that going into hospital is worrying apart from the operation itself. Women may be more anxious than men because they may be worried about their families at home, or it may be that they are more ready to admit that they are worrying. Johnston (1987) found that gynaecological patients were mostly worried about whether the operation would be a success, how long it would take to get back to normal and how they would feel after the operation. 'Worrying', as measured from a list of 25 possible worries, was closely related to the scores on an anxiety scale.

Healthy people go into hospital to give birth, but this experience may be very different from going in for an operation or investigation. Recently there has been an increasing demand for midwife care and home births, and more relaxed surroundings for hospital births (see pp. 2–3).

STRESSFUL MEDICAL AND SURGICAL PROCEDURES

Many people undergo minor, but potentially stressful, medical procedures in hospitals as inpatients. A diagnostic procedure such as a laparoscopy or a mammogram may be the cause of anxiety because of the fear of what might be found. Some procedures can be very painful, e.g. pelvic floor repairs or endoscopies, and in most surgical procedures a general or local anaesthetic is given. However, although this alleviates the pain it also means that there is a loss of control.

Some studies of preparation for stressful procedures in adults have shown benefits (Mathews and Ridgeway 1984). Information given about the procedure beforehand can reduce anxiety. In a study of cervical screening anxiety was reduced by giving information, reassurance and the opportunity to ask questions (Foxwell and Alder 1993). Many women find the procedure of taking a cervical smear distressing and do not fully understand the purpose, or the meaning of a negative result. One group of 30 patients (the study group), was given routine care plus an extra 10 minutes of information, reassurance, and an opportunity to ask questions. The control group was given brief information and a leaflet. The two groups were no different in anxiety scores before the smear was taken, but when they received the results 3–4 weeks later, anxiety levels were significantly reduced in the study group, but not in the control group.

- Why are hospitals stressful?
- Talk to someone who has been a patient recently or has visited someone. How do their experiences relate to the above?
- Do you think there are gender differences in patient behaviour? What are they?
- Contrast your experience of hospitals with a recent television drama.

RESEARCH INTO ANXIETY

Janis (1958) suggested that people differ in their approach to surgery. Some people worry a great deal, feel very vulnerable and have difficulties sleeping. A second group show moderate levels of anxiety. They are somewhat anxious, worried about specific procedures, but ask for information. The third group are unconcerned about the operation. They sleep well and deny that they feel worried.

Although these early studies claimed a *curvilinear* relationship between fear level and outcome, this has not been confirmed by other studies. There is more likely to be a *linear* relationship between anxiety and recovery. The greater the level of fear before surgery, the poorer was the recovery. Those who are anxious beforehand have more pain, more medical complications and slower recovery.

Case study

Mrs McNab, aged 75, had never been into hospital before. Her two children had been born at home, delivered by the local midwife. She was frightened by the ambulance ride from her remote croft into the city, although the paramedical staff were kind and gentle. On arrival she was undressed and given a hospital night-gown. The hospital bed was in a large ward full of strangers. Mrs McNab had never before slept in a bed outside her own home. The operation to remove her appendix was explained to her and she signed a consent form, although she had not brought her reading glasses with her. Following the successful operation she experienced great pain but did not ask for pain relief because she thought this would damage her brain. She missed her family acutely and was frequently found weeping.

- What could be done to alleviate her distress?
- How might her distress affect her recovery?

The experience of hospitals

- Hospitals are changing as more medical care takes place in the community.
- The experience of being a patient may be stressful, and not all patients react in the same way.
- Loss of control may occur in hospital patients.
- Stressful aspects of hospitals include lack of privacy, the ward environment, identification of professionals, worry about surgery, worry about the outcome, and anxiety about the family at home.
- Many medical and surgical procedures are stressful, but the stress can be alleviated by preparation.

PSYCHOLOGICAL PREPARATION FOR SURGERY

Psychological preparation for surgery has been developed to reduce patients' anxiety and to improve recovery in the post-operative period.

ANXIETY

Anxiety is an unpleasant emotion associated with threatening situations or thinking about threat (see pp. 112–113). People differ in their propensity to experience anxiety; those with anxious personalities generally tend to have higher levels of anxiety, but are also more likely to experience heightened anxiety when exposed to a threatening situation such as exams, surgery or speaking in public. Increased anxiety is associated with changes in cognition, behaviour and physiology.

Cognitive effects are shown both in terms of how attention is directed and deficiencies in tasks requiring sustained attention or speed in decision-making. When anxious, people pay more attention to threatening aspects of their environment and interpret ambiguous events as threatening — for example they might interpret the word 'stroke' to mean a cerebrovascular accident rather than gentle touching. Deficiencies in attention and speed of thinking can result in failure to take in important information, and patients are likely to have greater difficulties in taking in medical information. The cognitive deficiencies may affect behaviour, but in addition, anxiety leads to poorer motor control and so one may experience shaky hands when attempting very important tasks. Anxiety is associated with physiological changes associated with sympathetic arousal, including increased palmar sweating and increased

heart rate; other changes such as catecholamine release and changes in platelet aggregation time may affect recovery processes.

Thus anxiety in surgical patients should be avoided not only because it is unpleasant for the patient to experience, but also because, by focusing on the threatening elements of the situation, the patient may exaggerate the dangers involved. Anxiety is likely to make it more difficult for the patient to understand information given or to cooperate fully with instructions. In addition, physiological processes associated with anxiety may interfere with recovery.

ANXIETY IN SURGICAL PATIENTS

Patients are anxious before surgery for a number of reasons, as they experience various threats. They are anxious because they have an illness requiring surgery, because they have to undergo the surgical procedure, and because there may be uncertainty about the outcome and the likely speed of recovery. In addition, patients worry about being away from home and how the family is coping, as well as continuing to worry about their usual preoccupations such as money, relationships, etc.

Using standard measures of anxiety which have been developed to deal with the problems of subjective reporting, patients are found to have high levels of anxiety both before and after surgery. For example, Figure 1 shows daily anxiety levels from 4 days before to 14 days after major gynaecological surgery. Compared with normal levels of anxiety as measured 5 weeks after surgery, patients

show high levels both before and after surgery.

Anxiety before surgery has been found to relate to many post-operative outcomes, including:

- distress
- pain
- use of analgesics
- physiological functioning
- return to normal activities
- length of hospital stay.

Therefore methods of reducing anxiety are likely to improve patient outcomes.

METHODS OF PSYCHOLOGICAL PREPARATION

A variety of methods of preparing people for surgery have been developed and typically they are administered on the day before surgery, although some have been used in outpatient visits prior to admission. Some methods have been used with groups of patients, and others incorporate the use of booklets, audio and video tapes.

Methods used include:

- information-giving: procedural and sensation information
- behavioural instruction
- cognitive coping
- relaxation/hypnosis
- emotion-focused or psychotherapeutic discussion
- modelling.

Information-giving — procedural and sensation

Procedural information Patients are informed about the procedures they will undergo, when they will happen, and where they will be. For example, they

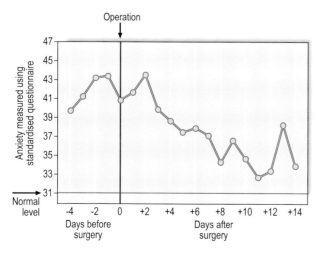

Fig. 1 **Anxiety levels before and after surgery.** (Reproduced with permission from Johnston M 1980 Anxiety in Surgical Patients. Psychological Medicine 10: 145-152)

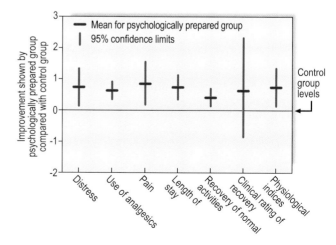

Fig. 2 **Benefits of psychological preparation for surgery.** This is a summary of 40 clinical trials. (Diagram based on data from Johnston and Vogele 1993)

would be told about waking in the recovery room and the possibility of having a drip or catheter.

Sensation information As well as procedural information, patients are informed about the sensations they are likely to experience. For example, they might be told that pre-medication will not necessarily make them feel drowsy or that following major abdominal operations they may experience pain due to wind.

Behavioural instruction

Patients are instructed and may be encouraged to rehearse things they can do post-operatively to reduce pain and facilitate recovery. For example they may be taught how to cough without pulling on the wound incision or how to turn over in bed without causing unnecessary pain.

Cognitive coping

Based on the assumption that patients' thoughts about what is happening may serve either to raise or reduce their anxiety, interventions have been designed to encourage more adaptive cognitions. For example they may be trained to reinterpret events in a more positive manner — e.g. a patient who is thinking that the doctor passing the end of his bed is a sign that his condition is giving rise to concern may, after training, propose that this is a sign that he is making progress. Or they may be trained to use cognitive coping techniques that they have found useful in other situations — e.g. if a patient says that distraction has been useful in previous anxiety-provoking situations she may be advised on how to use such a technique before and after surgery (see pp. 122–123).

Relaxation/hypnosis

A variety of general relaxation procedures and hypnotic techniques have been used which patients can practise in bed before surgery, sometimes using taped instructions.

Case study

For most patients, pre-operative anxiety is unpleasant, but not disabling. The following case describes a man whose anxiety interfered with his ability to have surgery.

Mr Aspell was admitted to a surgical ward, for abdominal surgery on the day after admission. He was anxious about the whole procedure, but particularly in anticipation of undergoing anaesthesia. After receiving his premedication on the morning of surgery, he could not contain his anxiety and took his own discharge. Since there was nothing further the hospital could do, he returned to his GP who was now faced with a patient who required surgery but could not tolerate the procedures.

The GP referred Mr Aspell to a psychologist who used psychological preparation procedures involving relaxation training and cognitive techniques. He was particularly trained to use relaxation as a distraction technique, especially when experiencing worrying thoughts. He was taught to recognise negative thoughts such as 'What if I die during surgery?' or 'What if I am still aware of what is going on even if the doctors think I am unconscious?', and to deal with them by thinking of counteracting thoughts, such as 'I've never heard of that happening to anyone I know — why should it happen to me?' or 'These doctors are experts — I am in safe hands.'.

Mr Aspell was able to return to the surgeon and to proceed with treatment without further interruption.

Emotional focused/psychotherapeutic discussion

Patients are invited to discuss their worries, either on their own with a therapist or in groups. There are no very clearly specified instructions for this type of intervention.

Modelling

This method, which is most commonly used with children, shows the patient a film of a similar-aged patient going through various stages of the surgical procedures. The method communicates a considerable amount of procedural information and may demonstrate use of any of the other methods.

RESULTS OF PSYCHOLOGICAL PREPARATION

The first properly controlled trial (Egbert et al 1964) randomly allocated 97 patients to special preparation or normal care. The specially prepared group had less pain and used fewer analgesics post-operatively and their hospital stay was on average 2.7 days shorter than for patients in the control group.

Since then, there have been approximately 40 controlled trials involving comparison of groups randomly allocated to psychological versus normal care. The results of these studies have been aggregated using special statistical (meta-analytic) techniques. Clear benefits for patients have been demonstrated. Figure 2 shows the mean difference between the psychologically prepared and control groups, expressed in units of standard deviations, and the 95% confidence intervals, for each outcome.

The group receiving psychological preparation shows statistically significant benefits where the mean difference is greater than zero and where the confidence interval does not pass through zero. So there is evidence of benefit on measures of distress, pain, use of analgesics, physiological indices such as heart rate and blood pressure, behavioural indices including resumption of normal activities, and length of hospital stay. Clinical ratings of recovery do not show a reliable difference. One might expect to find improved patient satisfaction, but too few studies have examined this variable to draw conclusions.

 STOP THINK   While the benefits of psychological methods of preparing patients for surgery have been known for at least 20 years, they have not been widely implemented. Why might this be?

The limitations in implementing these techniques may be due to the lack of appropriately trained staff. The development of booklet or taped instructions may facilitate the use of these techniques, but needs to be more fully evaluated.

Psychological preparation for surgery

- Patients are anxious before and after surgery.
- High pre-operative anxiety is predictive of poor post-operative outcomes.
- A variety of methods has been developed for preparing patients for surgery.
- These methods have been shown to improve post-operative outcomes in well-controlled clinical trials.

INSTITUTIONALISATION

The term 'institutionalisation' refers to a form of behaviour which has sometimes been observed in health care settings. It is also seen in places like prisons, homes for elderly people, and even university halls of residence. It means that the occupants become so used to living in an environment in which the institution provides for their every need, that they become incapable of functioning successfully or appropriately outside it. It is sometimes accompanied by depersonalisation, where the individual loses a clear sense of themselves as an individual and develops a social identity that is defined entirely by the institution.

ROLES

During the average day an individual will encounter many social environments and play different roles in each. These different roles not only provide for variety, they also provide for an expression of different aspects of the person's character and self. People may literally feel different in each setting and certainly the behaviour of others will be different depending on the role being played. A computer engineer will behave very differently and be seen by others to be behaving differently when he is with his young son, his golfing partner or a commercial rival from another company. There is considerable role diversity within any one individual. The critical skills which accomplished role players possess are to move comfortably from role to role as circumstances dictate.

The idea of role, therefore, encompasses flexibility and continuity. Roles also carry certain rights, expectations and responsibilities as well as understandings in the minds of others about appropriate behaviour. A useful way of describing this process is to imagine a distinction between self and identity (Fig. 1).

Where the self is broadly congruent with identity, the two aspects of the person are mutually reinforcing. So when the computer engineer goes to work, his colleagues treat him as a computer engineer, not as the window cleaner or typist. When the computer engineer goes into the supermarket to do his shopping, however, he is treated as a customer and is not asked to repair the computerised bar code system on the checkouts. For most people, most of the time, diversity and continuity present few problems in the roles they play, and the texture of their life is determined by the variability in what they do. Problems arise when self and identity in one, or many, or even all social roles become discordant. Problems also arise when the potential to express different aspects of self is limited, when role diversity becomes narrowed and when expectations from others become focused on the fact that the individual is principally an inmate in an institution.

INSTITUTIONS AND INSTITUTIONALISATION

For someone in an institution like a hospital, the situation is very specific. The potential range of roles they can play becomes tightly controlled. They only have one set of companions and to the other people with whom they share their environment, they are mainly a patient. Their identity is that of a patient and other people respond to them as a patient. At the same time not only is the range of potential roles limited, but also the rights and freedoms to control the way those roles are expressed is curtailed (see also pp. 98–99). The forms of behaviour that are observed in people who have spent a long time in institutions seem to stem from the fact that the range of what they can do is limited and rather one-dimensional, and that they are separated from varied contact with others. In these circumstances identity has become very narrow, and gradually the person's sense of self, of who and what they are, will become narrowed too. People's very sense of personhood is eroded in such a narrow and confining environment, yet they have to learn to survive in the very restrictive world of the institution. For the patient, the long-stay institution is an experience in which social skills atrophy by disuse and become focused on a very small fraction of their potential as a human being. Self and identity become focused on the role in the institution and surviving the experience (Fig. 2).

However, institutionalisation is more than simply a narrow range of social contacts. Where institutionalisation becomes well established and habitual it produces a level of dependency of the patient on the institution. Living in an environment in which independence is taken away, self and identity are constrained and where the kinds of choices which most adults take for granted are removed, reinforces dependency and depersonalisation. This removal of choices occurs because the rights which attach to social roles outside of institutions are controlled

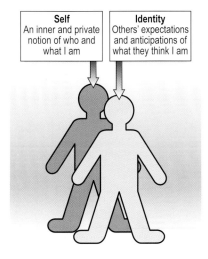

Fig. 1 **Self versus identity.**

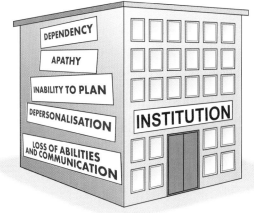

Fig. 2 **Features of institutions and their effects.**

within institutions. For example, in many hospitals, including general hospitals, the time at which lights are put out, the time at which patients may get up, the time when lunch is served and, in some traditional institutions, the clothes people can wear are all clearly defined. While such rules are drawn up so that the institution can function effectively, they take away the power and control that individuals have over their own lives. What is important to understand is that it is the removal of the little things in life that characterises life in institutions as much as the denial of freedom itself. It is often those little things in life which are actually the way in which our individuality is expressed and our sense of personhood defined.

- Are social roles scripted very rigidly or can people interpret the way they play particular roles?
- To what degree is institutionalisation a feature of the patient experience in General Hospitals?

TOTAL INSTITUTIONS

'Total institution' describes an organisation in which inmates are regimented together and spend most of their time in the company of other similar inmates, eating, sleeping, relaxing and working. One of the most influential studies of the ways in which patients survived in such places was conducted in a large American state mental hospital in the 1950s by Erving Goffman (Goffman 1968). A Total Institution for Goffman was one in which personal privacy was virtually non-existent. Goffman argued that the key task facing an individual in a Total Institution

was survival, or what he called 'making-out'. Making-out was about trying to reassert individuality and control over some very limited aspects of personal life. Goffman noticed that little things like hoarding bits of paper, of clinging desperately to possessions like combs or toothbrushes, or simply withdrawing into an inner mental world were common behaviours.

Goffman's conclusion was that many of the behaviours which patients in mental hospitals exhibited were explicable in terms of the structure of the institutions themselves and the way patients tried to survive in them, rather than a consequence of illness. At the time, Goffman's work constituted a startling critique of organizations which, while allegedly providing care and rehabilitation, turned out to be making matters worse. They made matters worse because the withdrawal, the obsessiveness over little things, the pacing up and down, could be and were easily interpreted as signs of psychiatric illness, rather than a consequence of incarceration. But not only did the institutions make matters worse, they seemed to be organised in ways which also encouraged high degrees of dependency among the patients — which meant that the longer they were in hospital, the harder it was to make any kind of transition to normal non-institutionalised life. Similar observations have since been made about prisoners, ex-members of the armed forces and indeed anyone exiting from a Total Institution.

Goffman's work has been very influential, and general and psychiatric hospital care is now organised, in theory at least, around principles of respect for the individual. However, while the most rigid kinds of hospital organisation have mostly disappeared, the processes of institutionalisation and dependency remain important for inpatients and more particularly for people in hostel accommodation, old people's homes and nursing homes, and long-stay psychiatric and geriatric wards.

Notwithstanding attempts to protect people's dignity and the desire to treat the whole person, the dynamics of care are sometimes such that patients find it easier to cope with their institutional experience by adopting a passive, depersonalised and dependent response and going along with the imperatives of the institution. Sometimes they are not in a fit state to do anything else. For example, patients in intensive care units, patients undergoing major surgery, children, and many kinds of long-stay and elderly patients who are not physically well enough to return home may find themselves undergoing the social and psychological pressures towards institutionalisation. While not on the same scale as Goffman's inmates, the life of any hospital patient is about coping with the experience of being a patient as well as the experience of being ill, and the focus and dynamics of the institution define in large measure what has to be coped with.

Case study

Mavis is 61 and has spent the last 40 years in psychiatric care. She cannot remember why she was admitted, and indeed never speaks about life before her admission. None of the other patients know anything about her other than that she has been in hospital a long time. She sits quietly most days in an armchair in the dayroom. She stares out of the window. She is not very particular about her appearance, but she is very concerned about the few possessions she has accumulated. A little while ago a new staff nurse was appointed to the ward and she threw away an old magazine cover that she found under Mavis' mattress. When Mavis discovered that it had gone she caused a terrible commotion. No one could understand why Mavis made such a fuss, it was after all only an old magazine cover. Mavis had had it for 5 years and she particularly liked to look at the picture on the cover. It was of a pub in a village in England somewhere. It reminded her of something nice, although she couldn't recall what it was. The doctors are convinced that Mavis's condition will not deteriorate further and indeed she could probably be discharged. However, she has nowhere to go — no one knows or remembers any living relatives. And Mavis does not want to go. She is entirely dependent on the institution. It is her world. Her identity and her self are intrinsically bound up with the institution. Without the institution she would have no social identity and without the institution she would lose her sense of who and what she is. She cannot really remember what she was.

Institutionalisation

- Large institutions such as psychiatric hospitals have been termed total institutions.
- In total institutions all aspects of life are regimented and controlled in a single setting.
- In total institutions social role opportunities become narrowed.
- The structure of total institutions generates particular forms of social behaviour which are as much a consequence of the institution as of illness.
- Total institutions tend to encourage dependency rather than independence. This frequently makes the transition to the normal world quite difficult.

HEART DISEASE

Coronary heart disease (CHD) describes a number of conditions including angina pectoris (sensation of tightness or chest pain because of brief obstruction or constriction of an artery) and myocardial infarction (MI, death of heart muscle — myocardium — as a result of blockage of the arteries which prevents oxygen reaching the myocardium).

The main medical interventions are:

- pharmacological (medications to reduce blood pressure, prevent clotting, etc.)
- re-vascularisation: percutaneous transluminal coronary angioplasty (PTCA); coronary artery bypass grafts (CABG)
- coronary care
- cardiac rehabilitation
- risk factor reduction (primary and secondary).

PREVENTION

CHD is the most common cause of premature mortality and a frequent cause of morbidity in Western industrialised societies. Major well-established risk factors are smoking, hypertension and high serum cholesterol. Additional lifestyle risk factors include lack of exercise, obesity, hostility and stress. The Type A behaviour pattern (hard-driving, time urgent, hostile) was identified in the 1960s as the typical coronary-prone individual but recent research has indicated that high hostility alone is the factor most associated with greater risk of CHD. The best evidence that stress causes heart disease comes from animal rather than human studies (Fig. 1). In surveys of patients and healthy populations, 'stress' is the most commonly reported cause of MI (see pp. 50–51).

CHD is related to socioeconomic disadvantage (see pp. 44–45). This may in part be due to patterns of smoking, diet and work experience as working class men smoke more, have a poorer diet and are more likely to have jobs where they have little control and high demands compared with middle class men. While some have argued that socioeconomic disadvantage is an important risk factor and that reductions in CHD require greater socioeconomic equality, others have suggested that individual risk may be reduced by changes in behaviour and lifestyle.

Thus changes in behaviour and lifestyle offer opportunities for prevention (both primary and secondary) and countries such as the USA where there have been major changes in lifestyle have shown significant reductions in CHD. Nevertheless, even though we can identify those people most at risk of CHD, because it is so common, most of the people who actually suffer from CHD are those at average or low risk. This is known as the prevention paradox.

RESPONSE TO SYMPTOMS

Individuals may misinterpret symptoms. A large number of patients referred to cardiology departments present with non-cardiac chest pain probably due to anxiety about physical symptoms. Equally, many patients experiencing an MI do not recognise the symptoms as those of an MI and therefore delay in seeking help (see pp. 84–85). Average delay between first symptoms and arrival at hospital is 3–4 hours in the UK (Birkhead 1992). Given the importance of early thrombolysis, such delays may critically determine the patients' treatment and survival (see Case study). A rapid response ensures more effective treatment and therefore better outcomes.

Case study
Delay to treatment for symptoms of a myocardial infarction

On the way home from their wedding anniversary meal, Mrs MacDonald feels pressure in her chest. She thinks it unlikely to be anything more serious than indigestion at her age (51). She does not like to mention it as it would spoil the evening. Going upstairs to bed the pain intensifies and she comes out in a cold sweat, so she lies down to see if she feels better. Her husband worries that it is a heart attack but Mrs MacDonald says 'I don't think so — women don't have heart attacks. It's more likely to be the menopause!' After some hours of increasing symptoms, she calls her GP. By the time the ambulance takes her to hospital, she is too late for the full benefit of thrombolytic drugs.

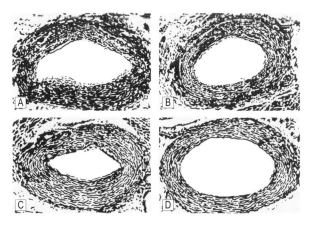

Fig. 1 **Effects of social stressors on coronary artery in cynomolgus monkeys.** The diagrams show cross-sections of coronary artery of monkeys subjected to different living conditions. Greatest occlusion of the coronary artery was found in (c), dominant monkeys subjected to the stress of having the group they lived with broken up regularly. Less occlusion was found in those living in stable groups (a and b) or in subordinate monkeys in unstable social groupings (d). (Drawing based on photograph in Manuck et al 1983)

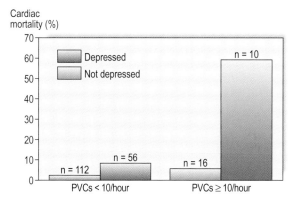

Fig. 2 **Outcome for depressed and non-depressed MI patients.** Depressed patients were more likely to die than those who were not depressed. This was true for both those with a low rate of preventricular contractions (PVCs) and those with a high rate. (Source: Frasure-Smith et al 1995)

RESPONSE TO MI

MI (heart attack) is a sudden life-threatening event and many patients experience high levels of anxiety and depression. Significant family members may be even more distressed than the patient in the early period, while the patient is in hospital. These high levels of distress are unrelated to the severity of the MI and may persist for months or years after the MI.

In addition to its immediate debilitating effects, depression is associated with higher mortality rates. In a study of 222 MI patients, depressed patients were over 3 times as likely as non-depressed patients to die within 18 months. These results still held when other factors such as severity of MI were controlled for (Fig. 2, Frasure-Smith et al 1995).

Early cardiac rehabilitation programmes can reduce the emotional distress of patients and their families. Cardiac rehabilitation programmes have been shown to:

- reduce mortality
- improve cardiovascular fitness
- reduce psychological distress
- increase rate of return to paid employment
- reduce health service costs.

Benefits from such programmes have persisted for years. Programmes may involve education, exercise, dietary and vocational counselling, and psychological components such as stress management. The addition of psychological components to exercise and education-based programmes results in greater patient benefit.

In a randomised controlled study, 862 cardiac patients were allocated to an educational programme or to this programme plus an additional psychological programme (see Case study).

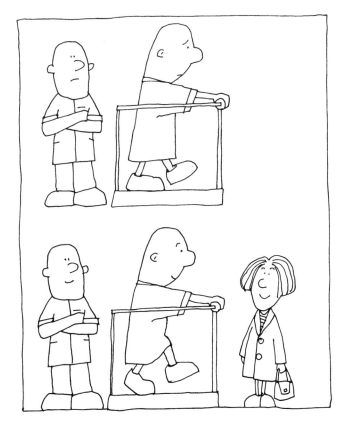

Fig. 3 **Following MI, patients whose rehabilitation exercises were observed by their spouses did better than those only seen by the rehabilitation team.**

Case study
Psychological cardiac rehabilitation programme

Patients in the Recurrent Coronary Prevention Project (Friedman et al 1986) met weekly in small groups and were trained to make the following changes.

- **Cognitive**, e.g. 'I must always arrive first at work' may be reconstrued as 'As long as I arrive by 9 a.m., I can complete a good day's work'
- **Behavioural**, e.g. learning to walk at a more relaxed steady pace
- **Emotional**, e.g. learning to relax in response to early signs of anxiety or anger.

After 4.5 years, the latter group had experienced significantly fewer non-fatal cardiac events and fewer deaths — 12.9% versus 21.2% (Friedman et al 1986).

Rehabilitation may be enhanced by involving spouses or lay carers in routine medical procedures. For example, allowing spouses to observe routine treadmill testing of cardiovascular fitness (Fig. 3) increases both patient and spouse confidence in the patient's ability to engage in energetic activities, with resulting greater activity levels at home in the time following the test.

RESPONSE TO STRESSFUL MEDICAL PROCEDURES

Medical procedures may be stressful due to the discomfort or pain experienced as well as the uncertainty about the outcomes. Psychological preparation can reduce the stressfulness of the procedures and improve the outcomes (see pp. 100–101); for example, compared with patients receiving normal care before CABG, patients receiving cognitive and behavioural preparation were less distressed and recovered more quickly. In addition, they were less likely to suffer from acute post-operative hypertension, a life-threatening condition (Anderson 1987).

 STOP THINK Psychological factors are involved in many aspects of coronary heart disease. How might members of a cardiology department wish a psychologist to contribute to their work?

Heart disease

- CHD may be prevented by changes in behaviour and lifestyles.
- Socioeconomic disadvantage is associated with a high incidence of CHD.
- Patients may fail to recognise the symptoms of MI, with resulting delays in medical treatment.
- Anxiety and depression are common responses to MI of both patients and their spouses.
- Depression following MI is an independent predictor of mortality.
- Cardiac rehabilitation, including psychological components, enhances patient outcomes and survival.
- Psychological preparation for medical procedures reduces their stressfulness and improves post-operative recovery.

SOCIAL ASPECTS OF HIV / AIDS

HIV (Human Immunodeficiency Virus) appeared at a time when it was widely believed that science had brought infectious diseases under control, and it seemed that all of a sudden a new incurable disease presented itself. It is only possible to treat some of the secondary effects of HIV and AIDS (Acquired Immune Deficiency Syndrome — the disease stage of most infected people) and since the infection is currently not curable the main remedy lies in prevention. Since the virus can be transmitted in different ways (Table 1), prevention requires targeting different types of behaviour.

Although HIV is widespread (over 140 000 AIDS cases were reported in Europe by March 1995) it is clear that the infection is not equally spread amongst members of society or between societies. Even within the UK (Fig. 1) we see great differences in the proportion of people infected through sexual intercourse between men and intravenous drug use (IDU). The figure for women as a percentage of the total number of people diagnosed with AIDS differs considerably between Scotland and England and Wales (Fig. 1). The proportion of women among the people diagnosed with AIDS in Scotland (19.9%) is nearly twice that in England and Wales (12.6%). Thus certain groups of people have a far higher infection rate than others.

The disease has distinct social aspects. At a social level it involves several taboos, such as sex, drugs and death and dying, and consequently it is heavily stigmatised. Secondly, at a personal level, the acceptance of being diagnosed as HIV positive can be very difficult. People can feel isolated, shocked, frightened, panicked, guilty, profess denial and become depressed, but some also display a sense of coming to terms with themselves, and even acceptance. Such emotions are understandable, as awareness of one's own mortality will be increased.

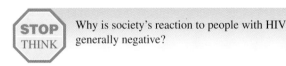

Why is society's reaction to people with HIV generally negative?

DOUBLE STIGMA

HIV has what is called a 'double stigma' attached. Stigma refers to the identification and recognition of a bad or negative characteristic in a person or group of persons and treating them with less respect or worth than they deserve due to this characteristic (see pp. 120–121). The double stigma refers to 'terminal illness' and 'sexually-transmitted diseases'. The former stigma is also applicable to cancer and other terminal diseases. The latter refers to stigma attached to 'deviant', 'unnatural', or socially undesirable activities, such as men having sex with men, injecting drug use, or prostitution. Alonzo and Reynolds (1995) explain that stigma is 'identification of some sort of moral contamination that causes others to reject the person bearing it'. Thus people living with HIV are regarded as 'dangerous, dirty, foolish and worthless' in comparison to descriptions of cancer or stroke patients.

Experiencing stigma (stigmatisation) may lead to low self esteem in the infected person, reduced willingness to seek medical and social help, and increased difficulty in sharing worries with friends, relatives and neighbours. At a societal level widespread fear of HIV/AIDS still exists despite the fact

Table 1 **Routes of transmission of HIV**

- Unprotected penetrative sex (vaginal, oral or anal)
- Unsterilised needle/syringe which has been used by someone infected with HIV
- Mother to child during pregnancy, labour and breast-feeding
- Infected blood or tissue transfer
- Receiving semen from an infected man for artificial insemination

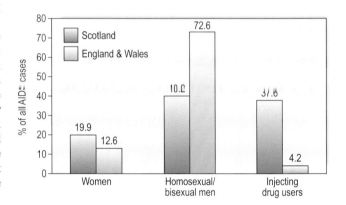

Fig. 1 **Percentage women, homo/bisexual men and injecting drug users among cumulative number of AIDS cases in Scotland and England and Wales to 30 June 1997 (SCIEH 1997).**

that it has been scientifically demonstrated that AIDS is not communicable by day-to-day social contact. This fear and stigmatisation can easily be translated into discrimination and victimisation of people with HIV. HIV/AIDS is branded a plague, which implies that people living with HIV are threatening and dangerous rather than threatened, because they carry the potential to contaminate the healthy through transmission of a contagious disease. This led to some dentists and doctors refusing treatment even when safe procedures were available.

Society also often makes a distinction between 'innocent' and 'guilty' victims. It is believed that the people with HIV bring it on themselves through their own doing, and they are blamed for their disease, and as a result are branded as 'guilty' victims. In contrast, 'innocent' victims are infected through mistakes by the medical profession or infected blood. Babies of HIV infected mothers are included as innocent, while their mothers may be seen as guilty.

The use of the phrase 'risk group' reinforces the idea that HIV can only happen to certain people. The idea of stressing risk behaviour is far more meaningful both in terms of reducing the stigma attached to being HIV positive and in terms of preventing the spread of the infection. It is not what people are that gives them a higher risk, but what people do.

HIV AND THE MEDIA

The media are a major source of information for people, as well as influential in forming or at least confirming people's opinions. Many people in industrialised countries will not personally know anyone who is infected with HIV; consequently the perception of the disease is likely to be mediated or even formed by mass media. This includes 'facts' in, for example, newspapers and television news programmes, and 'fiction' in soap operas and cinema films.

In an interview with The Independent newspaper (3 November 1993, p. 23) Suzanna Dawson, who in a soap opera played the wife of a character who had AIDS, said:

'... I've had some terrible experiences of the kind of prejudice HIV-positive people face ... I've been slapped and spat at in the street, booed off the field in a charity match ... it makes you feel so alone, so scared ... I've picked up the phone at 2 a.m. to hear some guy screaming: "You're a dirty bitch, spreading disease throughout the world."'

Ms Dawson suffered this level of abuse even though she was merely the actress playing that role.

One of the most irresponsible headlines in the British tabloid press was found in The Sun. Lord Kilbracken was quoted as saying that the chances of receiving AIDS from heterosexual sex were 'statistically invisible'. The headline in The Sun read:

'Straight Sex Cannot Give You AIDS — Official!'
(Snodden 1992).

The Daily Telegraph of 20 May 1983 had as its headline:

'Alarm as Lethal Plague spreads to Non-Homosexuals'
(Wellings 1988: 87).

PSYCHOLOGICAL ISSUES

One key set of psychological issues centres around the question: 'Who do you tell?' Being diagnosed HIV positive may involve having to adapt one's behaviour and outlook on life. Telling a partner or family could mean having to admit to injecting drugs, or having sex with another man, or being sexually unfaithful. Telling employers might mean losing a job, not necessarily because the employer wants to get rid of you, but because your colleagues do not want to work with you any longer. Bringing up the issue of using safer sex methods can also be problematic. It is a difficult enough issue for most, especially at the time of first sexual intercourse. However, people with HIV might find suggesting the use of condoms with prospective sexual partners difficult, because of the fear of being rejected, emotionally or physically (see pp. 50–51).

Case study

Andrew (age 20) is a third-year medical student. He took an HIV test together with his new partner when they started a sexual relationship. He felt it was a waste of time, a fashion, and really went along to please his partner. Although he was counselled at the time, he was very shocked to be told that he tested HIV positive. His thoughts jumped back and forth between his new partner and what would happen to the relationship, his study and his career. He wondered: 'Who gave me the virus?' and 'Which private habits do I have to disclose, and to whom? Will I die young and horribly?'

STOP THINK   What other issues might this medical student face after his recent diagnosis?

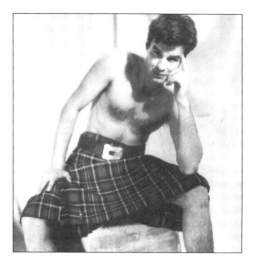
Fig. 2 **One HIV health promotion in Scotland.** The slogan read, 'What should a real Scotsman wear under his kilt?' (Courtesy of Scottish AIDS Monitor and Lothian Health)

HEALTH PROMOTION AND HIV

HIV health promotion activities have often focused on the sexual transmission of the virus. Since (a) people with HIV are generally not recognisable until the end stages of the disease, and (b) the virus has a long incubation time, the health promotion message had to be aimed at all men and women who are sexually active, not just the high-risk groups.

Figure 2 shows one of the posters/postcards with a safer sex message targeting the general population. The message is clearly aimed at men, unlike previous health promotion activities for condoms, when condoms were 'only' contraceptives, and often seen as a woman's responsibility (see pp. 54–55).

HIV/AIDS IN DEVELOPING COUNTRIES

The majority of people with HIV live in the Third World. Many of these developing countries have poor economies, and consequently underfunded public health systems. In Africa HIV is transmitted mainly by heterosexual contact; in Europe and the USA homosexual contact is still the leading factor, although heterosexual transmission is increasing. Many areas of Africa do not have the means to screen blood consistently, which means that HIV is still being transmitted through blood transfusions, and very few medicines or social services are available for people with AIDS. It is worth remembering that for some African nations hit hardest by AIDS, the entire national health budget is equal only to that of one large hospital in the USA.

Social aspects of HIV/AIDS

- Prevention is the main, the only approach to stop the spread of HIV/AIDS.
- People living with HIV/AIDS often suffer from a double stigma.
- Mass media have played an important role in influencing public perception of the disease.
- We should move away from thinking in terms of risk groups to risk behaviour. It is not important who you are, but what you do.
- The majority of people with HIV live in the developing world, where much less funding is available for prevention and care.

CANCER

Despite differences in the progress of different cancers and the increasing effectiveness of medical treatments, cancer continues to be the most widely feared group of diseases. It creates greater anxiety than coronary heart disease, which has approximately double the fatality rate. Psychological and social factors are involved in the aetiology and response to the disease and its treatment.

AETIOLOGY

In a review of the preventable causes of cancer, behavioural factors were implicated in the majority of cancers (Doll and Peto 1981). These behavioural factors include:

- smoking (involved in 30% of cancers)
- diet (35%)
- reproductive and sexual behaviour (7%)
- alcohol use (3%).

Other psychological factors, such as stress, may also be important. Animal studies have shown that tumour growth is faster and resulting death is earlier in mice subjected to uncontrollable stress (electric shocks), compared with animals receiving a similar amount of controllable shock. It has been proposed that Type C personality (characterised by lack of emotional expressiveness and resigned acceptance of negative events) increases the risk of cancer, but there is little scientific support for this proposal. There is some evidence that depressed individuals are more cancer-prone.

Primary prevention has focused on the behavioural and lifestyle factors, while secondary prevention has also directed attention to emotional factors.

COMMUNICATION ABOUT CANCER

The topic of cancer is associated with many social and clinical taboos. In popular language and in medical settings euphemisms such as 'growth', 'tumour', 'lump', 'shadow' are used to avoid the word 'cancer'. These communications may arise from the fears and misconceptions surrounding cancer, but they also give rise to such fears. Thus patients with benign disease sometimes suspect that they have malignant disease but that their doctor is withholding the information.

Doctors may refrain from using the word 'cancer' because they believe patients prefer not to be given a potentially terminal diagnosis. However, research studies show that members of the general public were more likely to say that they would wish to be informed of a terminal diagnosis than doctors estimated they would be. Further, these individuals were more likely to believe that they would *personally* wish to be told than that other people should be told. Nevertheless, they may not take these opportunities when offered, for example in medical screening. Screening for the detection of precancerous cells or for the early diagnosis of treatable cancers has often resulted in poor uptake rates (see pp. 66–67).

Reticence about communicating about cancer may also be associated with unduly pessimistic views of the impact of the disease. Doctors' rating of the quality of life of cancer patients was significantly worse than the patients' own rating. Communications about cancer are fraught with problems due to these negative attitudes of patients, their families, health professionals (including doctors and nurses), other hospital personnel and the wider lay community (see pp. 92–95).

RESPONSE TO DIAGNOSIS

Even when the term 'cancer' is used in giving the diagnosis, patients may subsequently report that they have never received such a diagnosis or they may simply fail to recall information given in stressful and emotionally charged consultations.

In order to ensure that patients can recall the full description of their condition and the potentially reassuring communication about treatment and prognosis, some clinicians have provided patients with an audio-taped recording of the diagnostic consultation. Initial results suggest that these tapes may help patients to communicate information about their condition and its treatment to their family, and patients have responded favourably to receiving the tapes.

Patients have varied ways of coping with a cancer diagnosis. Kubler Ross has proposed a sequence of staging of the response to a poor prognosis ranging from shock and denial through anger, depression and finally acceptance. While there is considerable doubt about the actual sequence of stages, this range of response is commonly observed in patients with cancer. Researchers have investigated whether some coping methods may result in better adjustment or prognosis. In general, coping strategies which focus on emotional aspects of the response are associated with poorer emotional adjustment. By contrast, patients whose strategies focus on thinking about the issue in a different way, e.g. by acceptance of the condition, or on seeking solutions to problems, show better subsequent adjustment. Coping strategies may also influence prognosis: patients showing 'denial', 'fighting spirit' or 'stoic acceptance' were found to survive for longer than patients whose coping responses were of 'helplessness/hopelessness' (Greer et al 1979 — see Fig. 1).

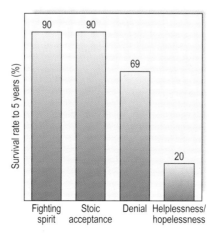

Fig. 1 **Initial psychological responses to breast cancer by 5-year outcome** (Adapted with permission from Greer et al 1979.)

Case study
Psychosocial treatment and survival in cancer

Spiegel et al (1989) randomly allocated 86 patients with metastatic or advanced breast cancer to either a control group which received normal care (N = 36) or an experimental group (N = 50) who additionally participated in a weekly small group led by professional staff and run over 1 year (see Fig. 2). The experimental group showed the following benefits:

- decreased emotional distress
- decreased pain
- increased survival time (mean survival time for experimental group = 36.6 months, for control group = 18.9 months).

The divergence in survival rates began 8 months after the intervention ended.

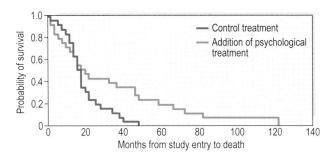

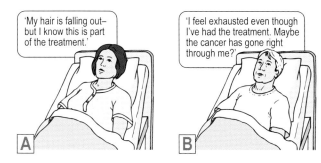

Fig. 2 **Patients with metastatic breast cancer receiving psychological treatment showed longer survival.** (Reproduced with permission from Spiegel et al 1989.)

Fig. 3 **Which patient is likely to be more depressed — A or B?**

PSYCHOLOGICAL INTERVENTIONS

Various patient support groups and psychological interventions have been designed. Professional-led groups, provided in clinical settings, have aimed to

- provide emotional support
- allow expression of emotion
- enhance self-esteem by being able to support others
- increase the range of coping strategies and
- enable patients to learn from successful coping attempts by others.

There are now a number of controlled clinical trials which show that these groups improve the emotional adjustment, reduce pain and increase survival.

RESPONSE TO TREATMENT

Where two medical treatments are thought to have a similar prognosis, patients may be offered a choice of treatment. While doctors originally expected patients to prefer the less mutilating cancer surgery, e.g. lumpectomy rather than mastectomy, this has not been borne out in studies. In patients with advanced prostate cancer, orchidectomy (surgical removal of testicle) or bi-monthly hormonal injection (synthetic luteinising hormone) with minimum side-effects gave similar medical results. When given the choice of treatment, a large proportion, 23 out of 50 men, opted for the mutilating surgery rather than the minimally invasive injections (see pp. 98–99).

Just as patients' choice of treatment may be unexpected, their response during treatment may also be somewhat surprising. In a study of outpatients receiving chemotherapy, levels of distress were found to be associated with some side-effects of treatment but not others. Distress was associated with tiredness and lack of energy rather than with hair loss or nausea. The authors argue that patients had been informed that the treatment would result in hair loss and nausea, and were therefore less concerned by those side-effects. By contrast, they had not been told to expect general tiredness and therefore attributed this symptom to advances in the disease rather than to the chemotherapy (Nerenz et al 1982 — see Fig. 3).

One side-effect of chemotherapy has been studied extensively. Many patients experience anticipatory nausea and vomiting as the course of treatment progresses. For the initial treatments, nausea is experienced during and after the treatment. With later treatments, the nausea can occur before treatment, on arrival at the hospital or even on the journey to hospital. This effect has been explained in terms of classical conditioning (see p. 20) — the patient learns to associate the visit to hospital with the administration of chemotherapy and therefore responds as if to chemotherapy, with nausea and vomiting. Considerable success has been achieved in training patients in relaxation techniques, to practice in anticipation of and during chemotherapy, thus obviating the need for antiemetic drugs.

 STOP THINK

To what extent is fear of cancer, in patients and in the general public, increased by the following:

- taboos on using the word 'cancer'
- poor communications with cancer patients
- mass media images of cancer.

Case study
Providing test results in an oncology clinic

Miss Browne returns to the oncologist for test results following biopsy for a breast lump.

Doctor *The tests on your breast lump are negative...*
Miss Browne *So there's nothing you can do...*
Doctor *Oh yes. Don't worry, we don't leave things like this. We'll be proceeding with local excision of the necessary tissue. It's all quite routine, and under general anaesthetic.*
Miss Browne *That means I'll have to have the operation after all. What's the point?*
Doctor *That's how these lumps are always managed. Everything will be fine. Try not to get upset. We'll fix a date for doing this as soon as possible. What about Wednesday next, coming in on Tuesday evening. OK?*

What did the doctor understand by the word 'negative'?
What did Miss Browne understand?
What are Miss Browne's thoughts as she comes into hospital for surgery?

Cancer

- Cancer is the most widely feared of all diseases.
- Behavioural factors are important in the aetiology of cancer and therefore offer opportunities for prevention.
- Communication about cancer may be limited by social taboos, concern to avoid upsetting patients, and undue pessimism about the impact of the disease.
- Patients' coping strategies can affect subsequent adjustment and survival.
- Psychological interventions can reduce emotional distress and may prolong survival.
- Patients' choices of, and response to, treatment may be unexpected from a medical point of view, but may be psychologically meaningful.

INFLAMMATORY BOWEL DISEASE

Inflammatory bowel disease (IBD) illustrates how social and psychological processes impact on the response to and the experience of illness, and some of the issues which these processes generate for medical care. Ulcerative colitis (one type of IBD) will be used to demonstrate some of these features.

CLINICAL FEATURES

Ulcerative colitis is a disease of the lining layer of the large gut. It occurs mainly in late childhood or early adulthood. Its principal symptoms are chronic unpredictable diarrhoea accompanied by heavy anal bleeding, weight and appetite loss and abdominal pain. Its causes are unknown at present, but an autoimmune action is suspected. There is no medical cure and treatment with steroids, although initially useful, becomes less effective with time. Salazopyrin/sulphasalazine is used as an anti-inflammatory agent.

The complications of colitis can be severe. There may be perforation of the bowel, and the effects on the overall health of the patient can be very marked. Where the disease is present for more than 10 years there is a very greatly enhanced risk of the development of bowel cancer. At present the best treatment option available in the face of unremitting symptoms and/or the development of cancer is the surgical removal of the bowel. This involves creating either an internal pouch to collect the waste matter of digestion with normal anal evacuation, or simply redirecting the faeces through the abdominal wall via a stoma. The operations are major and have a profound effect on one of the body's major systems.

The importance of social and psychological issues is best demonstrated by considering the natural history of the illness from the patient's point of view.

ONSET

When the first symptoms — usually diarrhoea — appear, the most typical response by the sufferer is to minimise them. Diarrhoea is quite common, so the sufferer often makes the not unreasonable assumption that the symptoms will remit of their own accord. This may continue until such time as blood appears in the motion. This is usually taken as a critical and frightening symptom by the patient. Whereas diarrhoea is common, anal bleeding is not. Contact with the medical profession is frequently made some time after the appearance of blood.

> *'I was working. I had two children ... I began to feel, y'know, unwell. Went to my GP. Didn't examine me at all, and told me I was suffering from piles, haemorrhoids, and gave me some medication. The piles wouldn't go away, and I was back there. And by this time it was terribly painful. And I started to get really worried because I was losing blood. So I made another appointment with another doctor in the practice, and she took me into the examination room, examined me straight away, and within a week I was up at St George's Hospital. And I remember it, y'know I have an awful thing about eye contact. She was in here with the nurse and she examined me, and of course she saw there was something wrong, and she looked at the nurse, and she looked away again.'*

> 38-year-old teacher (Kelly 1992)

The important social-psychological concept involved here is help seeking (see pp. 84–85). Diarrhoea comes well within the range of the normal experience of most people, who will wait and see whether it passes in a day or two ('temporising behaviour'), but for most people the appearance of blood will trigger the person to consult the doctor. From a medical point of view a patient consulting for the first time with rectal bleeding would also be seen as having a significant symptom requiring investigation, but it would possibly not engender the same degree of anxiety as experienced by the patient, and as far as colitis is concerned bleeding does not necessarily indicate an exacerbation of the illness. Thus the patient's estimation of the seriousness of the symptom may not necessarily correspond to the doctor's. However, in order to manage the patient's symptoms and anxieties successfully the doctor must be aware not only of the physical symptoms but also how they are being interpreted by the patient. The fact that the patient believes a symptom to be grave is what is important in understanding why the patient has consulted, and consequently has implications for present and future management.

DIAGNOSIS AND TREATMENT

Confirming the diagnosis will involve inspecting the patient's colon with a colonoscope — a fibreoptic instrument inserted via the back passage. Alternatively, a barium enema will provide radiologic confirmation. From the patient's perspective both procedures are undignified, uncomfortable, frequently painful, and often highly stressful, as this patent described:

> *'So I got the appointment for the X-ray Department, went in, without a care in the world. I came out absolutely devastated ... it was terrifying. I just didn't know what to expect, y'know, previously I'd had chest X-rays, things like that; and this barium enema, really I hadn't a clue what it was, what was going to happen. And you go into this place, which had this revolving table and everything and this room, and they pump all this stuff into you. It was ghastly'.*

> 33-year-old female school teacher (Kelly 1992)

The patient is taken into the darkened X-ray room. Barium is emptied into the bowel directly via the back passage. This causes pain. Then a series of X-ray photographs are taken while the radiographers retreat behind leaded screens. Most X-ray departments have little or no time to prepare people for these procedures and the fear and anxiety which may be generated are considerable because the patient is uncertain as to what is happening. The stressfulness of these kinds of experience has been shown to be significantly reduced if patients have been well prepared in advance (see pp. 98–101). Furthermore, recognising the indignity of the procedures can also be reassuring for the patient.

Having made the diagnosis, the physician faces a dilemma. If the disease can be brought under control, all well and good. However, what the physician also has to convey is that this may only be a temporary respite and that the patient may face a long period of chronic illness of varying severity. This raises some very important ethical and legal issues about how much information a patient needs to know. If doctors do provide a full account of the potential seriousness of the illness, the patient can be terrified and lose hope. If the doctor keeps the information from the patient and the illness takes a grave turn, and surgery has to be recommended, the patient may feel angry and may feel they have legal grounds on which to sue their doctor.

'And really, I don't think my family, I think they thought like me, it wasn't a serious thing. Cos nobody had ever said to me, 'It's like this and it'll get worse and you'll maybe have to get surgery'. Nobody ever mentioned the word ileostomy or anything: well, I suppose they didn't want to scare me.'

33-year-old manual worker (Kelly 1992)

In a disease like colitis, the patient's sense of self has to change towards being a person who has an illness. This process can be emotionally painful because we invest heavily in psychological terms in our sense of self.

It is usually the case that the patient enters treatment for this disease in the expectation of a cure. Even if the physician has not explained all the likely complications and difficulties, eventually the patient will come to realise that they are not going to recover fully. This is further complicated by the fact that if the patient is trying to live as normal a life as possible, they face a tension between the demands of fulfilling usual social responsibilities and accepting the limitations imposed upon them by the illness.

Although this is not easy, people do manage to cope with their illness in spite of the difficulties it presents. Doctors can help here, by encouraging the patient to live as normal a life as they can, but also by helping them to recognise the limitations the illness can produce.

STOP THINK — To what extent might there be a conflict between the medical and psychological management of colitis? Is the refusal of some patients with colitis to have surgery adaptive or maladaptive?

LIVING WITH THE ILLNESS

Many aspects of life are likely to be affected by the illness. The chronic unpredictable diarrhoea means that things like travel, shopping, walking, eating, socializing are interrupted as

the sufferer has to go off and find a toilet. The nature of the symptoms are such that the patient usually has very little warning (perhaps less than 30 seconds) of the need to evacuate. Sufferers become highly skilled in breaking off from social interaction, arranging journeys and trips so that toilets are always with easy reach, and carrying a change of clothes for the occasions when they self-soil.

'I didn't enjoy shopping or anything. I was always wanting to be near a toilet; I, well, always felt nauseated with it. I didn't have the energy to go shopping like everybody else ... we couldn't plan anything ...'

46-year-old housewife

It is sometimes remarked that patients suffering from colitis exhibit odd behaviour: obsessive attention to detail, concerns about personal cleanliness. However, the general consensus is that this behaviour is an adaptive product of the struggle with the illness, rather than a cause of it, which allows them to survive and function in the world, in spite of their illness.

SURGERY

For some patients with colitis, the prospect of surgery has to be confronted. There are two important behavioural issues. First, the patient has to deal with the prospect of major body-altering surgery which will leave them with a stoma. Second, the patient now faces a new psychological threat. While the medical decision may be relatively straightforward, it is not automatically viewed in that way by the patient. Some will refuse surgery believing that the threats arising from the illness are preferable to the threats arising from the surgery. Helping the patient adapt to surgery is therefore a key problem in this procedure. Preparations for surgery should not involve trying to make the patient 'accept' their illness or the fact that they need an appliance. Helping the patient prepare for surgery should be about allowing them to acknowledge the psychological pain and distress and the associated feelings of loss that this surgery engenders. It should aim to help them work through their feelings of hurt. This is a difficult and traumatic procedure from the patient's perspective and one which requires considerable social and psychological skills on the part of the people caring for that patient (see pp. 100–101).

Case study

Gillian is 52. She was first diagnosed as having colitis when she was 46. She is married with two teenage children. Her doctor has just told her she needs to have a total colectomy and ileostomy. She is completely distraught at the prospect. She thinks of herself, and always has, as an attractive woman. She is horrified at the prospect of wearing a bag. Yet, she is very ill. She has not had a proper night's sleep for nearly 3 years. She has to get up in the night three or four times to go to the toilet. During the day it is even worse. She usually cannot go for longer than an hour before she has to open her bowels. Her work as a secretary is becoming increasingly difficult. Her boss is very understanding but the fact that she constantly has to leave the office has made things very awkward. Her appetite is poor, and when she does eat she sticks to a diet of minced breast of chicken and white bread. She and her husband used to go out a lot, but they stay at home all the time now. Her doctor has told her that the operation will make her better. Gillian, however, is resolute in her refusal to have the operation.

Inflammatory bowel disease

- The process of making decisions about seeking help are governed by social and psychological factors as well as the degree of medical seriousness of the condition.
- Symptoms which are regarded as critical by the patient will not necessarily be the same ones as those identified as medically serious.
- In a disease like colitis social and psychological symptoms may be evident, but they are usually a consequence rather than a cause of the illness.
- The treatments for colitis, as with many illnesses, are frequently viewed as more psychologically threatening by the patient than the illness itself. These threats condition patient behaviour as much as the threats from the disease and its symptoms.
- The surgery performed to cure colitis is often associated with very powerful feelings of distress and loss.

ANXIETY

Anxiety is part and parcel of daily life. It is adaptive: it provides the motivation to study for exams and it prompts the rush of adrenaline that gives a certain sparkle to a public performance, whether this is sport or presenting a seminar paper. Most of us have experienced episodes of unpleasant anxiety. Usually these are time-limited and resolve themselves. But even when they do not warrant treatment, their physiological effects can still interfere with health by making other conditions worse (e.g. asthma or eczema), or by confusing the clinical picture (e.g. in diagnosis and management of heart disease).

WHAT IS ANXIETY?

Anxiety refers to an emotional state, which can usefully be divided into three components:

- **Thoughts**. Thoughts often act as the trigger for creating the state of anxiety, e.g. 'What if my foot slips off this ledge and I fall down the rockface?', 'What if I can't answer key questions at the interview?' or 'What if we split up and I'm left on my own?'
- **Physical symptoms**. These are numerous. Most commonly they include an increased heart rate, increased blood pressure, feelings of tension in the muscles, sweating, nausea or indigestion, trembling, blushing, tightness or dryness in the throat, dizziness.
- **Behaviour**. Behaviour is what you do in order to reduce anxiety, for example refusing to go on up the rockface, or avoiding interviews, or doing deep breathing in order to ease the physical symptoms of anxiety in an interview. Behaviour which reduces anxiety without spoiling your health or welfare is adaptive, but many of the ways in which we respond to anxiety are often maladaptive, e.g. avoiding social occasions, or using alcohol for relief.

HOW IS ANXIETY MAINTAINED?

The three components listed above can interact to maintain anxiety and can also make it worse. The case study illustrates how anxiety can escalate.

Whatever the initial cause of Andrew's symptoms (see Case study), whether it was residual symptoms of 'flu, or the overheated shop combined with his thick clothing, he had interpreted the sensations as potentially threatening (the risk that he would faint in the shop and how embarrassing this would be). These anxious thoughts set off further symptoms (through the release of adrenaline and noradrenaline) which were interpreted as increasingly threatening. The only way of reducing them was to escape, as before. The pattern has thus been learned: 'If I enter the shop, I will experience very unpleasant symptoms causing loss of control and potential disaster. The only way to stop it is to avoid going into busy shops.'

TYPES OF ANXIETY

Phobia

A phobia is a fear that is out of proportion to the potential threat. Being afraid of a pit bull terrier dog would not be classed as a phobia, but being afraid of a moth would. There is a significant risk to your safety in the first, but not the second. Many people assume that these simple phobias are the result of a traumatic event in childhood which set up a conditioned response (see pp. 20–21) but this can be established in only a minority of cases. Furthermore, with phobias, the fear is usually that of panic, or loss of control, rather than any harm that the animal or object could cause (McNally and Steketee 1985). Simple phobias often appear in early childhood.

There are two 'phobias' which are different. One is the phobia for blood or injury. Research suggests that there may be a genetic component, since Marks (1986) found that 68% of sufferers had first-degree relatives with the same condition. It is also characterised by a *decrease* in heart rate, often causing fainting, whereas other phobias are associated with an increased heart rate. Agoraphobia is also different since it is a more generalised fear of circumstances, usually being in a crowded place with no easy means of escape. The onset tends to occur in the late teens or early twenties. Physiologically it is also more like generalised anxiety (see below) with more persistent and diffuse arousal. There are often other symptoms, such as depression.

Social anxiety

Social anxiety is common and refers to the anxiety felt in the presence of other people. A degree of social anxiety might be experienced on being asked a question in a lecture theatre. Severe social anxiety can be crippling, when the sufferer feels under constant scrutiny.

Generalised anxiety

Generalised anxiety refers to the experience of all-pervasive anxiety, not apparently linked to any specific situation, event or object. The person experiences a high state of arousal for much of the time and a general sense of dread.

Panic attacks

Panic attacks are sudden waves of acute anxiety that seem to come out of the blue.

Case study

Andrew was recovering from 'flu when he went into a supermarket on a Saturday afternoon to stock up on food. He was dressed in warm clothing to combat the winter weather outside. Inside the shop it was hot and crowded and he had to wait in a long queue for the checkout. While waiting he began to feel very hot himself, slightly faint and nauseous. He broke out in a sweat and thought that he might actually pass out in the shop. He put down the basket and went straight to the entrance for fresh air. He began to feel better, but decided just to go home.

The next time he went to the supermarket, he thought about his last visit, and wondered if it might happen again. He thought that people might notice if he looked flustered or nervous, and this would be embarrassing. Thinking and imagining the scene was accompanied by a quickening heart rate, and then sweating and a feeling of dizziness and nausea. He thought again that he might faint and that this would be terrible. He made straight for the door and on getting outside, began to feel better again.

Think of the last time that you sat a difficult exam. When did your anxiety peak? Was it a week before, the day before, the morning of the exam, waiting outside to go in, sitting down at the desk, looking at the paper, or answering the questions? It differs from person to person, but commonly the anxiety peaks at some point *before* the exam, rather than during it. This is a common feature of anxiety: anticipation of an event is often worse than the actual event. Anxiety-provoking thoughts initiate and maintain the anxiety while waiting, but are replaced by the thinking necessary to actually tackle the feared situation itself. It may help to remind yourself of that when you are next anxious.

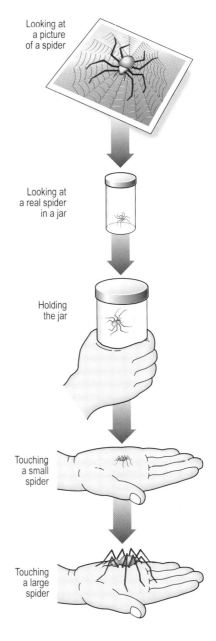

Fig. 1 **Graded exposure to a spider.**
(From Puri 1996)

TREATMENT

Methods of treatment depend on the nature of the anxiety and the individual's preference.

Drugs

These work by reducing the physiological symptoms of anxiety. The most commonly used group of drugs are the benzodiazepines, but these can cause dependence, and with prolonged use, subsequent withdrawal from them can cause rebound effects: symptoms similar to the original anxiety. The beta-blockers, which control heart-rate, are sometimes used to reduce symptoms for a one-off occasion, e.g. a musician giving an important performance. If the anxiety is more general, anti-depressants may be used, partly because there are often depressive symptoms associated with the condition.

Psychological therapies

Psychological therapies might take various forms, e.g. counselling (see pp. 126–127) or cognitive-behaviour therapy (see pp. 128–129). As a general principle, they would aim to identify the cause and maintenance of the problem and then break the cycle of anxious thoughts, physical symptoms and maladaptive behaviour. For a simple phobia, graded exposure is most effective: the patient learns coping strategies (not to be afraid of the fear itself) then confronts the feared stimulus in a series of stages. In this way the patient learns that it is tolerable (Fig. 1).

Many aspects of health care are anxiety-provoking in themselves. Waiting to see a doctor makes most patients anxious because they often feel ill and therefore vulnerable. They are dependent on the doctor for help, do not know what to expect and may find it difficult to say exactly what they want to say. Coming into hospital produces the same effect, but has the added stress of being taken into a strange institution and having loss of control imposed upon them (see pp. 98–99). It is easy to underestimate the degree of anxiety that patients often feel when faced with a doctor. They may react in maladaptive ways: by not giving the right information, or by being defensive, hostile or tearful. They are frequently too anxious to listen or remember what is said to them. They may show clinical signs of anxiety which may be mistakenly attributed to some other cause. Every effort should be made to reduce anxiety in order to get the most out of a clinical encounter.

Case study

Mr Crawford had a hip replaced and was recovering well from the surgery. He was anxious to get out of hospital and was due to be discharged but had persistent high blood pressure. Extensive investigations could reveal no explanation. He said that he wanted to go home anyway and was not bothered about the blood pressure. Medical staff were concerned about the inexplicable hypertension and wanted him to stay in until it resolved. He became agitated and insisted that his blood pressure would go down if they let him go home. They felt that this was too great a risk, and kept him in hospital overnight. The following day he was more agitated and the blood pressure remained high. Anxious to get home, he discharged himself against medical advice. The general practitioner was notified and he paid a home visit that evening. Mr Crawford's blood pressure was almost normal. Although the medical staff had no way of knowing it in this case, it appeared that hospitalisation per se was enough to cause anxiety that maintained the abnormally high blood pressure.

Anxiety

- Anxiety is common and usually time-limited.
- Persistent anxious thoughts, physical symptoms and maladaptive behaviour can interfere with healthy functioning.
- The same three components can maintain and increase anxiety in a feedback system.
- Some drug treatments for anxiety run the risk of dependency.
- The prevalence and effects of anxiety among patients are underestimated.

DEPRESSION

Depression is a common illness. The prevalence ranges from 5 to 18% of the general population depending on the location and method of the survey, and it is often associated with other illnesses. It is also disabling, and patients may be unable to function effectively for several months. Although many people experience temporary periods of low mood and may describe themselves as depressed, a depressive illness has a constellation of signs and symptoms that make it rather different.

WHAT IS DEPRESSION?

Depression is characterised by low mood and a loss of interest in all usual activities. It is persistent. The patient suffers appetite and sleep disturbance, a loss of energy, tiredness and reduced activity, an inability to concentrate, and feelings of worthlessness. They have a negative view not just of themselves, but of the world and the future. It can be a chronic or recurring condition, but most people suffering primary depression will not have a recurrence.

TYPES OF DEPRESSION

At one time it was common to distinguish between two sub-types of depression: endogenous (coming from within the individual) and reactive (where an external event precipitated the illness) but the more recent view is that no such neat distinction can be made.

There is a continuum of depression. Mild depression is likely to be treated in General Practice, but severe depression, which may have psychotic features such as delusions, requires hospitalisation for medical and nursing care, and to protect the patient from the risk of suicide.

WHO IS AT RISK?

Gender

Women suffer depression more commonly than men. In adulthood, they suffer approximately twice the rate, although at older ages the rate for men increases. Depression is often a factor in the development of alcohol problems, particularly in middle-aged men.

Social factors

Working-class women with children have considerably higher rates of diagnosed depression and admission rates to psychiatric hospitals than middle-class women, whether or not they have children (Table 1).

Brown (1978) has argued that working-class women are more at risk for two reasons. Firstly, they are more likely to experience one or more vulnerability factors (Table 2) leading to low self-esteem. They are also more likely to experience a provoking agent: a severe life event or major difficulty, particularly in relation to housing, partner's job, finance or marriage (Table 3). A major life event is unlikely to be the sole cause of depression, but will combine with vulnerability factors, such as the loss of a mother in childhood, the lack of a confiding relationship and the stress of isolation at home with small children, to precipitate the onset of illness (Table 4).

For working-class mothers, a number of other factors lead them to be at greater risk of chronic depression (lasting more than 12 months): the increased likelihood that they have experienced violence or abuse in childhood, or parental indifference or unstable relationships in adulthood, combined with material deprivation (Brown and Moran 1994).

Genetic factors

It seems that some types of depression tend to run in families. The concordance rate for affective disorder (severe mood disorder) in monozygotic twins is 40%, compared with 11% for dizygotic twins. In one large study of patients with affective disorder, 23% had mothers with a similar history, and 14% had fathers with the same problem, compared with 1% and 2% in control patients (Winokur and Pitts 1965).

Personality factors

Some personality traits make a person more vulnerable to depression. Setting very high standards for one's own behaviour makes it difficult to feel satisfied.

The desire for perfection may have arisen through a strict upbringing where parents expected high achievement. When this is combined with relationships which were not close or supportive, it is hard for the individual to develop and maintain high self-esteem. One long-term study on doctors indicated that those who showed high levels of self-criticism as students were more likely to suffer depression in their thirties (Firth-Cozens, 1996).

Table 1 **Percentage of women developing psychiatric disorder in year** (Source: Brown 1978)

	Severe event/ major difficulty	No severe event
Women WITHOUT child		
Middle-class	22%	0%
Working-class	10%	2%
Women WITH child		
Middle-class	8%	1%
Working-class	31%	1%
All women		
Middle-class	15%	1%
Working-class	25%	3%

Table 2 **Specific 'vulnerability' factors for women**

- Lack of intimate or confiding relationship
- Loss of mother before age 11
- 3+ children aged < 15 years old at home
- Unemployed

Table 3 **Severe events/difficulties**

Events Long-term (> 1 week), marked threat focused on woman, or woman and partner

- Deaths
- Illness/accidents to subject
- Relationship changes
- Important news, decisions, disappointments
- Crises involving lost pets, burglaries
- Illness/accidents to others
- Change of role of subject
- Job change
- Residence change

Difficulties Problems that had gone on for at least 4 weeks

Table 4 **Percentage of women developing psychiatric disorder in the year, by severe event or major difficulty, by vulnerability factors** (Source: Brown 1978)

		With event/difficulty	Without event/difficulty
Has intimate relationship	employed	9%	1%
	not employed	11%	1%
No intimate relationship but no other vulnerability	employed	15%	0%
	not employed	30%	11%
No intimate relationship AND other vulnerability	employed	63%	0%
	not employed	100%	0%
(n)		(33/164)	(4/255)

Life events

The loss of someone or something important can precipitate depression. It is easy to see how this could happen in bereavement, but it can also be due to the loss of a partner through divorce, the loss of friends through moving to a new area, or the loss of a role through unemployment or children leaving home.

 STOP THINK A study of 12 500 Amish people of Pennsylvania (Egeland and Hotstetter 1983) revealed a prevalence of only 1% for affective disorder. Why should this rate be so much lower than for other studies? The Amish live in a culture where there is a strong family and community support. Current social problems such as drug and alcohol abuse, violence, or family disintegration rarely occur. Perhaps this accounts for the lack of depression. But theirs is also a comparatively closed community and the Amish marry within it, making their genetic pool stable and separate from the rest of the USA. Perhaps they are genetically less prone to depression. A third explanation is that coping strategies, learning to be resourceful, to solve problems, to make use of support is culturally transmitted. It would be hard to separate these three factors.

TREATMENT

Many patients with less severe depression will be treated by their general practitioners, using counselling (see pp. 126–127) and/or anti-depressant medication such as selective serotonin reuptake inhibitors or tricyclic anti-depressants. It usually takes some weeks before any benefit will be noted by patients and they may need to be encouraged to persist with treatment.

Cognitive-behaviour therapy (see pp. 128–129) has also been shown to be effective. It is helpful for patients without psychotic symptoms who are able to engage in the learning process involved. It focuses on the negative thinking that is characteristic of depression. By enabling patients to see the effect of this thinking on their mood and behaviour, they can develop the ability to think more objectively, with associated benefits to the way they feel and behave. A number of studies have indicated its superiority to drug treatments (Blackburn et al 1981). For some patients, a combination of drugs and psychotherapy is required. This is presumed to be because the chemical treatment provides a boost to increase activity and aid concentration, enabling the patient to take an active part in a 'talking' therapy.

Electro-convulsive therapy (where electrodes are placed at the side of the head and a current passed through) has been shown to be effective in controlled clinical trials. It is not usually given as the first method of treatment, but can be helpful for people who have not responded to any other approach. Patients often complain of memory loss following ECT, but the evidence for this is not conclusive.

All treatments for depressed patients tend to have high dropout rates. This is likely to be due to a number of reasons: depressed patients lack energy and concentration and will find the effort of attending therapy difficult. They are also likely to have a pessimistic view of the treatment (one of the symptoms is a sense of hopelessness). No therapy offers an instant cure, so they get little positive reinforcement for coming to the first few treatment sessions.

HEALTH AND SOCIAL POLICY IMPLICATIONS

Apart from the importance of treating depressed patients, it is also important to consider possible preventive measures at the individual, family, community and population levels. Giving GPs resources and training to identify depression may help to reduce the high rate of untreated depression. Similarly, the provision of readily accessible facilities for psychiatry, clinical psychology and counselling would direct resources to where they are needed. Local community health projects reduce the stigma attached to seeking help for mental health problems and can help in primary prevention: by building self-esteem and social support, income support, employment opportunities and good housing. These would all alleviate what is a common and treatable disorder.

Case study

Angela Barber was 29 and had been living with her partner, Jim, for 6 years. Their children were aged 5, 2 and 3 months. Jim's new job as a long distance driver took him to continental Europe. She had relied heavily on him for practical help with the children, as well as emotional support. When he was away, she found it difficult to cope. In winter she remained indoors in their flat with the children, sometimes for days at a time. She became increasingly miserable, feeling exhausted and irritable. When Jim did return home, they argued frequently and he usually stormed out. She lost interest in food and could not be bothered cooking for the children. She found them excessively demanding, and sometimes resorted to hitting them to gain control. She went to her GP, complaining of insomnia.

The GP assessed her and diagnosed depression. He prescribed anti-depressant medication but also asked the Health Visitor to visit the family. Although initially very hostile, Angela acknowledged that there were difficulties. The Health Visitor referred her to a day centre. It provided an indoor play area, and the opportunity to meet other parents. Angela attended once, but found the effort of getting there and speaking to strangers too much. She had to be persuaded to return by a social worker, who went with her. After several weeks, the effects of the medication helped her sleep, energy and concentration, and the day centre was less daunting. She got to know one other mother whom she met at other times. After 3 months she noticed an improvement in mood, and things settled down at home. She still found it difficult when Jim was away but got some support from friends and was more tolerant of the children.

Depression

- Depression is a common and serious illness.
- Symptoms lie on a continuum from mild to severe.
- Increased likelihood of provoking factors and greater risk of vulnerability factors put working-class women more at risk of depression.
- Effective treatments are anti-depressant medication and cognitive-behaviour therapy.
- Primary prevention includes alleviating material and emotional deprivation.

PHYSICAL DISABILITY

Physical disability is the inability to perform activities due to impairments resulting from disease or disorder. Disabilities include being unable to walk, stand, eat, hear and see, and can be the result of such diverse conditions as cerebral palsy, rheumatoid arthritis, stroke, multiple sclerosis or accidental injuries. Given the prevalence of chronic disabling disease in current Western industrialised cultures, disability is an important issue in modern medicine, especially in older populations.

WORLD HEALTH ORGANIZATION MODEL

In the World Health Organization definitions, physical disability is contrasted with physical impairment, which refers to loss of structure or function due to disease or disorder, and with social handicap, which refers to social disadvantage or inability to engage in normal social roles as a result of disability or impairment (WHO 1980) (see Fig. 1).

According to this model, impairment is a direct consequence of disease or disorder, disability arises as the result of impairment and handicap may result from impairment, either directly or indirectly as a result of the disabling aspects of the impairment. For example, a person having a stroke might have disorder of cerebrovascular and brain tissue in the left hemisphere, which results in limited functioning of the right arm and leg (impairment), leading to inability to walk (disability) and therefore restrictions on the ability to get to work or to social events (handicap). An impairment, such as facial scarring, may not cause any disability but the individual may still be handicapped if he/she feels unable to attend social events due to embarrassment.

ASSESSING DISABILITY

It is important for clinical staff to assess the patient's level of disability in order to evaluate improvement or deterioration in his/her condition. For example, in someone with multiple sclerosis, it may only be possible to assess improvements in the individual's ability to perform movements or tasks, rather than changes in the underlying disorder. Such assessments can also be important in assessing recovery from injuries such as a fractured wrist or neck of femur, or from surgical procedures, especially orthopaedic procedures.

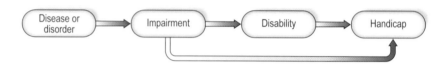

Fig. 1 **World Health Organization model.**

These assessments are used to determine further medical care, referral to rehabilitation therapists (especially physiotherapists, occupational therapists, speech and language therapists), provision of aids or adaptations to the home, or recommendations for absence from work, pensions or welfare benefits. Further assessment occurs in rehabilitation settings; for example, occupational therapists assess the individual's range of abilities and disabilities before suggesting adapted methods of performing Activities of Daily Living (ADL). Disability is typically assessed by measures of ADL, which assess the person's ability to perform everyday self-care or mobility. These measures assess activities which virtually everyone would wish to perform and therefore do not include activities which may be important for particular individuals. For example, the Barthel Index includes:

- personal toilet (wash face, comb hair, shave, clean teeth)
- feeding
- using toilet
- walking on level surface
- transfer from chair to bed
- dressing
- using stairs
- bathing.

There are two main methods of assessment: *self-report* and *observation*; the first requires the individual to describe difficulties experienced and in the second they must perform defined activities while a trained observer notes successes and failures. Using self-report methods allows the clinician to assess a wide range of activities, occurring in home and private situations, covering all times of day and night, and over a period of days, weeks or months. Observational methods are restricted to what can be assessed in the limited setting of the hospital or in the limited period available in a home visit; patients who can use the toilet independently in the hospital setting may not be able to do so at home if there is less space to manoeuvre or no support to lean on, and they may be even more disabled if they need to go to the toilet during the night if this involves additional flights of stairs.

CONSEQUENCES OF DISABILITY

Social handicap
As indicated in the WHO model, disability contributes to social handicap, preventing the individual from participating in normal social roles and increasing the likelihood of social disadvantage. The handicap experienced may depend on the type of disability. If the disability is present from birth, e.g. in cerebral palsy or cystic fibrosis, then the individual may experience disadvantage throughout their lifetime and affect school, employment, marital, parenting and other social opportunities. By contrast, an injury as a young adult, a myocardial infarction in middle age or a stroke after retirement will have very different impacts both on the individual and on his/her family.

Depressed mood
There is plenty of evidence that people with disabling conditions are on average more depressed than people without disabilities. However, the level of depression is not simply a function of the severity of the disability. Other factors such as the individual's coping strategies also affect mood (see pp. 114–115).

Individuals vary in the way that they think about their condition. *Coping styles* can affect the impact of the disability. Avoidant styles, such as pretending there is no problem or avoiding situations where the problem might be apparent, can be useful in the short term in maintaining a positive mood. However, such styles tend to be maladaptive as a long-term strategy, and more accepting, problem-solving approaches tend to be associated with better long-term adjustment.

FACTORS INFLUENCING DISABILITY

The WHO model presents disability as the consequence of disease and impairment, but clearly other factors influence the level of disability, as illustrated in Figure 2 (and on page 118, Fig. 1).

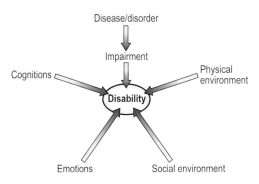

Fig. 2 **Factors influencing disability.**

Physical environment

The physical environment both within and outside the home can be important. Someone using a wheelchair will be less disabled living in a single-level, open-plan house than in a cosy cottage with an awkward staircase; but the reverse might be true for another individual with a balance problem who gets around by holding on to furniture or other supports. Outside the home, buildings without ramp access or which have many changes of level may be inaccessible to people with mobility difficulties. In any situation, someone with arthritis may be unable to wash their hands if the taps require the grip which their joints cannot perform. The extent to which the individual is disabled can therefore be determined by the physical environment as well as the underlying impairment. Disability can be remedied by altering home and public facilities. Thus the degree of disability may be indirectly influenced by the individual's financial position which enables him/her to purchase or adapt their home facilities, by social and welfare provision of appropriate aids and adaptations, by legislation which requires public buildings to be appropriately designed, and by public awareness of the need for such provision.

Social environment

Disability is also affected by the behaviour of other people, in the form of emotional or practical support. A spouse, nurse or care-attendant who is fearful of falls will give little support to the individual trying to overcome disabilities, whereas a carer who rewards every effort will enable the person to do more. Similarly, making the arrangements necessary for the disabled person to attempt the task independently is more likely to result in progress than solicitously ensuring that the individual gets everything done for them. In a study of elderly residents in a care facility (MacDonald and Butler 1974), it was noted that residents received more attention if they used a wheelchair to get to lunch and the researchers proposed that this attention was reinforcing wheelchair use. For an experimental period, attention was not given when residents used wheelchairs but was given when they walked to lunch. This resulted in less use of the wheelchair and more walking. Thus the degree of disability displayed was influenced by the behaviour of those caring for the disabled residents.

Emotional state

People with impairments who are depressed tend to be more disabled. Depressed mood lowers the individual's motivation to try to overcome difficulties or to engage in exercise which might help to regain function. Thus one may observe a vicious circle whereby the disability causes depression which results in greater disability; this circle can be broken either by dealing with the depression pharmacologically or psychologically or by creating highly motivating conditions in a rehabilitation environment.

Anxiety may also exacerbate disability, by reducing the individual's confidence to tackle activities within their physical ability. For example, following a myocardial infarction, a patient was so anxious about having another MI, and so sensitive to chest pain, that she restricted her activities to within 30 yards of her home; psychological treatment using a programme of graded exercises to increase her confidence enabled her to overcome the anxiety and reduce her disability.

Cognitions

What the person thinks may also affect disability. Individuals who have high beliefs in their ability to control the situation (perceived control) or to perform a task (self-efficacy) achieve more than those with similar impairments but less confidence in their abilities. In a study with patients with chronic pain, increasing perceived control by rehearsing situations in which they had been successful led to lowering of disability, while decreasing perceived control by recalling failures resulted in greater disability.

STOP THINK
Mr Harrison was disabled as the result of a spinal cord injury incurred by falling from a lorry. From being an able-bodied lorry-driver, he was now confined to a wheelchair. However, he felt his quality of life had improved as he was now studying for a degree rather than being a manual worker. The clinical team believed that Mr Harrison could learn to walk again but seemed unmotivated. What factors are likely to be influencing Mr Harrison's degree of disability? What would be the appropriate clinical approach?

Case study

Mrs Craig was interviewed when she had symptoms of motor neurone disease which meant that she could not contain her saliva and she had difficulty in speaking and eating. She had been born with only one eye and had started to become blind in this eye as a result of diabetes, a condition which had resulted in her losing a leg. Despite this accumulation of disabilities, Mrs Currie did not appear down-hearted and scored in the normal range of a test assessing mood disorder. She had good social support and coped by concentrating on the positive aspects of her life-style. Her mental representations and coping style appeared to protect Mrs Currie from becoming depressed.

Physical disability

- Disability is assessed by ADL measures, using both self-report and observational methods.
- The consequences of disability include social handicap and depressed mood.
- Disability is influenced by impairment due to disease or disorder, the physical environment, the social environment, emotions and cognitions.

LEARNING DISABILITY

The implications of a learning disability for the health of individuals who are affected and their families can be far reaching, and they may need considerable clinical, social and psychological care and support. Learning disabilities are relatively rare and often doctors in hospital and the community can feel uncertain how best to respond to people with learning disabilities and their carers. This section introduces you to some of the issues and should help you to develop an interest in and empathy for people with learning disabilities, their families and carers.

DEFINITIONS

It is important to recall the WHO definition of disablement which distinguishes between impairment, disability and handicap (see pp. 116–117). These definitions of disability and handicap should be contrasted with the view of some groups of disabled people that 'disability' is created by society through various physical, social and psychological barriers (Fig. 1): the 'social model' of disability.

- Look out for posters and advertisements — how do they portray people with a disability?
- Is the social model of disability simply an extension of the concept of social handicap (see pp. 116–117) or is it fundamentally different?
- In what ways do you think that medicine and research contribute to disability?

PREVALENCE

Learning disability is commonly divided into two categories:

- *mild* — where the person has an intelligence quotient (IQ) (see pp. 30–31) of between 50 and 70
- *severe* — where the person's IQ is < 50 (it is difficult to measure IQs below 30).

Approximately 3% of the UK population (1.4 million people) have a mild learning disability, and about 3 per 1 000 (160 000 people) are severely disabled. This implies that GPs with 2 000 patients on their lists will have approximately 30–40 people with mild learning disabilities and 6–8 with severe disabilities. About 50 000 severely disabled adults and children are in long-stay hospital care, so this figure reduces to about 4–6 people in the community.

There have been significant advances in neonatal care, and in screening for learning disabilities (particularly Down's Syndrome) before birth to enable parents to choose whether or not to proceed with the pregnancy. Both of these have reduced the incidence (number of new cases per year) of children with learning disabilities. Medical advances have also enabled children with learning disabilities to survive into adulthood and middle age. So, although the overall prevalence has not changed over recent years, the age distribution of people with learning disabilities is showing a shift towards a larger proportion of older people, and they are likely to make relatively heavy use of community and hospital services.

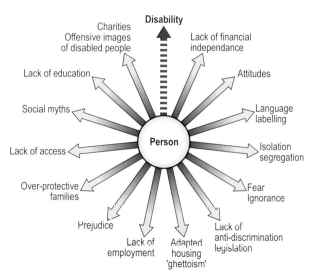

Fig. 1 **It is the 'barriers' present in society that truly disable people.**

CAUSES

In the case of people with mild learning disabilities, the cause is generally multifactorial and the precise mechanisms are unclear. It is generally found that environmental problems like poor housing, poor nutrition, excessive smoking, alcohol and drug abuse can retard foetal and infant development, as can premature birth, difficult delivery, low birth weight and infections. It is, therefore, not surprising that mild learning disabilities are more commonly found in working class families (9 times higher). There is less of a class association with severe learning disability where the casual agents are more specific.

RELATED DISABILITIES AND PROBLEMS

It is relatively common for severely mentally disabled children to experience other disabilities, and for disabled children and adults to experience higher than average episodes of ill-health. A study in East Sussex of people with learning disabilities living at home, and known to a national charity, found that 26% experienced fits, 15% found walking difficult and 10% could not walk at all (Holland & Youngs, 1990). 10% were blind or partially sighted and 7% were deaf or partially deaf. 63% of these disabled people had a speech impairment which created communication difficulties. For many people, difficulty in communicating caused frustration and anger which contributed to behaviour problems. Table 1 illustrates the problems that parents

Table 1 **Problems faced by parents of child with learning disability in previous year**

Incontinence	19%
Giving continuous care	18%
Lack of fredom, social isolation	14%
Strains in the family	14%
Worry about injury, illness, surgery	12%
Night care	12%
Lifting, carrying	10%
Mental/physical illness, fatigue	8%
Bathing, washing, personal hygiene	8%
(Source: Holland & Youngs 1990)	

had faced over the preceding year. Of particular importance are their feelings that they have to provide continuous supervision to prevent something negative happening to their child. This can lead to social isolation, to deterioration in the principal carer's own mental and physical health and to strains on family relationships. The study concluded that there was a need for improvements in both the quantity and quality of sitter/minder services, respite care, and someone accessible to talk to about problems: a role that an empathetic general practitioner can fill.

THE EXPERIENCE OF HAVING A CHILD WITH A LEARNING DIFFICULTY

It often takes some time for a baby to be identified as having a learning disability, and it is often the mother who begins to realise that something is wrong. She is likely to be very anxious (see pp. 112–113)) and to have many, often confused, concerns which she may find difficult to express. It is very important that doctors take these concerns seriously and do not dismiss them as the product of an over-anxious mother's worries.

Parents are very likely to experience strong feelings of loss, in many cases similar to the loss associated with bereavement (see pp. 16–17). They will need time and support to grieve for the child they had been looking forward to, and to adjust to the implications of having a child with learning disabilities.

As the child grows older, particularly when it is time for school, the extent and implications of cognitive impairment become clearer, and parents have difficult decisions to make about schooling. The decision will be strongly influenced by how vulnerable they feel their child to be, his/her social abilities, emotional adjustment and physical abilities, and their own feelings of protectiveness. Both the family GP and the paediatric specialist can be helpful in listening to parents, and in helping to identify and mobilise appropriate support and services.

NORMALISATION AND COMMUNITY CARE

Normalisation is an approach or philosophy which has pioneered the integration of people with learning disabilities into society. It is difficult to summarise but in essence the approach recognises that services set up to care for people with special needs, particularly long-stay institutions, often develop negative characteristics (see pp. 102–103). These need to be recognised so that, where possible, they can be transformed into positive characteristics. Table 2 summarises some of the main principles of the 'normalisation' philosophy.

A key component of normalisation is the development of *community care* (see pp. 146–147). A review of 46 studies of various types of community care development and people with learning disabilities in Britain reported that community care which was well structured and resourced did result in improvements in material standards of living, more satisfaction with life, and people became more competent and made more constructive use of their time. However, some people continued to show serious challenging behaviour and some experienced isolation, little integration into the local community, and experienced restrictions and problems similar to those experienced in institutional care (Emerson and Hatton, 1994).

Case study

Jill's first child, Sarah, was not an easy birth, but there was nothing in her pregnancy or delivery to suggest that anything might be wrong with Sarah. It was only some months later, when Jill felt that Sarah was not developing as she had expected, that she decided to check with her doctor. Although he reassured her that there was nothing to worry about, she felt that she was being dismissed as an over-anxious, first-time mother. Her husband, too, tried to reassure her that Sarah 'would soon catch up'. Some weeks later, and still concerned, Jill took Sarah to see another doctor in the practice who suggested that Sarah should see a paediatric neurologist. Although this confirmed her fears, Jill at least felt that her concerns were being taken seriously. At the hospital, the specialist reassured Jill that Sarah would not be severely disabled, a reassurance that she now strongly resents as it turned out to be false.

Jill says that coming to terms with Sarah's disability has been like losing the healthy child she was expecting. Aged 5, Sarah started to have fits but drugs help to control them. Sarah cannot speak but uses a basic sign language. She finds sudden noise frightening and can throw tantrums. Sarah has no sense of danger so Jill feels that she requires constant supervision, either from the special school, her parents, or the family that takes Sarah every other weekend to 'share the care'.

Over the years, Jill feels she has had to 'fight all the way' to get the services that Sarah and her family need. Her GP has been a key person, not in terms of expert knowledge, but as a support and an ally in getting things done.

Table 2 **Principles of service delivery to people with a learning disability**

- Enable people, where possible, to live ordinary lives by using means which are common, accepted and valued in their local community and culture
- Enhance the status of disabled people
- Acknowledge and respect disabled people as individual human beings with their own needs, preferences, abilities and social networks
- Work with disabled people, letting them retain, where possible, the initiative, choice and direction of their own lives
- No segregation from the rest of the community in housing, work, education or recreation
- Special, easily accessible services to meet needs inadequately served by ordinary means
- High professional standards in management, staffing and co-ordination of services

Learning disability

- Although the prevalence of people with learning disabilities is relatively low, the impact on the family of having a child with learning disabilities is considerable.
- Doctors can be a great support to a family if they listen carefully and work with the family to obtain the services the family needs.
- Speech impairments often contribute to a person's feelings of frustration, and can precipitate difficult behaviour.
- Parents often worry about what may happen to a child with learning disabilities and feel that they have to provide continuous surveillance.
- Community care for people with learning disabilities needs to be well structured and appropriately resourced.

LABELLING AND STIGMA

Labelling and stigma are terms used to describe negative evaluations made by individuals or groups about other individuals or groups. The terms are significant for medical practitioners for two reasons. First, negative labels are not infrequently applied by the public at large to people with particular diseases such as epilepsy or schizophrenia. Second, medical practitioners act as important labellers in much of what they do.

DOCTORS AND LABELLING

A psychiatrist has a pivotal role in diagnosing mental illness. When such a diagnosis is made it may result in institutional care (see pp. 102–103). General Practitioners sign sick notes and declare people unfit to work. A chest physician may be called upon to assess the degree of loss of lung function in a man with asbestos-related illness who is making an insurance claim against his former employer. In each of these three examples the medical diagnosis is also an important social label. The medical diagnosis is a biological or medical explanation of some underlying pathology in the body or mind. However, that diagnosis has social effects which go well beyond biology and may have profound social consequences for the person so labelled.

Social reaction

The behaviour of people at large may be strongly influenced by medical labels. For example, knowing that someone has epilepsy, or has been a patient in a psychiatric hospital, can strongly affect the way others respond to him/her. They are responding not just to the biological pathology, but to what they regard as its social significance. When the social significance of the label carries a strongly negative quality, this is referred to as stigma. The two terms — labelling and stigma — are not interchangeable because certain labels are highly positive. However, in the context of medical work, it is the negative attributions by self or others that are of particular significance.

The case study shows that an important distinction needs to be made between the presence of some deviation from normality — the presence of unrecognised coronary heart disease, and the social reaction to the diagnosis — the change in the man's behaviour and the response

of his wife and the insurance company. Sociologists have called this distinction *primary* and *secondary deviation* (Lemert 1951). Primary deviation is some kind of physical or social difference of an individual or a group. Secondary deviation is the response of self and others to the public recognition — the label — of that difference.

This idea of primary and secondary deviation was originally developed in the context of crime by Edwin Lemert (1951). He noted that many people commit crimes. He also noted that for the vast majority of people this is only a brief excursion into things like petty shoplifting or speeding in their car. The point was that these activities did not lead to a life of crime. Indeed, the vast majority of people who have at one time or another transgressed the law actually regard themselves as morally upright citizens. For most people, in other words, their law breaking has no long-term effects because it is not detected and it is not punished. Their law breaking is primary deviation since a deviant act has been committed. Secondary deviation occurs if and when the general public, the courts, and the police respond to an individual *as*

a criminal and that person's whole life gets caught up in that social role.

There are many examples of this process. People who are HIV positive will look no different from the way they did before they acquired their positive status (see pp. 106–107). However, once they themselves have the knowledge that they are HIV positive, their whole life may change. They may ruminate on their own mortality and perhaps alter their sexual conduct. If their HIV status becomes publicly known, or they choose to disclose it to others, then this in turn may alter the behaviour of others to the person doing the disclosing. It is not just patients with HIV or CHD who may experience the social consequences of illness. Insurance companies and employers, for example, frequently enquire into the health status of prospective customers/employees and effectively refuse to do business or employ people on the basis of the diagnosis. It is not so much that companies or employers do not have reason to protect their interests; it is rather that in so doing, they may produce profound social and psychological consequences among those whom they refuse to do business with and to employ.

Case study
Negative labels applied to self: the case of coronary heart disease

A middle-aged man has begun to experience the early symptoms of angina. He does not know what the pains are and he merely assumes they are caused by his playing vigorous games of cricket with his grandson. So long as he believes his pains are harmless, he will do nothing to alter his behaviour; indeed he continues to smoke and to drink alcohol as he has done for the last 40 years. A biological abnormality is present which could be medically detected but has not been. Therefore, it has had no social consequence for the man or his family.

However, let us assume this man goes for a routine insurance medical because he wants to alter his pension plan. He describes his symptoms and the doctor suspects heart disease. Following investigation, coronary heart disease is diagnosed. The medical label is applied and treatment can begin. But let us also imagine how the man feels. He is now a patient who thinks of himself as a cardiac case. He is very frightened. He immediately stops smoking. He also gives up drinking and goes onto a low-fat diet. He becomes extremely concerned about over-exertion and gives up playing cricket with his grandson. His wife also becomes anxious and discourages him from digging the garden and insists that he sit in an armchair at home. Finally, he is unable to get additional insurance and alter his pension. We can see that this man's life has been transformed, even though biologically speaking his angina is no worse now than it was before he had his medical check-up. However, his own behaviour, that of his wife and indeed that of his insurance company have all changed as a consequence of the medical label.

STOP THINK What are likely to be the primary and secondary deviations as a consequence of screening for disease? **Note**: no screening test is 100% accurate.

STIGMA

The term stigma is most usually associated with the work of Erving Goffman (1968), who was particularly interested in the public humiliations and social disgrace that may happen to people where highly negative labels are applied. He made the distinction between *discreditable* and *discrediting* stigma. A discreditable stigma is one which is not known about by the

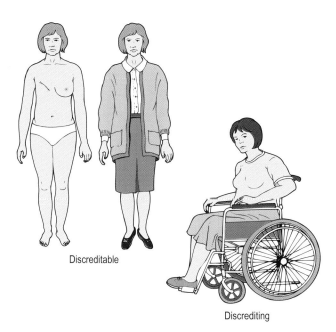

Discreditable

Discrediting

Fig. 1 **Discreditable and discrediting stigma.**

STOP THINK
- Not all medical conditions carry negative labels. Patients with the common cold, chickenpox, measles, and influenza, or who fracture their legs playing soccer, do not generally attract stigmatising labels and the social response of the general public is usually unremarkable. Indeed, such illnesses may attract sympathy. Why do these illnesses attract sympathy?
- Problems such as alcoholism, schizophrenia, syphilis, HIV/AIDS, and epilepsy, however, frequently do attract highly negative labels. What is the reason for these conditions attracting negative labels?
- Will smoking-related diseases and diseases related to poor diet and lack of exercise come to carry stigmatising labels in years to come?
- What are the implications of the existence of groups of illnesses which are stigmatised for the provision of care?

world at large. Only the person with the stigmatising condition and a few close intimates will know about it. A discrediting stigma, on the other hand, is one that cannot be hidden from other people because it is obvious and visible. People respond to the stigma rather than to the person.

A good example of a discreditable stigma is a patient who has had a mastectomy or an ileostomy (see pp. 110–111). To people in the street such patients look quite normal when they are fully clothed (Fig. 1). Apart from their closest intimates, their doctor and the few other people they might wish to inform, theirs is a hidden stigma. Other people do not react to it because they do not know about it. The person with a mastectomy or an ileostomy may go to great lengths to conceal it — say by not going to a swimming pool and never getting undressed in front of strangers. The existence of their mastectomy or ileostomy has an important effect on their own behaviour, but not the behaviour of others (Kelly 1991).

In contrast, someone with an amputation, or who is in a wheelchair, or who has lost an eye, does not have the option of concealing these things from others and people respond on the basis of the visible difference rather than the person (Fig. 1). What this means is that for some disabilities and disease conditions, the person has much less control over the publicly available information about them than is the case in other disabilities and diseases. As that information may be the basis of judgements, both positive and negative, and these judgements can have profound social and psychological effects, they are important medical issues.

Felt stigma and enacted stigma

A distinction that is sometimes made is between *enacted stigma* and *felt stigma*. Enacted stigma is the real experience of prejudice, discrimination and disadvantage as the consequence of a particular condition, say epilepsy. However, the research shows, at least in the case of epilepsy, that such frank negative stigmatisation and labelling is thankfully relatively rare (Scambler and Hopkins 1986). However, it is the fear that such discrimination might occur — which is defined as felt stigma — that can be so worrying. This is why the degree to which people feel able to be in control of information about themselves is so important. In epilepsy, for example, the worry may stem from the fact that the disease is not well controlled, and the concern is about having a seizure in public.

Labelling and stigma

- Labelling refers to the social response of individuals and groups to physical, psychological or social differences in others.
- Medical diagnoses are an extremely important example of labels, and doctors are key people in some labelling processes.
- Not all labels are negative but some medical ones certainly are.
- Primary Deviation refers to the fact of biological, physical or social difference.
- Secondary Deviation refers to the social response of the individual and others to the difference.
- Stigma is a particularly negative form of labelling.
- The fear of stigmatisation is a very powerful force affecting people's behaviour.

ADAPTATION, COPING AND CONTROL

It has frequently been suggested that there is a link between the manner of adaptation to, and coping with, the external environment and physical and mental health. It is, therefore, of considerable importance that we understand the way in which humans respond to external and internal stimuli.

Coping can mean any general adaptive process. It can also mean the mastery or control of major events. The behavioural sciences have developed two complementary ways of describing coping and adaptation — the first concerned with how people manage ordinary everyday things, the second with the way they deal with major life events. These two approaches have been brought together in what has been called the stress–coping paradigm (see pp. 52–53).

THE STRESS–COPING PARADIGM

The stress–coping paradigm was originally developed by Lazarus (1980). Lazarus starts from the position that the social (and biological) worlds are ubiquitously stressful. People have to cope with and adapt to different things, large and small, all the time. The degree to which this produces stress is determined by the extent to which these external stimuli are perceived to exceed the ability of the person to deal with them and, therefore, to endanger well-being. People have to appraise the extent to which the stimuli do this. They then will act or react accordingly.

According to Lazarus, when confronted by a stimulus that is potentially stressful, an individual engages in two processes of appraisal. These are called primary and secondary appraisal. Primary appraisal is the means whereby the person determines whether a stimulus is dangerous or not. If that person decides it is not dangerous, they may conclude that it is irrelevant to them. Alternatively, they may view it as benign or positive. If the stimulus is appraised as irrelevant, or benign or positive, it is not regarded as a stressor (Fig. 1). So while person X perceives taking an examination as stressful, because of the possibility of failure, person Y might see it as positive because it offers him or her the opportunity to demonstrate how clever they are. Person Z, meanwhile, regards it as irrelevant because he/she does not care about the outcome anyway.

If a stimulus is regarded as stressful, this is because it is perceived to represent harm, or loss or threat (anticipated harm or loss). The secondary appraisal process is about mastering the conditions of harm or threat. This can take several forms: seeking out information; taking direct action to confront the stressor; doing nothing and attempting to ignore it; or worrying about it (see Fig. 1).

The importance of this model is that it recognises that stimuli are not in themselves stressful. Stress arises as a consequence of the cognitive or thinking process which people bring to bear on particular stimuli (the appraisal processes) and on the extent to which they can control these stimuli by doing various things. It is when they are not able to control things, because they do not have the resources to do so, that stress arises. This approach emphasises, therefore, the social context within which coping takes place. It is in sharp contrast to the more deterministic versions of coping and stress theory which hypothesise a direct link between particular types of stimuli and the responses of people to them.

One of the best-known examples of the latter is the 'life-events' approach. This approach holds that certain events like the death of a close relative, losing one's job and getting divorced

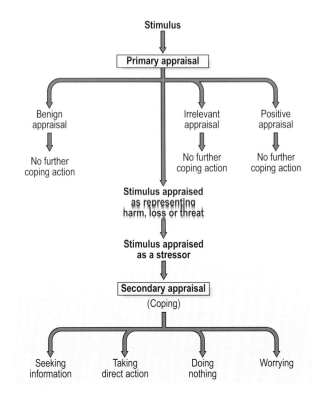

Fig. 1 **The stress–coping paradigm.** (Source: Kelly & Sullivan, 1992)

are of themselves stressful, and the levels of stress associated with them are predictable.

COPING AND ILLNESS

The view that particular events cause particular types of stress has been linked to the onset of ill health. It is argued that stress, and by implication the failure to cope or adapt, is responsible for the development of particular types of illness because certain biological responses in the individual lead to tissue damage (Seyle 1956). There is a good deal of research which focuses on specific illnesses which seem to follow stressful life events (Holmes and Rahe 1967; Fisher 1986).

While it is undoubtedly the case that exposure to external stimuli which are frightening and threatening may cause physiological changes in the human body, the question of the social environment in which this occurs is important. This is because coping is also related to the resources which people can bring to bear when they have difficult situations to deal with. Support of family and friends (a social network) and financial resources come into this category. These resources can and do have an important mediating effect on difficulties but cannot themselves prevent them. In the absence of social support, other life difficulties can be particularly damaging. A good deal of psychological morbidity can be accounted for in terms of combinations of low self-esteem, lack of financial resources and absence of social support (Brown et al 1975) (see pp. 114–115).

STRATEGIES OF ADAPTING TO CHRONIC ILLNESS

A number of typical strategies have been observed in the way people cope with, adapt to and try to gain some control over chronic illness. The responses are linked to the amount of threat

> ### Case study
> ### Childhood diabetes
>
> It is important to avoid defining coping as either good or bad. The manner of people's response to stimuli will vary and in some cases people may draw certain psychological or social rewards from the way they cope, even though others may regard their manner of coping as dangerous or self-destructive. This is sometimes observed in long-term chronic illness.
>
> In childhood-onset diabetes, for example, the family has to cope with illness and the difficulties presented by the symptoms and managing the self-medication and diet. However, it is perfectly possible for the young child to come to enjoy some of the benefits of being a sick person in the family: being spoiled and receiving special privileges in the family for example. Also the family may come to adapt to the illness in ways that they too find rewarding. Parents may receive psychological rewards from taking on the role of carer. This may work quite well while the child is young, but as the child grows up and tries to free him/herself from the control of the parents, successful earlier coping may become highly maladaptive. The child's attempt to grow and be independent may be seen as a threat by the parents, who may insist on the adolescent remaining in the sick role. The diabetic may respond by taking dietary risks in an effort to cope with parental control. Particular dynamics become established within the family, and these in turn may produce other things with which the family has to cope.

their illness presents to them, and what they are able to do about the threat.

Normalising

Here the patient acknowledges the symptoms, for example of asthma, but redefines them as part of normal experience and hence as nothing to worry about. By defining something abnormal as normal, the patient is neutralising the threat. This can present particularly difficult clinical management problems because the more successful the patient is in neutralising the symptoms, the more likely they may be not to comply with treatment (see pp. 90–91).

Denial

Here the patient denies the existence of the illness altogether. This may have profoundly beneficial effects especially in the early stages of a very worrying or threatening diagnosis. Denial may help the patient draw back, take stock and marshall help. In the longer run, however, denial prevents the patient from confronting the illness, will present particular difficulties for the treating doctor and may have considerable effects on the family or partner of the sufferer.

Avoidance

Patients who practice avoidance do not deny their problem. They set out to avoid those situations which might exacerbate their symptoms or lead to other problems. In this group of behaviours we find the person who suffers from claustrophobia and who therefore never lives or works anywhere where they may have to use a lift or get in an aeroplane. We find the reformed alcoholic who never goes to parties or social gatherings for fear that they might be tempted by the drink. We find the person with epilepsy who never applies for a job where they might have to reveal the fact of their illness. While individually each of these strategies is highly adaptive, they also contain within them certain maladaptive or potentially self-destructive elements. The person with claustrophobia or epilepsy may miss out on all sorts of opportunities while the reformed alcoholic may be cut off from a great deal of social intercourse.

Resignation

In resignation we find the person who has totally embraced their illness and for whom the most important thing about their life is their illness. Their whole being is consumed by their disease. They resign themselves to their fate. The illness is defined in such a way that instead of being something threatening, it grants certain psychological rewards. At certain times in a serious and grave illness, resignation may be an entirely appropriate way to respond. However, in many less serious conditions, total resignation leads to invalidism. The problem that this type of behaviour presents for the physician is that their best efforts to get the patient to attempt to take some control over their own life is resisted as the patient works hard to maintain their dependency on others.

Accommodation

Here the patient acknowledges and deals with the problems their illness produces — whether this is managing their symptom manifestations like pain, or managing a self-administered drug regime. The everyday work of handling the disease is seen as part of normal living. No attempt is made to build a special status out of the illness. Instead the person tries to deal with other people on the basis of his/her other characteristics, such as being a keen gardener, a football fan, a member of the church, and so on. They do not make their illness central to their life.

 STOP THINK While many disorders have been linked directly or indirectly to coping, the precise mechanisms whereby human behaviour in the face of stress produces psychological and biological consequences are very complex, and compared to many branches of medicine understanding of these mechanisms is limited. To what extent are coping and adaptation linked to psychological traits and psycho-sexual development on the one hand or to social factors, particularly availability of resources, on the other? Is it always going to be the case that what might be seen as maladaptive from a medical point of view would be bad for the patient?

Adaptation, coping and control

- Adaptation and coping refer to behaviours which involve dealing with everyday problems as well as major life events.
- It is the person who deals with these problems who defines them as everyday or major.
- Coping and adaptation are linked to a range of psychological variables and social resources.
- Stress results when the ability to deal with events is not equal to the events or stimuli.
- Failure to cope and adapt may have serious health consequences both at a physical and psychological level.
- Some strategies of coping seem to be inherently unstable or potentially self-destructive.

STRESS MANAGEMENT

Many people attribute their ill health to stress in their lives, and many occupations, including the medical profession, are stressful. Helping people to understand stress, and to manage it effectively, is important therefore to patients and to doctors themselves (see pp. 52–53).

INTRODUCTION

People from many professions and backgrounds claim to have the answer to managing stress, but there is no one technique which will suit all people in all circumstances. Managing stress is best seen in three stages:

- understanding what causes the stress
- developing appropriate behaviours (skills) to cope
- developing appropriate attitudes and beliefs (perceptions) to cope.

All this comes together to produce individual plans for stress management made up of a variety of techniques or coping strategies. Thus stress management can:

- focus on changing external causes of stress
- focus on changing the individual's response to stress
- focus on short- or long-term solutions
- be preventive or palliative.

INDIVIDUAL VERSUS ORGANISATIONAL STRESS MANAGEMENT

Most stress management focuses on changing the individual, or enabling the person to cope better, to 'fit' their environment. In some cases it is more appropriate that the environment should be altered to make more 'reasonable' demands on people. This is connected to beliefs and theories about what causes strain. In work situations, research suggests that employees see the causes of stress as relating to the job — be it environmental pollutants, excess demands or safety factors. Management, on the other hand, emphasises the individual, particularly personality and family problems. Not surprisingly, the two groups see the solution to stress in different ways. The 'worker' group see the solution in better working conditions, whereas management looks to stress management courses to enable the individual to cope with working conditions (see pp. 58–59). Thus, when looking at individual stress management, we should always be aware of the origins of stress and whether unrealistic demands come from the individual or the work/social environment.

 Consider stress in relation to junior doctors. Is the problem one of expecting junior doctors to function effectively and efficiently for more than 70 hours a week or is it that some junior doctors are not tough enough to do this? (See pp. 150–151.)

British general practitioners, for example, commonly report feeling stressed, much of which appears to be organisationally induced. Night work (comparable in some ways to shift systems), imposed administrative tasks which are perceived as a waste of time, busy and fully booked surgery sessions requiring faster working are all perceived and experienced as stressful. Whilst some of these are not immediately resolvable (for example, government-imposed requirements), the problem of night work is being addressed through the use of cooperatives, and inappropriately fast consulting through the selection of appointment times which are appropriate to the doctor's consulting style.

INDIVIDUAL STRESS MANAGEMENT

Some approaches (for example, relaxation) deal with symptoms and not the cause. For example, a person may feel they have too much to do and that too much is expected from them. They may see the part they play in contributing to this situation by their inability to be assertive. They describe themselves as 'a doormat'. To deal with the problem they need to learn assertiveness techniques.

Symptom management may be appropriate when someone needs to deal with anxiety before other coping strategies can be employed or when nothing can be done about the cause of stress and the person must learn to live with it. Another approach is to offset the negative effects of the situation by adding more positive things to the person's life elsewhere. Thus someone in a job they don't like, but can't leave, may find their stress reduced if they get involved in an activity outside work which gives them the rewards which work does not.

Generally we can look at coping and stress reduction techniques under the following headings:

- **Physical strategies**. These are usually aimed at symptom reduction and improving general health. They include relaxation (Box 1), yoga,

---

Case study

Dr G, recognising that he was often stressed because his surgeries/out-patient clinics always ran late, decided to increase each appointment slot from 7.5 to 10 minutes and to put a 10 minute space when he could 'catch-up' in the middle of the session. The result was that his surgeries/clinics ran more to time, he felt more relaxed, he prescribed less and his patients were, initially, more satisfied. However, after a few months of this new arrangement, the reception staff reported that patients often had to wait 3 or 4 days before they could get an appointment to see him. Why has this happened and what can Dr G do about it?

Box 1: Relaxation

There are many ways of practising relaxation and you should look around for one that appeals to you. Here's one simple approach: Make sure you have enough time set aside — some people find it useful to keep a particular time of the day free, when they will not be disturbed. Sit in a supportive chair, comfortable but not slouched. Begin by letting your shoulders fall/relax, and concentrate for a short while on letting your breathing come deep and slowly (see below). Then, beginning at your toes, slowly tense and then relax your muscles in each foot. Then work up through the muscles in your calves, thighs, bottom, abdomen, back, fingers, hands, arms, shoulder, neck, jaw and cheeks. If you don't have time to do this, then even as you walk, sit at meetings, study or drive, consciously relax your shoulders, neck, facial muscles and your breathing.

exercise, breathing techniques (Box 2), massage, aromatherapy and a healthy diet.

- **Skills**. The aim here is to identify what skills the person needs to cope with the causes of stress and includes everything from time management, assertiveness (Box 3), communication skills and problem solving, to study skills.
- **Cognitive techniques**. The objective is to look at what the person contributes to their problem by their beliefs, and to help them achieve more appropriate beliefs. For example, do they really have too much to do or are they adding to their work load by having inappropriate standards? Perfectionists often pride themselves in doing a good job, but it becomes a problem if they consistently miss deadlines by not finishing something because it could always be better.

Often these techniques involve looking for what the person gets out of the situation which is positive, before a change can be made. Thus many students say they work best under pressure and leave a project/essay to the last minute. They hand it in, saying, 'It would have been better if I'd had more time.' What they gain from this is the feeling that they are not being judged, and possibly found wanting, on their best work. It *could* have been better, if they'd had more time. They forget they did have longer, but chose not to use it. It protects them from doing the best they can and still not getting top marks.

Social support

Having someone who listens to you and offers support (and possibly advice) is extremely important in coping with stress. Most of us get this through mutually supportive relationships, whether this be with partners, friends or other family members As well as updating and advice giving, professional groups also offer the support of people dealing with the same circumstances. The social support derivable from self-help groups (see pp. 136–137) should not be underestimated.

Spiritual support

Although no-one can manufacture beliefs to order, a belief system (not necessarily religious) which helps answer existential questions such as 'Why am I here?' and 'What's it all for?' seems to be helpful in mediating stressors. Many people derive great help from behaviours or rituals associated with their religion or belief system, be it prayer, meditation or attendance at services, as well as from the belief itself.

Control and uncertainty

In the spread on Stress (pp. 52–53), it was said that lack of control and uncertainty were often underlying causes of stress. Any technique which enables the individual to gain (some) control over the situation, or believe they have ways of managing the uncertainty and plan for the future, will reduce their stress. This has sometimes been referred to as 'stress inoculation'.

Box 2: Breathing

As with relaxation, there are a lot of different approaches to breathing exercises to aid stress management. Breathing and muscle relaxation go together, so try and position yourself so that you can relax and feel comfortable. Then let your mind focus on the rhythm and depth of your breathing, letting the in and out breaths lengthen and deepen — but not forcing either. Stay relaxed and comfortable. Let your breathing come more from the bottom of your lungs, with the diaphragm doing the work. Sometimes it is helpful to count your breaths, slowly up to 10 and back down to 1, and some people find it helpful to concentrate either on the sensation of their lungs expanding or on the flow of air into their nostrils. It is generally more helpful if you can breathe in and out through your nose (Be careful not to hyperventilate.)

Box 3: Assertiveness

Some people find it difficult to say 'no', or to say what they want or how they feel. This can mean that their lives become very stressful doing what other people want them to do, or doing things to please other people. Being clear to others about your rights is a key element of assertiveness and does not mean that you have to deny their rights — which would be aggressive. Langrish (1981) has identified six basic rights which are worth thinking through and discussing with colleagues:

- the right to make mistakes (see pp. 150–151)
- the right to set one's own priorities
- the right for one's own needs to be considered as important as the needs of other people
- the right to refuse requests without having to feel guilty
- the right to express oneself as long as one doesn't violate the rights of others
- the right to judge one's own behaviour, thoughts and emotions, and to take responsibility for the consequences.

(From Langrish 1981)

If you do feel stressed, you might find it helpful to keep a daily stress diary — noting your stress levels, what you are doing when stressed, the activities you are doing for yourself and for others, and identifying other factors that contribute to feeling stressed. GPs who contributed to a study of stress (see p. 53) found completing a stress diary helpful in identifying factors that caused stress and could then address these factors.

STOP THINK

- What coping techniques do you already use to manage stress, and what do you need to develop?
- In a work situation, where should the emphasis in stress management lie — in changing the individual or the environment? For example: a hospital intensive care unit has a high turnover of nursing staff. Is it likely that this is due to job demands, staff characteristics or other factors?

Stress management

- There is no one universal way of managing stress that suits all people.
- Stress management can require the environment to change as well as the individual.
- Stress management involves developing appropriate behaviours and thoughts.

COUNSELLING

COUNSELLING AND MEDICINE

Counselling is about supporting people to make constructive changes in their lives. Patients may benefit from counselling when they need to consider a complex problem, make an important decision, adjust to a change in their lives or contemplate changing their behaviour. For example, counselling is used to help people decide whether or not they want to take certain diagnostic tests (e.g. the HIV antibody test), have particular treatments (e.g. radical mastectomy or lumpectomy for some breast cancers), or undergo medical procedures (e.g. the termination of an unplanned pregnancy). It is also used to support patients in adjusting to new life situations (e.g. leading a healthy life after a myocardial infarction) or changing their behaviour (e.g. reducing type A behaviour).

Counsellors may be professional or voluntary, and counselling may take place in one session (e.g. deciding whether to have an HIV antibody test) or over a series of meetings (e.g. helping someone to give up smoking). Some doctors are trained counsellors but many refer patients to others with counselling skills. Appropriate training in counselling skills is important because unskilled attempts at counselling can be harmful.

WHAT IS COUNSELLING?

Counselling is the use of interpersonal skills to develop a particular kind of supportive relationship. This may not be enough to help a client change an established pattern of behaviour. In such cases psychological therapies can be employed which have been specifically designed to facilitate behaviour change (see pp. 70–71).

Counselling aims to help people act effectively to achieve goals which they have chosen for themselves. This is likely to involve developing a better understanding of themselves, their abilities and the situations they find themselves in. Counsellors cannot change their clients' lives but they can support them in gaining the confidence, skills and self-efficacy required to make new choices and adopt new behaviours.

Counselling is often non-directive in the sense that it aims to support people in making decisions which take account of their particular circumstances and in setting goals which they can realistically achieve. For example, the aim of HIV

antibody pre-test counselling is not to advise patients on whether to take the test but to help them understand the risk which has led them to consider testing, to clarify the consequences of being tested and to help them make a decision which they will feel content about.

Counselling may become directive when it is clear that a particular course of action is very likely to have negative implications. As well as clarifying the consequences of various options, the counsellor may wish to advise on one course of action rather than another. For example, directive counselling would be appropriate when supporting post-myocardial infarction patients in identifying life changes which could make a second heart attack less likely.

Whether directive or non-directive, counselling involves more than advising, information giving or teaching. It also involves exploring: how a person can accept new information and relate it to their beliefs, hopes and desires, how they can develop plans based on this information, how they can gather the resources they need to translate those plans into action and how they can maintain new ways of behaving.

THE COUNSELLING RELATIONSHIP

Carl Rogers, an influential figure in the development of counselling practice, defined three essential characteristics of an effective counselling relationship: empathy, genuineness and unconditional positive regard.

Empathy

Empathy is the ability to understand clients' experiences and feelings in the same way as they do. It involves adopting the clients' own meanings and values when considering their experiences and communicating this so that they know the counsellor has an accurate understanding. An effective way of achieving this is to *reflect back* what the client has said, summarising what you think they *feel* and what they have *experienced*. For example, 'You feel anxious because the biopsy results aren't in yet'.

Genuineness

Genuineness is important because the client must be assured that counsellors are honest and genuine in their concern. This involves abandoning professional roles which may protect the counsellor

from becoming personally involved with the client's emotions. The counsellor must be sensitive to the clients' experiences and be able to share their own feelings when appropriate. Sharing personal experience may help a client realise that their problem is not unique and that other people have managed to overcome similar difficulties. For example, counsellors with appropriate experience might, in particular counselling circumstances, discuss the way in which work overload had previously damaged their personal relationships and how they had to consider the balance between work and leisure. Counsellors must, however, be careful to share their experience in a helpful manner. Seeking sympathy or counselling from the client will disrupt the counsellor–client relationship. Counsellors should also be able to acknowledge client complaints and share their concern that counselling is not working. This may initiate a new approach or lead to a more productive referral elsewhere.

Unconditional positive regard

This is an unselfish concern for clients that does not depend upon them behaving in a manner approved of by the counsellor. It involves avoiding pre-judgements which may follow from the counsellor's own stereotypes. Unconditional positive regard provides a non-threatening context in which clients can explore their self and situation. It is vital to the disclosure of things which clients believe are disapproved of by others. Positive regard for others is conveyed through *non-verbal communication* (see p. 92), including the way we sit and our tone of voice as well as what we say. If counsellors are unable to feel care and concern for a client (for whatever reason) they are unlikely to be the best person to offer help.

A fourth component of the counselling relationship is the establishment of *client responsibility*. Counsellors can help people clarify their options and support them in making decisions but they cannot take those decisions or act on a client's behalf. Counselling seeks to clarify what clients want to do, what they are choosing to do and how they view the consequences. Counsellors may, therefore, explore (and sometimes question) what is involved when clients say they want to do something for themselves but *cannot* or when they say they *have* to fulfil social obligations which they view as destructive.

STOP THINK   Write down how you would reflect back what this patient is saying, showing empathy.

Patient: *'I'm worried about my mother. I love her but she drives me mad. I don't know if she can go on alone and there's no one else to look after her. I don't know if I could stand having her live with me. I know I should look after her but I don't think I could go on if I couldn't get away. Do you think she'll be all right on her own? Can I get any help?'*

WHAT THE CLIENT ACHIEVES

Drawing upon Egan's (1990) model of helping we can identify five tasks which may be accomplished within a counselling relationship. These are described in terms of what clients achieve through the counsellor's help:

1. communicating a clear picture of his/her situation and feelings
2. constructing new ways of looking at the situation
3. defining goals and planning actions which could improve this situation
4. developing the motivation and abilities needed to implement change
5. becoming independent of the counselling relationship.

Not all of these tasks will be achieved (or given equal time) in any particular counselling relationship and a single counselling session may focus on one or all of them. Table 1 shows how these can be translated into specific gains in the case of bereavement counselling.

THE COUNSELLOR'S TASK

By attending closely to clients' verbal and non-verbal communication, asking open questions, guiding clients towards clarification and specification of their concerns and summarising and reflecting what is being said, the counsellor can assure clients that they are understood. The knowledge that someone else has a clear understanding of one's concerns is a considerable comfort even when nothing more is offered. It also deepens trust and encourages self-disclosure.

The counsellor may identify ways in which the clients' understanding of their world creates barriers to problem-solving and may question these understandings and explore new approaches or plans. Such intervention must be based on a trusting relationship and should be aimed initially at the problems causing the client most distress. Helping clients identify their needs and priorities is a key part of facilitating change and development.

Effective planning requires the identification of barriers which may prevent change and consideration of strategies

Table 1 **What could a counsellor offer a bereaved relative?**

- Enable the client to admit his/her loss
- Help him/her to express the range of feelings this gives rise to
- Encourage him/her to explore the prospect of life without the deceased
- Help him/her anticipate and understand his/her feelings over time
- Question destructive coping strategies (such as social withdrawal)
- Offer support while encouraging the establishment of alternative social supports.

See Worden 1991 (for details)

for overcoming them. This may involve focusing upon past successes to gain confidence, planning new approaches to achieving a goal, and learning new ways of interacting with people who are blocking the client's plans.

IS COUNSELLING EFFECTIVE?

Counselling is not effective for all problems and one of the counsellor's skills is to know when a client should be referred for further psychological or psychiatric assessment. However, counselling has been shown to be effective with many patient groups. There have been many quantitative assessments of the impact of counselling and psychotherapy (e.g. Shapiro and Shapiro 1983). Effectiveness has been measured in terms of reduced psychological distress, fewer symptoms or behaviour change.

There is convincing evidence that counselling can be of benefit to specific patient groups, including smokers who want to give up, post-myocardial infarction patients and those who have recently suffered a bereavement. Parkes (1980), for example, reviewed evidence on bereavement counselling (see p. 17) and concluded that it could reduce the risks of psychiatric and psychosomatic disorders. Bereavement counselling has been evaluated by comparing those who have received counselling with matched controls who have received no counselling. Counselled groups have been shown to report fewer symptoms, have fewer consultations with doctors and receive fewer drug prescriptions. Statistically significant differences of this kind in controlled studies provide good evidence that counselling can deliver health benefits.

Case study
Counselling in terminal care

John had been told he had terminal cancer. He reacted by becoming perpetually cheerful and denying that he needed any help. This protected him from talking about his illness but also prevented anyone from offering him help or making plans about his care. His consultant persuaded him to talk to a psychiatric nurse who was a trained counsellor. By gently talking to him about his feelings about death the counsellor gradually allowed him to express more negative emotions. Over a series of sessions John began to express fear, self pity, anger and sadness over his loss. During these sessions he recognised his feelings and accepted them as appropriate. He also began to talk about what was important to him now and clarified that relationships with his family were vital to his quality of life. This motivated him to talk openly to his wife and adult children about his cancer. He was also able to identify a number of decisions which he needed to make. Towards the end of his life John maintained that his nurse counsellor had 'opened his eyes to what really mattered'.

Counselling

- Requires skills developed through training and practice.
- Can be directive or non-directive.
- Aims to empower people to achieve goals which they choose for themselves.
- Can help people adjust to a new situation or change behaviour.
- Involves communicating clearly about feelings and experiences.
- Depends upon being able to communicate genuinely and empathetically.
- Involves helping people identify options and develop plans.
- Has been shown to be effective.

COGNITIVE-BEHAVIOUR THERAPY

Cognitive-behaviour therapy uses systematic techniques to enable people to think and act in a different way. It educates them to view themselves or their circumstances in a more adaptive way.

THOUGHTS, MOOD AND BEHAVIOUR

The theory behind the approach is that patterns of thinking influence both mood and behaviour. A habit of thinking negatively may arise from attitudes and assumptions which developed in childhood or from a major experience in adulthood. Many negative thoughts may arise from one basic assumption which colours all interpretation, e.g. 'I'm never any good at anything'. For some people, negative thoughts hinder healthy behaviour or prevent them from leading a full life (Fig. 1).

Applied to health problems, if people can change the way they think about themselves, they may change the way they behave: for example, cut down on drinking, alter eating habits, cope with pain, develop a social life or increase exercise.

WHAT IS THE RATIONALE BEHIND COGNITIVE-BEHAVIOUR THERAPY?

Cognitive-behaviour therapy arose out of behaviour therapy which had been shown to be effective in helping people change by means of classical and operant conditioning (see pp. 20–21). For example, people who are agoraphobic may be helped by building in rewards ('reinforcements'), for venturing out a little farther each day. This would be an example of operant conditioning.

In medicine, an example would be a patient in hospital who will not take part in physiotherapy following a hip replacement, because it is painful and difficult. A similar system of self-reinforcement could be used for each small step towards recovery: she might plan to buy new clothes as soon as she could stand unassisted for 30 seconds; or go home for a weekend as soon as she could take three steps; or to go out for a meal when she could walk 10 metres with the aid of a walking stick. The use of goals and rewards helps us all to achieve difficult tasks.

The addition of cognitive elements to behaviour therapy came about because it was realised that sometimes people hold such strong negative beliefs that these beliefs prevent them from behaving in a way which would help their condition. In

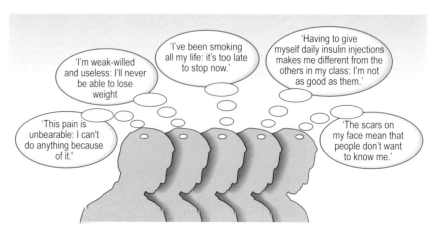

Fig. 1 **Some examples of thoughts that hinder healthy behaviour.**

Date	Mood 0–10	Dysfunctional thought	Behaviour	Alternative thought	Mood 0–10
Tues. a.m.	2	I'll never be able to do the things I enjoyed – hillwalking, gardening, swimming. It's hopeless	Asked Mary how long it took her sister to recover – she said it was about 2 months	I can't do a lot now, but I might be able to garden in 3 months' time	5

Fig. 2 **A thought diary showing the link between thought, mood and behaviour.**

the above example, the patient may not even attempt to stand up because she thinks, 'I'm so weak, I'll never be able to stand'.

THE TECHNIQUE OF COGNITIVE-BEHAVIOUR THERAPY

The answer is not to say to the sufferer 'Don't be silly, of course you'll be able to stand if you try,' as this may only antagonise. Instead, the aim is to lead the person to that conclusion by 'guided discovery'.

'You may be right, you may not be able to stand at the moment. Have you seen anyone else with a similar injury to yours? Have they made any progress? Is there any possibility that you might have the strength to do it? How can we test this out?'

The approach is collaborative: the patient is encouraged to gather evidence for and against particular beliefs and then to act on their conclusions in an experimental way. In this example data-gathering might include:

- attempting to stand for one second
- asking other patients with hip replacements how they felt at first and whether they made progress

- rating the probability in percentage terms of being able to walk again.

On the basis of results, she will revise her beliefs and will be asked to reflect on how she feels about the achievement. She learns actively about the role of negative thoughts in influencing both mood and behaviour.

Over time she will practise monitoring thoughts, challenging them, setting behavioural experiments and reviewing how these affect mood. Figure 2 shows a monitoring record. Work is carried out as 'homework' as well as within sessions. Having learned these skills, the patient is then in a position to be wary of negative thinking, to challenge it and to view circumstances and herself in a more objective way. Any basic assumptions which underlie negative thinking will also be elucidated and can themselves be challenged.

COGNITIVE-BEHAVIOUR THERAPY AND EMOTIONAL DISORDERS

Cognitive-behaviour therapy has been widely developed within the field of psychiatry where it has been shown in clinical trials to be effective with many disorders.

Dysfunctional thoughts tend to lead to emotional difficulties and problems in behaviour: when depressed, someone may feel tired and lethargic and have difficulty concentrating. They may think that they are lazy, incompetent and not likeable. This leads to a worsening of low mood and inactivity. This in turn makes the person more likely to think negatively about themselves and the depression is maintained in a vicious circle (see Fig. 3) (see pp. 114–115).

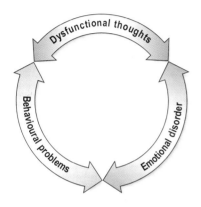

Fig. 3 **The link between dysfunctional thoughts, emotional disorder and behavioural problems.**

COGNITIVE-BEHAVIOUR THERAPY AND HEALTH PROBLEMS

Cognitive-behaviour therapy has been used increasingly in all fields of medicine where the same principles apply: the link between thought, mood and behaviour must be examined and any unhelpful aspects discussed critically. It has been shown to be effective in cardiac rehabilitation, the management of diabetes, asthma, chronic pain, epilepsy, irritable bowel syndrome and others. Pearce and Wardle (1989) outline a variety of applications.

ADVANTAGES AND DISADVANTAGES

There are advantages in using cognitive-behaviour therapy rather than medication: it avoids problems of adverse reactions, side-effects and dependency. The effects of the treatment are long-lasting. The patient has learned how to tackle problems as they arise. The main disadvantage is the time taken by a member of staff to carry out the therapy, as this is comparatively expensive when compared with pills. In many cases this will be outweighed by the long-term benefits since the patient is less likely to come back for further treatment.

In clinical practice, although cognitive-behaviour therapy looks like common-sense, and appears easy to apply, it takes much skill and there are pitfalls: one is 'Socratic questioning', i.e. the use of questions to lead someone to a different conclusion about themselves. This can easily turn into a seemingly aggressive cross-examination if the therapist is too persistent, or hasty, or selects inappropriate questions, or an inappropriate belief on which to target. Many people are trained in cognitive-behavioural techniques, including doctors, nurses, clinical psychologists and social workers, and it is likely that a patient with serious difficulties would be referred to one of these agencies for specialist help.

STOP THINK

If you were working in your first week as a junior doctor and were very anxious, were not sure how to put up an intravenous drip properly, had made two mistakes writing up histories, had been humiliated by your consultant and doubted whether you were bright enough or competent enough ever to make it as a doctor, how might you apply cognitive-behaviour therapy to yourself?

How could you gather evidence for and against your suitability to be a doctor?

Case study

A 47-year-old van driver suffered a heart attack 5 months ago while driving home from work. He had stopped the car, and flagged down a passing motorist who took him to hospital. On the day of his heart attack, he had felt unwell and had suffered chest pains when climbing stairs to make deliveries.

He made a full physical recovery and is not thought to be at great risk of another attack, but is now depressed, will not walk uphill or take much exercise at all, and thinks it unlikely that he will be able to return to work.

Figure 4 gives examples of the likely elements in the cognitive-behavioural cycle:

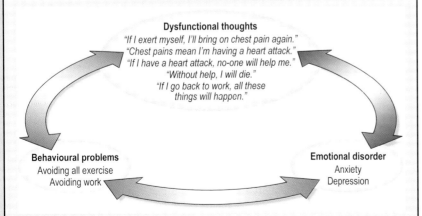

Dysfunctional thoughts
"If I exert myself, I'll bring on chest pain again."
"Chest pains mean I'm having a heart attack."
"If I have a heart attack, no-one will help me."
"Without help, I will die."
"If I go back to work, all these things will happen."

Behavioural problems
Avoiding all exercise
Avoiding work

Emotional disorder
Anxiety
Depression

Fig. 4 **Dysfunctional thoughts: the vicious circle.**

How would you begin to tackle this man's difficulties? What questions would you ask to enable him to examine his dysfunctional thoughts? Suppose that he agreed to try some gentle exercise, and he did experience chest pain. Are there any possible psychological causes? (See pp. 132–133.)

Cognitive-behaviour therapy

- Cognitive-behaviour therapy proposes that dysfunctional thoughts influence both mood and behaviour.
- The predisposition to have such thoughts may be laid down in experience from early childhood where particular attitudes were learned, but they may also result from experience in later life.
- Cognitive-behaviour therapy aims to help a person to change dysfunctional beliefs so that they view circumstances more objectively, and as a consequence feel and behave differently.
- The methods of cognitive-behavioural therapy include education, collaboration, agreed goals, homework, and monitoring and evaluation of progress.

MEASURING PAIN

Measures of pain intensity (or severity) can be used to monitor the effectiveness of pain treatments. Measures of the quality of pain can help distinguish between different types (e.g. pain due to a damaged nerve as opposed to pain caused by a pulled muscle) and so assist with diagnosis and treatment selection.

A MULTIDIMENSIONAL MODEL OF PAIN

Pain can be divided into four components:

- **Nociception**: the neural detection of noxious stimuli, for example, the response of sensors near the surface of the skin when the skin is cut.
- **Pain sensation**: the experience of pain, for example feeling pain in response to a cut.
- **Affective responses to pain**: emotional reactions to pain sensations, for example, feeling depressed in response to chronic pain.
- **Behavioural responses**: the response to pain sensation, for example crying out, holding an injured hand, complaining or reacting aggressively.

Nociception is not directly translated into pain sensation, emotional responses or behaviour. The gate control theory, for example, suggests that neural 'gates' in the spinal cord can amplify or suppress the transmission of nociception to the brain. This means that a person's psychological state can affect their pain sensation as well as their emotional and behavioural responses. This is the basis of psychological approaches to pain management (see pp. 132–133). Monitoring the effectiveness of such management may involve measuring aspects of pain sensation, types of affective response to pain and pain behaviours.

PAIN LOCATION

Patients can usually indicate where they feel a pain and this can assist diagnosis. There are also assessment instruments which include diagrams of the body on which patients are asked to draw their pain. These can be used with patients (for example, children) who find it difficult to describe their pain and to monitor changes in where the pain is felt.

PHYSIOLOGICAL MEASURES

Muscle tension, heart rate, skin conductance and electrical activity in the brain have all been used as indicators of pain experience. For example an electromyograph (EMG) is used to monitor muscle tension and it has been shown that some headache patients show different EMG patterns according to whether or not they are in pain. However, physiological measures are not regularly used in pain assessment because physical indicators can also be influenced by other psychological and physical processes such as mood, stress, diet and exercise.

SELF-REPORT MEASURES

The most frequently used measures of pain depend upon the patient's own description of his or her pain. Attempts have been made to standardise and quantify aspects of patients' reports so that they can be compared over time. For example, if we can say the intensity of a patient's pain has fallen from a daily peak of 5 points (before treatment) to a daily peak of 3 points on the same scale (during treatment) this is more reliable than the person's observation that her pain seems better.

When using self-reports it is useful to remember two key rules:

1. *Always believe the patient.* Research across medical specialities, including paediatrics and surgery, suggests that many patients suffer unnecessary pain. One reason for this is that health care professionals mistakenly think that patients exaggerate pain.
2. *Measure pain as it is experienced.* Pain recall may be unreliable. For example, a patient's present pain may distort his/her memory of previous pain.

We shall consider three commonly used types of self-report measures: visual analogue scales, simple rating scales and the McGill Pain Questionnaire.

Visual analogue scales

A visual analogue scale (VAS) provides a measure of pain intensity (Fig. 1). It consists of a 10-centimetre line with the ends labelled 'no pain' or 'worst possible pain'. The patient can simply draw a line through the VAS to indicate how bad their pain feels now.

The VAS is easily administered and correlates well with patients' verbal reports of pain intensity. It is also sensitive to change and can be used to monitor intensity fluctuations over time.

Simple rating scales

Rating scales are also used to measure pain intensity. They present the patient with a series of graded descriptions. For example, the 'present pain index' which is included in the short form of the McGill Pain Questionnaire (Melzack 1987) consists of five descriptions:

- 0, no pain
- 1, mild pain
- 2, discomforting pain
- 3, distressing pain
- 4, horrible pain
- 5, excruciating pain.

Other scales may use fewer descriptions, e.g. mild–moderate–severe–agonising. Category scales may also be accompanied by illustrations. The 'Wong/Baker Faces Rating Scale' (Fig. 2) for children uses five faces illustrating 'doesn't hurt at all' to 'hurts as much as you can imagine'.

Patients can learn to use these scales easily. After a little practice they can translate their present pain sensation into an intensity rating between 1 and 5 without referring to the scale. This can be very useful in keeping a pain diary. The main disadvantage of these scales is that they have a limited number of ratings and are, therefore, less sensitive to small changes than the VAS.

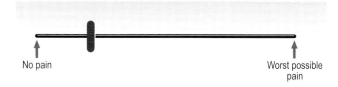

No pain   Worst possible
                                                  pain

Fig. 1 **The visual analogue scale.** The patient's pain rating can be scored out of 100: in this case, 21.

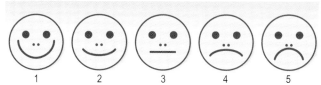

1   2   3   4   5

Fig. 2 **The Wong/Baker Faces Rating Scale for children.** (Adapted from Wong and Whaley, 1986.)

STOP THINK Mrs Barton is a new patient who arrives in her GP's surgery looking distressed and complaining of an intense headache.

If you were her GP, what kinds of questions would you want to ask her about her pain? What kind of measures might be usefully included in a pain diary for Mrs Barton?

The McGill Pain Questionnaire

The VAS and simple rating scales only measure pain intensity. The McGill Pain Questionnaire (MPQ) attempts to measure pain intensity, the quality of sensation (What does it feel like?) and the emotional impact this has on the patient (What does it make me feel like?).

In the short form of the questionnaire patients are presented with a VAS, the present pain index, eleven items using adjectives describing the sensory quality of the sensation and four items describing its emotional or affective impact. Two of each are shown below.

Sensory items
- Throbbing: none (1), mild (2), moderate (3), severe (4).
- Sharp: none (1), mild (2), moderate (3), severe (4).

Affective items
- Tiring-exhausting: none (1), mild (2), moderate (3), severe (4).
- Fearful: none (1), mild (2), moderate (3), severe (4).

The MPQ gives a range of information about the patient's experience and is widely used. One criticism of the questionnaire is that patients may not commonly use the descriptions offered in the questionnaires and may, therefore, not know how to use them. This may be especially true of the long form of the questionnaire which employs 78 pain adjectives. The Windowpain measure, however, attempts to simplify this.

Windowpain: a new pain measure

Self-report measures, such as the McGill Pain Questionnaire, have been criticised because they may be used differently by patients with varying reading abilities. A new computer-based measure has attempted to overcome this problem (Swanston et al 1993). Windowpain uses animations displayed on a personal computer to represent different qualities of pain sensation — for example, a vice for pressure pain and a needle piercing a flesh-coloured area for piercing pain. Patients can choose one or more animations which correspond to the quality/ qualities of their pain sensation. They can then indicate the intensity of the pain by adjusting the animations. For example the vice can be turned to squeeze a red ball and the needle can be moved to just touch the skin or plunge deeply into it (Fig. 3). Windowpain also includes an animated VAS. Patients prefer this measure to traditional questionnaire measures such as the short-form MPQ. It allows measurement of the quality and intensity of pain sensation but at present does not measure emotional or behavioural responses.

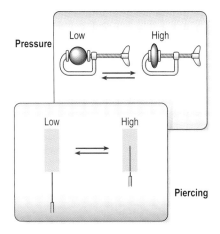

Fig. 3 '**Windowpain**'. One example of computer-based animation representing different qualities of pain sensation.

Measuring pain behaviour

Patients can be asked to perform simple tasks such as walking so that the extent of their pain behaviour can be observed. A series of rating scales from 'never' to 'very frequent' can be used to rate how often the patient expresses pain by, for example, groaning, grimacing, rubbing, stopping to rest or holding part of the body. The problem with such measures is that the patient's behaviour may change when different people are observing. For example, it has been found that some patients exhibit more pain behaviour when their spouse is present.

Pain monitoring may be most useful when undertaken by the patient themselves as part of a behaviour change programme which they want to be involved in (see Case study). These may be included in a pain diary.

Case study
Monitoring and modifying pain behaviour

George has had chronic back pain for almost 2 years. He tends to grimace, wince and groan frequently throughout the day and spends a lot of time telling other people how awful his pain is. His wife and others have been sympathetic but increasingly want to spend less and less time with him. He has become aware of this and wants to regain some of his previous social life. He and his wife talk to their doctor about the most effective pain relief for George and he begins this course of treatment. In addition they are taught to monitor George's pain behaviour so that he becomes conscious of it. This helps George to deliberately respond differently to pain in public and so change established pain behaviours which do not bring relief and tend to alienate those from whom he needs support. His wife also learns to help him by changing how she responds to his pain behaviour. Previously she has been most sympathetic when he expressed most pain. Now she rewards George with attention and affection when he is talking and involved in conversation but not expressing pain. She ignores him when he winces, grimaces, groans or complains too frequently. This approach may not reduce George's pain but it may improve his social life and the social support he receives, which is likely to enhance his overall quality of life.

Measuring pain
- Includes assessment of pain sensation (including quality and intensity), affective responses to pain and pain behaviour
- It is recommended that (1) present pain is measured and (2) patients' pain reports are believed.
- Two commonly used measures of pain intensity are visual analogue scales and rating scales.
- The McGill Pain Questionnaire attempts to measure pain quality and affective responses as well as pain intensity.
- New measures using computer animations, such as Windowpain (which measures pain quality and intensity) are being tested.

THE MANAGEMENT OF PAIN

There have been major advances in the medical management of pain in recent years, particularly in palliative care, and in acute pain after surgery, but many patients with long-standing pain, e.g. 'bad backs', have not derived much benefit from either drugs or surgery. Whether you accept the theory that pain is a psychological response, or is a physiological response mediated by psychological factors, it is widely accepted that pain includes a major psychological component. This being so, psychology should be able to help patients with pain, if not to eliminate it, then to reduce its disabling effects. Psychological treatments are described in this spread.

ASSESSMENT OF PAIN

'Measuring pain' describes how the nature and intensity of pain are defined and measured. For clinical purposes, other factors need to be included, especially discussion about the patient's model of pain. Patients may be reluctant to accept psychological components. One way of overcoming this is to ask the patient to keep a diary of pain. This provides an accurate record of activity and pain, which would not be available just from memory. A record like this, revealing fluctuations, can prompt a discussion of how circumstances affect pain. In the example shown in Figure 1, which is a day's record of low back pain, the diary indicates that pain is reduced when the patient is lying down, and when swimming or in the bath. Sitting for any length of time is associated with increased pain, although slightly less so when the patient is out with friends than when alone at home. This diary reveals not only the effect of physical activity but also social activity on the level of pain.

A description of onset, course, the patient's pain behaviour (what they can do, what they have to avoid), levels of anxiety and depression (common among those suffering chronic pain) and the patient's beliefs about the cause need to be discussed. On this basis, a shared model can be negotiated. Realistic goals have to be established, e.g. what activities the patient would like to resume, and whether these are feasible.

Assessment is carried out initially to establish a baseline, then repeated at intervals during treatment to monitor progress. This provides a record for both patient and staff to see how different aspects of treatment affect levels of pain.

PAIN MANAGEMENT TECHNIQUES

Pain clinics are likely to be multi-disciplinary and the treatment will be tailored to the patient. It may include, for example, pharmacology, physiotherapy and clinical psychology. Psychological approaches that have been shown in clinical trials to give significant improvements are outlined here.

COGNITIVE-BEHAVIOUR THERAPY

As with the other applications of this therapy (see pp. 128–129) the aim is to educate the patient to re-interpret events (in this case, sensations), to change behaviour and thereby improve mood. The three factors inter-relate, but in pain management, the starting point is often the thoughts ('cognitions') associated with pain. There are various techniques that are helpful:

- **Distraction**. Think of something else. Read aloud from a newspaper, count the number of trees outside, or count backwards from 100.
- **Imaginative distraction**. Imagine that you are somewhere else, so pleasant that you might temporarily ignore the pain. You might be in a beautiful garden, or lying on a tropical island in a warm breeze.
- **Change the context**. Imagine that the chronic pain in your back as you walk home has just occurred in the middle of a game of football, and being essential, you will carry on to the end of the match despite the pain.
- **Re-label the pain**. Think of the contractions in childbirth not as 'pain' (a distressing concept), but the 'opening-up' of the cervix and evidence of progress towards the birth.
- **Distance the pain**. Think of the pain objectively, rather than subjectively, so imagine writing about it and describing it for a magazine article: it is a phenomenon to be observed.

To go with the cognitive techniques, there are behavioural techniques which aim to interrupt the physiological processes involved in pain or to alter the behavioural response to pain.

Day/time	Activity	Level of pain (0–10)
8.00–11.00	Lying in bed	4
11.45	Had a long, hot bath	3
12.45	Went to 'Ship Inn' to meet friends	5
2.30	Walked along the beach	5
4.00	Went for a swim in the swimming baths	2
5.30–11pm	Sitting watching TV at home	7

Fig. 1 **A pain diary.** Note decreased pain when lying down or swimming, and increased pain when sitting alone. Sitting with friends is reported as slightly less painful.

Date	Where you were/what you were doing	Level of pain (0–10)	How you dealt with the pain	Pain afterwards (0–10)
7th August Morning	Sitting ironing	8	Stood up to iron	7
	Sitting reading the paper	7	Went to meet friend: sitting on bus reciting poetry in head as a distraction	5
Afternoon	Sitting over lunch	9	Imagined pain in hip was wave of icy sea water, coming and going	7
	Arrived home	8	Put on music, did relaxation exercises	5
Evening	Lying on the floor watching TV	5	Tried to keep concentrating on film—not think about the pain in my hip	4

Fig. 2 **A pain diary showing circumstances, level of pain, response to pain, and outcome.**

- **Relaxation**. Patients learn in a series of relaxation exercises how to reduce overall tension in muscles. Tension often exacerbates pain and may sometimes be the cause of it. This is particularly helpful for those with headache.
- **Biofeedback**. This can help people to identify and reduce tension in specific muscles by providing an auditory signal which feeds back the level of tension. Electrodes are attached to the target site (e.g. frontalis muscle for headache) and the patient learns how to selectively let go of tension in the muscle. In clinical trials this method has not been shown to be superior to general relaxation, but some patients who have difficulty identifying the difference between tension and relaxation may find it useful.
- **Operant techniques**. Behavioural methods can alter pain behaviour. This approach (see pp. 20–21) is intended to reduce disability caused by pain. The patient and therapist agree realistic goals of increasing activity and then rewards are built in to increase the probability of the goals being reached.

HOW DO YOU CHOOSE A TECHNIQUE?

In clinical practice, pain management usually includes many techniques which are taught to patients who then choose which strategy is likely to work for them. Pearce and Erskine (1989) describe different types of treatment. All cognitive and behavioural techniques include assessment and monitoring of progress to enable the patient to learn the connections between thought, behaviour and feeling. Figure 2 shows an example of a pain diary for a day.

DO PSYCHOLOGICAL TREATMENTS WORK?

Clinical trials conducted have often been of cognitive-behavioural packages and it is difficult to tell which are the active ingredients. In general, combined packages tend to be superior to either approach on its own. For example, Turner (1982) compared two group therapies for patients with chronic low back pain and found cognitive therapy combined with relaxation to be slightly better than relaxation on its own. Both were better than the control group who were assessed over the same time, but remained untreated on the waiting list.

Case study

Fergus worked on an oil rig until he crushed his knee falling from an upper to a lower deck while moving heavy equipment. The orthopaedic consultant declared surgery to have been successful, but 4 months later Fergus still complained of limited mobility in the joint and a constant gnawing pain that disrupted sleep, made him irritable, permanently tired and depressed. His girlfriend confirmed that he was considerably disabled.

He went to a pain management clinic. The anaesthetist reviewed his case and considered that his medication ought to be reduced rather than increased. The cause of the pain was discussed, and although Fergus still wanted further surgery, he was willing to try to reduce pain by other methods. He was keen that staff realise his pain was genuine and was reassured that this was not disputed. He started in a group run by a clinical psychologist.

He found relaxation quite helpful in coping with the pain when he was getting off to sleep, but when it was acute, he used to imagine that the pain was a ball of hot metal that was gradually cooling down. He reduced medication but wanted to keep the option of being able to take something if his pain was really bad at night.

His progress was monitored by a pain diary, and from this he saw that there were times when he had less pain. These were when he was out walking the dog. This surprised him, since he thought exercise made the pain worse. He decided to increase exercise, and was more conscientious about his physiotherapy.

At the end of eight sessions in the group, he said that the pain was more manageable, but was still nagging and he wanted a second orthopaedic opinion. He acknowledged that he was sleeping better and that average pain ratings for a week had reduced from 8.5 in Week 1 to 4.5 in Week 8. His girlfriend said that he was less irritable and was going out much more. When he looked at the change in his own ratings of pain, sleep, mobility and social activity, he realised that he had made substantial improvement and felt in greater control.

At follow-up 6 months later, he had seen his original orthopaedic surgeon again and reluctantly accepted that further surgery would not help. But he had maintained the gains made in the group and although he did not feel fit to return to the rigs, was seeking other work. He went out socially two or three times a week, walked the dog daily and had taken up archery.

 Chronic pain and disability are sometimes the result of an industrial accident or an unsuccessful medical procedure, and patients may sue for negligence. Cases can take years to come to court. During this period, what are the factors involved in terms of operant conditioning?

Think of the potential reinforcement for pain-related behaviour.

While waiting for a settlement, it is not in the patient's financial interest to show any improvement. It is often very difficult for independent medical opinion to determine just how much the person is affected by pain, and it is hard for those trying to help the patient: in fact it may not be appropriate to attempt rehabilitation or pain management until a case is over, yet the assessment of compensation needs to take into account how much the person is affected, once they have recovered as much as possible.

Consider Fergus's case history above. If he were suing the oil company for compensation, do you think he would have taken part in the pain management programme?

The management of pain

- Pain management involves a multi-disciplinary team who assess a patient and design an appropriate treatment package.
- Psychological treatments include both cognitive and behavioural techniques.
- Cognitive techniques aim to work by changing the interpretation of pain sensations.
- Behavioural techniques are used by patients to alter responses to pain.
- Cognitive-behavioural techniques include records of treatment, progress and outcome on a range of measures for review by both the patient and staff.

THE ROLE OF CARERS

Doctors need to be aware of informal carers for two reasons; firstly, because caring for an elderly, chronically sick or disabled relative may affect the health of the carer, and secondly, because community care (see pp. 146–147) relies on families to take on the role of carer.

Caring has been divided into responsibility for the person (as may be the case for example when caring for an adult with schizophrenia) or carrying out of direct care tasks (as when caring for an elderly parent no longer able to care for him- or herself).

ROLE OF CARERS

Different models of care give carers different roles. Twigg and Atkin (1991) have suggested four models: carers as a resource, as co-workers, as co-clients, and when superseded.

Carers as a resource

This is probably the most common view: that it is the natural order of things for a family to be responsible for the care of its members. This is the background against which current British community care policies are set. The focus of services is on the dependent person and the aim is to maximise the level of informal care. There is little concern for the well-being of carers, who are only doing their duty. The White Paper 'Caring for people — community care in the next decade and beyond' (1989) clearly states this policy:

'The greater part of care has been, is and always will be provided by families and friends.' (Foreword)
'The government acknowledges that the great bulk of community care is provided by friends, family and neighbours. The decision to take on a caring role is never an easy one... However, many people make that choice and it is right that they should be able to play their part in looking after those close to them...' (Paragraph 1.9)

Carers as co-workers

This model also aims to maintain and increase informal care, but acknowledges that to do so the needs of carers must be recognised — both psychological and physical needs such as domestic help, aids and time away, including holidays. Support for relatives may be provided along with education and advice, the latter aimed at making 'caring' more

appropriate. This raises questions of how far relatives are being turned into quasi-professionals, and the appropriateness of this. In the mental health field psycho-education groups for relatives of people with schizophrenia are popular. These give information, offer advice about coping and problem solving and often aim to alter the emotional atmosphere of the family and thus reduce relapse (Lam 1991).

Carers as co-clients

Here the carer becomes an indirect client and is thus a legitimate focus for support and services. This may cause confusion in the health service where the formal status of 'patient' is clear, but may prove less of a problem for social work where the definition of 'client' is more accommodating. Thus carers may find it easier to get help and support in the social services than through the NHS unless such services can be seen to have a direct clinical outcome. Family therapy treats all members as 'patients' or 'clients'.

Superseded carers

The last model looks to the future of the dependent person, aiming to make him or her independent and thus not (or less) reliant on the support of the carer. This model may be most appropriate for those dependent on parents. Not only is it better for disabled persons to have greater independence for themselves but it helps answer the question of who will look after them when their parents are themselves unable to cope.

IMPACT OF CARING ON THE FAMILY

The impact on the family is usually referred to as 'burden', being either objective (that which can be objectively measured and externally validated) or subjective (that which is perceived by the carer). It should be noted that objective burden and subjective burden are not necessarily correlated (Platt 1985).

Objective burden

Objective burden comprises the things which are externally observable and objectively quantifiable.

Financial problems include loss of earnings if the carer has to give up their job, as well as additional costs ranging from extra laundry or heating to special aids and trips to hospital. The loss of employment not only affects finances but deprives the carer of outside contact and a role other than that of carer.

The disruption of household can be severe, particularly in terms of loss of freedom and privacy, which includes the difficulty couples may have in spending time alone together. Children may be affected through restrictions on their lives, particularly if they become carers for parents.

The tasks vary, depending on the needs of the person being cared for. For elderly dependants care may focus on physical

---

Case study

Mrs McLeod (65) lives alone with her son Alex (34) who has had schizophrenia since he was 19. He has lived with his parents apart from a few short stays in hospital. Mr McLeod died 8 years ago. They are visited occasionally by Alex's sister, but an older brother has moved away and doesn't want any contact.

Alex hears voices, spends most of the day in bed and is up at night wandering round the house, smoking and playing music loudly. Mrs McLeod asks him to turn the sound down because of complaints from neighbours, but this leads to bitter arguments. At other times Alex gets very anxious and depressed and wakes his mother to talk to her. She gets very little sleep and is constantly tired. Although she had smoke alarms fitted Mrs McLeod still worries about the risk of fire as Alex often leaves cigarettes burning. All the furniture has burn marks.

His only trips out of the house are to the clinic for medication and to buy cigarettes. He refuses to attend a day centre. He used to go walking at night but since being mugged he has stopped this.

Mrs McLeod also rarely goes out as she does not like leaving Alex alone, both because she fears what might happen and because she feels guilty when he is alone. Because Alex doesn't like anyone coming into the house and because of his sometimes bizarre behaviour she has stopped inviting anyone. Her two great worries are whether she did anything that might have made Alex schizophrenic and what is going to happen when she dies.

tasks, and the drudgery of the unremitting tasks involved in caring for someone who can do little for him- or herself should not be underestimated. Where the dependent person has a mental illness, care may focus more on supervision and taking responsibility, perhaps for finances or medication. Behaviour which causes most concern to families is usually that which is socially disturbing or embarrassing, or which puts the person at risk.

The effect on the carer's health, both physical and mental, is both an objective burden and the consequence of objective and subjective burdens. Green (1988) reports that approximately two-thirds of carers are themselves in poor health, with about half at risk of a psychiatric illness (depression, anxiety). Many suffer physical injury, predominantly to their backs, from lifting. Social isolation is a problem both in terms of its own impact on the life of carers and because it contributes to other problems. The majority of carers receive no help from outside sources, and the amount of time spent caring can severely restrict the carers' involvement with the world outside the family.

Subjective burden

Subjective burden is difficult to measure objectively and is, to some extent, how the carer feels about caring. Thus social isolation is not just the absence of outside contacts, but the extent to which the carer feels isolated and withdrawn. Carers may feel their independence is eroded, together with their freedom and their sense of identity.

Stigma is experienced both by people with particular conditions (see pp. 120–121) and by their carers, and reflects society's negative view. It may be a feature of being made to feel that they have contributed to the problem (e.g. a child's

mental illness) or it otherwise reflects on them, as the following quotes suggest:

> *'How can I tell anyone my husband's schizophrenic? They'll think there must be something wrong with me to have married him in the first place.' (wife)*
> *'My mother-in-law blames me. Said there was nothing wrong with him before he met me.' (wife)*
> *'Sometimes I just want to kill us both. I'm getting on … can't go on like this much longer … what's to become of him? If I did it … we'd both be at peace.' (mother)*

The emotional impact includes everything from anxiety, depression, despair, hopelessness and helplessness to resentment, frustration and anger. Stress results when the carer is unable to continue coping with the demands being made. This may be exacerbated by guilt and worry that they aren't doing enough or that they have somehow contributed to the problem. Concern about the future is especially important for elderly carers who worry about what will happen when they die.

Lastly, the role of carer has an impact as it changes the relationship between two people. For a woman, it is often expected and becomes an extension of the role she had been performing all her life, especially if caring for a child who has now grown into an adult. Roles are reversed when caring for parents, and when caring for a spouse the mutual support in the relationship may be lost. The role of carer usually falls on one person in a family, most commonly a woman (see Fig. 1, Table 1).

Research has tended to concentrate on the negative aspects of caring and it is easy to ignore that caring for a loved one can bring rewards and pleasure as well as burdens and sorrow.

- As a general practitioner, how does your responsibility to the ill or disabled person (the dependant) conflict with your responsibility to the carer (who may also be your patient)?
- Should relatives have the right to choose whether they care, or to what extent, for a dependent relative? What happens (and who pays) if they choose not to?

Carers' complaints

Not being recognised as providers of care is central to other problems such as lack of adequate services, support and lack of information and advice. This may be particularly strong where people feel they had no choice in taking on the caring role.

CURRENT POSITION

Both social work and the health service now have to take account of carers' views when planning services. The Carers (Recognition and Services) Act 1995 gives carers their place in the provision of care. No new resources, however, have been forthcoming to implement the Act.

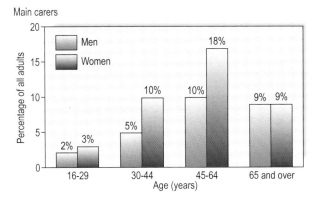

Fig. 1 **Percentage of all adults who are main carers.** (Source: Green 1988.)

Table 1 **Percentage of adults (aged 16 and over) who were carers by sex, age and marital status**

Sex and marital status	Age				
	16–29	30–44	45–64	≥ 65	Total
	Percentage who were carers				
Men					
married	6	11	17	16	13
single	6	12	16	9	8
widowed, divorced or separated	[4]	10	16	7	11
Women					
married	8	16	24	18	18
single	7	14	29	15	10
widowed, divorced or separated	9	20	20	8	13
All adults					
married	7	14	20	17	16
single	6	12	22	13	9
widowed, divorced or separated	10	17	19	8	12
Source: Green 1988					

The role of carers

- The first line of care for most people with chronic illness/disability.
- There are four models of care: carers as resources, co-workers, co-clients and superseded carers.
- Burden can be objective or subjective.
- Major problems are lack of recognition, lack of services and lack of information.

SELF-HELP GROUPS

No doctor or health professional can afford to ignore the rise of the self-help movement in the management of illness, disability and social problems. Self-help ranges from the large, national organisations to small, unique local groups. All have arisen from people wanting to take more control of their lives and responsibility for the management of their illness/ disability. Probably the largest and most famous self-help organisation is Alcoholics Anonymous (AA) (see pp. 78–79) with its 12-step programme (Table 1). This is a model followed by other organisations such as Gamblers Anonymous, Narcotics Anonymous and Overeaters Anonymous. The concepts behind the 12-step programme have been incorporated into some professionally-run services.

Table 1 **Twelve steps of Alcoholics Anonymous**

1—We admitted we were powerless over alcohol — that our lives had become unmanageable.

2—Came to believe that a Power greater than ourselves could restore us to sanity.

3—Made a decision to turn our will and our lives over to the care of God *as we understood Him.*

4—Made a searching and fearless moral inventory of ourselves.

5—Admitted to God, to ourselves and to another human being the exact nature of our wrongs.

6—Were entirely ready to have God remove all these defects of character.

7—Humbly asked Him to remove our shortcomings.

8—Made a list of all persons we had harmed, and became willing to make amends to them all.

9—Made direct amends to such people wherever possible, except when to do so would injure them or others.

10—Continued to take personal inventory and when we were wrong promptly admitted it.

11—Sought through prayer and meditation to improve our conscious contact with God *as we understood Him,* praying only for knowledge of His will for us and the power to carry that out.

12—Having had a spiritual awakening as the result of these steps, we tried to carry this message to alcoholics and to practise these principles in all our affairs.

TYPES OF SELF-HELP GROUPS

Self-help groups divide into two broad categories — those whose aim is to help members and those with a primarily campaigning role, aiming to change public attitudes and policy, although many include both aims.

In the health field, self-help groups exist for practically every condition whether defined as illness or some 'deviation from the norm'. There are groups for people with life-long conditions (e.g. Association of Cystic Fibrosis Adults), chronic medical conditions (e.g Ileostomy Association), mental health problems (e.g. MIND), and people who define themselves as survivors — of the system (e.g. Survivors Speak Out) or of abuse (e.g. Incest Survivors Group). Groups exist for relatives (e.g. National Schizophrenia Fellowship). Other groups exist for those experiencing traumatic life events including bereavement (e.g. Compassionate Friends).

FUNCTIONS OF SELF-HELP GROUPS

Support

The emotional support, acceptance and understanding that comes from others in a similar position cannot be overestimated and the importance of social support has been discussed elsewhere (pp. 52–53). For particularly stigmatised or disadvantaged groups their main source of social contact and friendship may come through such groups. Some people may feel more stigmatised by being expected to socialise with such people, or see it as a sign of weakness. A study of bereavement

support groups (Levy and Derby 1992) suggested that joiners were viewed as less self-sufficient. Members of the British Council of Organisations of Disabled People (BCODP) who organise the 'Rights not Charity' demonstrations are more likely to view themselves as political than those who do not join.

Role models

Those who have overcome or learned to live with the problem provide a powerful model for others in the same position and can offer a hopeful and optimistic view of the future.

Information and advice about coping

Both patients and relatives complain of lack of information; this is collated and disseminated by self-help groups, and ranges from public lectures to specially written booklets (Fig. 1) to discussion groups. Information can shade into advice about coping, and even counselling. One study showed that as well as support, gaining information was the main reason women attended a Breast Cancer Support Group. They received information on specific and supplementary treatments, and general information on breast cancer. The authors conclude 'surgeons, oncologists… have neither the time nor sometimes the awareness of the need to deal with the problems expressed' (Stevenson and Coles 1993).

Coping strategies

Those with the problem usually have more to offer in the way of practical

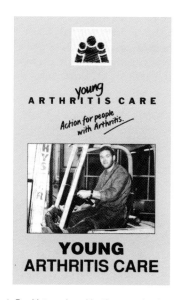

Fig. 1 **Booklet produced by the organisation Arthritis Care.**

advice about day-to-day management of the disorder and general strategies for coping than do most professionals.

Ideology

Self-help groups have their own philosophies with which members identify and which may or may not be in line with current professional thinking. When alternative views are put forward there is likely to be tension, if not hostility between and within groups. People may seek out groups which support their position; thus it is suggested that carers' groups such as the National Schizophrenia Fellowship (UK) and the National Alliance of the Mentally Ill (USA) focus on schizophrenia as biological illness whereas the users' organisation MIND (UK) takes a more personal/social/political view of mental illness. The recognition of shared beliefs is an important part of support.

Mutual aid

In self-help groups, help is reciprocal and the giving as well as receiving of help is fundamental. Giving help has a range of benefits including increased meaning and purpose to one's own life, increased feelings of self-worth and confidence, the positive reinforcement, both personal and social, that comes from helping and even the rehearsal of coping strategies by advising others. AA is explicit about this reciprocal help, its twelfth step requiring members to take the message to other alcoholics (Table 1).

Most self-help groups engage in face-to-face contact, although the number of support groups springing up on the Internet suggests this is not always necessary.

Empowerment

Patients frequently feel powerless in the face of both their illness and the medical profession. Self-help groups foster empowerment in two ways. One is through information, education and advice about the illness and coping, thus giving the individual some sense of mastery and control. Secondly, self-help groups may seek to influence service delivery and policy both nationally and locally and educate the public with the aim of changing public attitudes. This can be seen as a more consumer-oriented approach to empowerment. Some groups specifically challenge the media portrayal of their disability. Disability rights groups, for example, picket the 'Children

in Need' appeal to make people aware of their views and their objection to charity.

Self-help and service provision

Small local self-help groups which aim to do nothing more than offer support and advice within the group will continue to flourish although individual groups may wax and wane, dependent largely on the health of those who run them. In Britain as elsewhere, the development of community care (see pp. 146–147), has pushed many self-help groups to become service providers. Groups have gained grants to provide services directly (to client groups rather than just members) and the distinction between self-help groups and voluntary organisations is sometimes not clear. In some areas, particularly mental health and physical disability, the user movement is strong and overlaps with self-help groups.

Although this has positive aspects, as services are more likely to be tailored to users' needs and those most involved have a say in the running of services, it can also have some less desirable consequences. Self-help projects usually suffer from insecure, short-term funding and can be used to plug gaps in services rather than adequately resourcing statutory agencies. Groups may lose their 'mutual aid' orientation and the centrality of the user's experience may be diminished as staff are brought in to run the organisation and its services. In the chase after money to fund services some of the campaigning and more 'political' aspects of the group may be lost in an attempt not to offend potential funders.

Case study
National Schizophrenia Fellowship (NSF)

The template for many relatives'/carers' groups in mental health world-wide is the NSF which was founded in November 1972 as a charity. On 9th May 1970 John Pringle published a letter in *The Times*, 'A case of schizophrenia', describing what it was like to live with someone with schizophrenia. The response was overwhelming and today there are over 160 branches in Britain. Strong regional development in the 1980s led to NSF (Scotland) being established in 1984 and the Northern Fellowship and the North-West Fellowship in the north of England.

At its heart the NSF is an organisation which offers support to carers of people with schizophrenia, and 90% of its membership are carers. Local groups, usually run by a relative, meet regularly to share information, advice, problems, experiences and feelings and to gain support, acceptance and help with coping. Professionals often give lectures and participate in discussion; although some groups have ongoing professional support to maintain them, the focus is on carer experience and control.

The Fellowship has always had a campaigning role and, although not opposed to the closure of mental hospitals, it campaigns for this not to exceed the rate of replacement community services and also emphasises the need for asylum. The NSF, both locally and nationally, responds to consultation documents and community care plans. It is frequently viewed as *the* voice of carers of the mentally ill, despite being predominantly white and middle-class. It has always been active educationally, running local and national conferences for members and professionals, and in many areas carers speak to groups of nurses, social workers and doctors in training, giving their perspective on life with schizophrenia, the role of relatives as carers and their response to services.

The NSF is now firmly in the arena of service provision, running drop-in centres, employment projects, cafés, housing projects and respite care. The rapid expansion in service provision can be seen simply by looking at the accounts. In 1988–9 the turnover was £769 143 but by 1992–3 this had expanded by £6.1 million.

The NSF has spawned similar organisations throughout the world which meet together as the World Schizophrenia Fellowship. Founded in 1982, its membership includes Australia, Austria, Canada, Colombia, France, Germany, Great Britain, India, Indonesia, Ireland, Israel, Japan, Malaysia, Netherlands, New Zealand, South Africa, United States and Uruguay.

STOP THINK

- What can professionals gain from being involved with a self-help group?
- Is there a danger that self-help could be seen as a 'cheap alternative' to other services?

Self-help groups

- Provide an alternative to the traditional approach.
- Value personal experience.
- Seek to empower members.
- Have roles as service providers and campaigners as well as offering support.

PALLIATIVE CARE

SPECIALIST CARE FOR THE DYING —WHY IS THERE A NEED?

In the latter half of the last century, as families grew smaller and hospitals became more accessible, the process of dying shifted from the home to the institution. Refuges, founded mainly by religious orders, were dedicated specifically to the care of the dying. These were known as hospices. With the development of modern medicine and its emphasis on diagnosis and cure, death became less acceptable. As a result, it is argued, patients with incurable disease became isolated in large acute wards and their physical and emotional problems were neglected. The need became apparent, therefore, to develop hospice care as an alternative approach to caring for the terminally ill (Naysmith and O'Neill 1989).

THE DEVELOPMENT OF PALLIATIVE CARE

The main pioneer of the hospice movement in Britain was Dame Cicely Saunders, who worked both as a volunteer nurse and social worker and later as a doctor at two of the first London Hospices, St Joseph's and St Luke's. This experience made her aware of the need for a centre which would specialise in pain and symptom control in the terminal stages of disease but also provide an environment that would allow people to adjust emotionally and spiritually to their approaching death (Saunders and Sykes 1993). Her subsequent foundation of St Christopher's Hospice in London as a centre of excellence provided the cornerstone of the modern hospice movement in both Europe and America. Its rapid expansion over the past two decades has been accompanied by the recognition of the care of the dying as a medical speciality. The term 'palliative care' has replaced the older term 'terminal care' to describe the care of the person in the final stages of life (Doyle, Hanks et al 1993). In 1990 the World Health Organization defined it as 'the active care of patients whose disease is not responsive to curative treatment'. It also developed guiding principles for practitioners (WHO 1990) which stated that palliative care:

- affirms life and regards dying as a normal process
- neither hastens nor postpones death
- provides relief from pain and other distressing symptoms
- integrates the psychological and spiritual aspects of patient care
- offers a support system to help patients live as actively as possible until death
- offers a support system to help the family cope during the patient's illness and their own bereavement.

Although the advent of hospice care has dramatically improved the care of terminally ill people, particularly in the area of pain control, evidence suggests that these guidelines are still not being met in every setting in which the terminally ill are cared for. There is therefore an increasing drive to make hospice standards of care available for all dying patients and not an exception for a small minority.

SETTINGS

In the past, hospice care has largely been confined to those patients who were dying from cancer because most were funded by charitable contributions. An important consequence of the expansion of the hospice movement however has been the spread of its principles and goals to other places of care. Palliative care services now exist in a wide variety of forms ranging from autonomous centres funded by charity, to hospital support teams, to designated palliative care wards in large acute hospitals. In addition, specialist palliative home care teams can assist general practitioners in caring for patients who choose to die at home.

TOTAL PAIN

The philosophy of the hospice movement is the alleviation of total pain and the affirmation of the quality of life remaining. This means tackling not only physical pain (see pp. 132–133) but also any emotional, psychological, social or spiritual problems the patient has which might contribute to the patient's total distress (Fig. 1).

As Figure 1 shows, the extent of a patient's pain may be affected by a whole range of physical, psychological, social and situational factors which may influence his/her ability to cope with it. Physical effects of the disease process and treatment, for example radiotherapy or surgery, may therefore be exacerbated or precipitated by other complications of the illness. These may include anger at medical staff over unnecessary delays in diagnosis, lack of communication from them or failure to provide a cure, anxiety about other family members, finances or prognosis, or depression resulting from the loss of job, role, or function, which the illness may have entailed.

The concept of *spiritual pain* is often the most difficult aspect of pain for doctors and other carers to manage because it is less tangible and sometimes not easily distinguishable from psychological pain. In addition, it may be present in patients who have no strong religious beliefs. Guidelines from The World Health Organisation state that the spiritual aspect of human life is concerned 'with meaning and purpose and for those nearing the end of life, this is commonly associated with a need for forgiveness, reconciliation and affirmation of worth'.

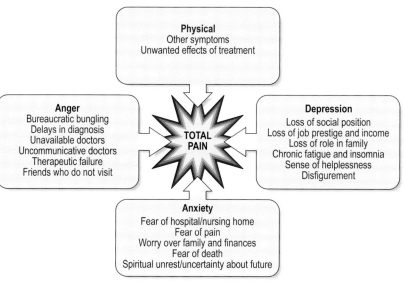

Fig. 1 **Composition of total pain, and factors influencing sensitivity.** (Source: Twycross, 1994)

The degree to which individuals are free from total pain will therefore depend on the ability of their carers to understand and treat its many causes.

THE MULTI-DISCIPLINARY TEAM

The need for a multi-disciplinary team of health professionals who will work together and as individuals is therefore essential to the concept of tackling total pain. Core members will include medical and nursing staff, social workers, chaplains, physiotherapists and occupational therapists.

However, the individual needs of the patient and his/her family will dictate which member of the team plays a central role. For example, in the case of a patient with persistent nausea it may be the doctor who directs the patient's care. On the other hand, a patient who is facing severe financial difficulties due to loss of work as a result of the illness may need most help from the medical social worker. The team should delegate tasks amongst its members to ensure that its resources are mobilised effectively and care prioritised in order to meet each individual's needs as efficiently as possible. Specialist nurses are often employed to provide a link between the hospice/hospital and the patient's own home. These nurses are specially trained in palliative care. They act as a resource for other community staff like general practitioners to allow patients to stay at home for as long as possible, and by helping to control difficult and problematic symptoms. In Britain, they are called Macmillan or Marie Curie nurses after the charities which fund them.

Case study

Jane was a 49-year-old woman with cancer of the breast and bony metastasis. She was married to Adam, a lawyer, and had two teenage daughters, Sara and Louise. Her prognosis was poor and after receiving a course of palliative radiotherapy, she had come home to spend her remaining time with her family. Neither daughter knew how serious their mother's condition was, though both suspected that it was not good because of the number of health professionals constantly visiting the house. Both Jane and her husband thought that in protecting their daughters from the truth they were shielding them from unnecessary anxiety and grief. As a result, relationships in the family were strained, both girls were doing badly at school and Jane was experiencing uncontrolled pain and nausea which prevented her from sleeping and eating properly. At this point the General Practitioner, after consulting the District Nurse, decided to refer Jane to the Macmillan Nurse for advice on pain control and help with improving communications among the family. As her visits to the family progressed, Jane and Adam were encouraged to share their knowledge of Jane's prognosis with their daughters. Both learned that instead of protecting their daughters they were in fact alienating them, causing them to feel confused and isolated. Gradually, through open communication, Louise and Sara came to accept that their mother was dying, but that as a family they could still make the most of the time that was left. Jane was also given a different form of pain relief: a syringe driver which administered analgesia continuously while allowing her to remain as mobile and unrestricted as possible. In the end Jane died peacefully and comfortably at home surrounded by Adam and her daughters.

COMMUNICATION

The effectiveness of the team will largely depend on good communication between its members and between itself and other health professionals as well as patients and their families. The hospice philosophy stresses the importance of open communication between the patient, carer and professional. Open awareness and truth telling with cancer patients are now becoming accepted practices, but the extent to which the patient and carer are fully informed will depend on their understanding of the information imparted by health professionals and their willingness to confront their diagnosis and prognosis as well as the ability of health professionals to provide clear messages (see pp. 92–93).

 STOP THINK Write down how you think Jane's daughters felt when initially they were not told of the seriousness of her condition. Think of how you would go about breaking down the barriers to communication between the family. Imagine that you were the Macmillan Nurse in this situation, and plan what you would say to Jane and Adam. Think how you might negotiate between them and Sara and Louise.

THE FUTURE OF PALLIATIVE CARE

As with every other medical speciality, practitioners of palliative care are increasingly having to be accountable for the care they provide. New measures are now being developed to assess the physical and psychosocial well-being of patients with advanced cancer and other terminal illnesses. One of the most common measures used is quality of life. Quality of life scales, which conceptualise the physical and psychosocial needs of patients in multi-dimensional instruments, provide outcome measures of care which go beyond the traditional end-points of tumour size, side effects of treatment, and survival (see pp. 40–41). These can enable doctors and researchers to evaluate the care patients receive more holistically and allow comparisons of care to be made across settings, between patients with different types of cancer, and between patients at different stages of the disease process.

Palliative care

- The provision of terminal care has been revolutionised by the modern hospice movement, particularly in the area of pain control.
- With the growth of the hospice movement has come the recognition of the care of the dying as a medical speciality known as palliative medicine.
- The philosophy of the hospice movement emphasises the alleviation of total pain and the patient and his/her carer as a unit of care.
- Palliative care is provided by a multi-disciplinary team of health professionals including doctors and nurses, physio and occupational therapists, social workers, pastoral staff and nurses specifically trained to be advisors in palliative care (e.g. Macmillan or Marie Curie nurses).
- Quality of life measures are now being developed to enable doctors and researchers to measure and evaluate the physical and psychosocial well-being of patients. These conceptualise patients' needs in multi-dimensional instruments and provide outcomes of care which allow comparisons to be made across settings and between patients with different types of cancer and at different stages.

ORGANISING AND FUNDING HEALTH CARE

The organisation and funding of health care affects patients as well as health care providers. Doctors, as health care providers, might be restricted in their own actions owing to the existing organisation of health care, or they might feel that their patients' access to certain expensive tests or interventions is restricted.

 In what ways is the government of your country involved in the provision of health care?

Health care systems all over the world seem to be facing a funding crisis. The main issue here is the allocation of scarce resources. This is not simply a question of money but also of political decision-making and priorities. In order to understand the current organisation and funding of health care, we have to look at historical developments and the underlying political decision-making process.

We concentrate on three countries, the UK (with a predominantly state-run welfare system), the USA (with a predominantly free-market system), and Germany (with a mixed health economy), representing the major ways health care is organised and funded (see Case study). Total expenditure on health (including private and public health expenditure) in these three countries differs considerably, as does the proportion of the gross national product spent on health care.

UNITED KINGDOM

All citizens of the UK are included in the NHS. The NHS is a universal, tax-funded health care system (Judge and Mays 1994). Doctors, nurses and hospitals are paid by the state for the provision of care. The NHS requires some additional payments from patients, for example for prescriptions and dental check-ups, but the overwhelming majority of care provision is free of charge. Treatment is decided on (mostly) by doctors. General Practitioners are gate-keepers in this system, selecting patients and referring patients to the appropriate specialist. Medical care is available to all, thus also without stigma to the poor. However, there is a problem of waiting lists in certain areas of medical care (see pp. 144–145). This has stimulated an increase in the small (about 12% in the early 1990s), but growing, private health care sector, which is often provided by the same doctors in the same hospitals as the standard NHS care.

USA

The American system, compared to the NHS or other European health provision systems, is predominantly commercial insurance-based (Navarro 1989). Most people take out their own private health insurance. These insurance companies reimburse doctors, hospitals, and others, for care provided. Most people have the freedom to go to the medical professional or hospital of their choice. A limited number of people are covered by state-organised schemes, such as Medicaid, which provides health care for the poor, but eligibility is incomplete and coverage usually excludes dental services and prescribed drugs, and Medicare, for all people over 65, which provides limited coverage. Over 20 million people are not insured or are seriously under-insured.

GERMANY

Of the German population, 90% are insured by one of 1300 sick funds, which are funded by income-related contributions and are self-governing and self-financing institutions. The average contribution rate is approximately 13% of an employee's gross income. Half of the contributions are paid by the employers and the other half by the employees. Self-employed persons and employees earning over a certain ceiling are allowed to opt out of the statutory insurance scheme and join one of the 66 private health insurance companies. As in the UK, family doctors are gate-keepers in this system, selecting patients and referring patients to the appropriate specialist. Patients receive comprehensive coverage which entitles them to unlimited primary and hospital care. The sick funds reimburse the doctors, hospitals and pharmacists for delivery of their services. Privately insured people pay the doctor or pharmacist and their insurance company reimburses the patient. Legal restrictions and government regulations limit the freedom of the sick funds to control cost, prices and the quantities and range of provisions.

 What are the main differences in the way health care is organised in the USA on the one hand, and in Germany and the UK on the other?

WHAT ARE THE ADVANTAGES OF EACH SYSTEM?

The German national insurance-funded and the British tax-funded systems have many similarities as predominantly universal and comprehensive systems. The two are more similar to each other than either is to the American system. Therefore the European collective system will be compared with the American private system.

Case study — three different ways of funding and organising health care provision

United Kingdom
- State-run national health service funded mainly through taxation
- Every citizen covered
- Per capita spending on health US$ 1039
- 5.7% of GNP spent on health services

United States of America
- Mainly private health insurance system with market-based health care provision
- 10% population not covered
- Per capita spending on health US$ 2354
- 13.6% of GNP spent on health services

Germany
- National health insurance-based system with a market-based health care system
- Every citizen covered
- Per capita spending on health US$ 1511
- 8.7% of GNP spent on health services

Table 1 **Collective systems of health care: advantages and disadvantages**

Advantages	Disadvantages
Social citizenship/cohesion	Reduces individual responsibility
Combats the Inverse Care Law[1]	Increases deference towards the doctor
No fee results in less over-doctoring	Free care encourages trivial complaints
More scope for coordinated planning	Impedes search for market-solutions
Bargaining-power economies of scale	Vote-catching discourages quality
Tax-revenue is cheap to collect	Higher public spending
Easier to meet emergencies: e.g. AIDS, war	Makes health a political football

[1] The Inverse Care Law argues that the provision of health care in a market economy is inversely related to the need for it; in other words poor facilities are to be found in depressed areas characterised by high morbidity, and better facilities in affluent areas characterised by low morbidity (Tudor Hart 1971: 405).

Table 2 **Advantages and disadvantages of private systems of health care**

Advantages	Disadvantages
Liberal citizenship/choice	Choice only for those who can pay
Market: best mechanism for regulating any distribution	Health insurance market does not equate health care market
Similar quality care for low price; better care for higher price	Many cannot afford the higher price
Direct service and short waiting lists	Inverse Care Law: services concentrated
Improvements stimulated by market	Improvement stimulated by profit, not need
Patients = consumers, i.e. know their rights	Patients still depend on doctors' opinion

Table 1 lists some of the main advantages and disadvantages of collective health care systems. Some of the listed issues are political, others more clearly medical. For example, the first advantage is obviously political: it expresses ideals of shared citizenship and enhances social cohesiveness in society. On the other hand, the issue that 'free care encourages trivial complaints' has a direct impact on the doctor. If care is free for the patients we might expect that more people will come forward with relatively minor complaints.

Table 2 shows some of the main advantages and disadvantages of private health care. For example, in the first advantage, 'liberal citizenship/choice', Americans have the freedom to shop around for their health care; they can decide to have an all-inclusive insurance or only insure for hospital treatment. They are not told by the state what they must do; this is a very political argument. The first disadvantage 'reduction of individual responsibility' refers to the fact that the American way of organising has resulted in a health insurance market, not a health care market. Consequently people who have a good medical insurance cover have little incentive to seek lower prices for health care. This is one of the reasons why the system is so expensive. Finally, an issue concerning doctors directly is the extent to which patients have a choice. For example, whether they opt for brain surgery, chiropractic or psychiatric treatment is not completely a free choice, since most patients will be unable to judge the quality and the usefulness of the services on offer. Furthermore, the increase in patients' complaints and litigation indicates that patients are dissatisfied with the services provided. However, this is not completely a problem of private medicine, since the number of complaints and court cases in the UK is also on the increase.

PAYING THE DOCTOR

These are observations of imperfections in the different ways of organising health care, not judgements about these systems. Take for example the remuneration of the doctor's fees. There is no right way of fixing the doctor's payment. Every method of payment has significant disadvantages: a fee-for-service payment may have the effect of encouraging some doctors to advise more treatment than is really necessary, whereas payment on a capitation basis, i.e. number of patients on the roll, may mean that doctors are in too much of a hurry to give adequate individual attention to each patient.

CONVERGENCE

There appears to be a tendency for the different models of health care provision to converge. In the 1990s the Clinton Administration pushed for reforms in the health care system that would increase the role of the state, while in countries with a national health care system (e.g. the UK) or national health insurance system (e.g. Germany) governments are trying to increase the role of the market.

Case study

In Britain, the Conservative government (partly on the advice of an American health economist) introduced in 1990 an 'internal market' into the National Health Service (Fig. 1). The intention of the reforms was to encourage greater cost-effectiveness and value-for-money by introducing competition. 'Service providers' (local hospital and community trusts) compete with each other to win contracts from 'purchasers' (health authorities and GP fund-holders) to provide services to patients at an agreed standard of quality and cost. There is considerable debate as to whether or not the internal market is achieving its object of greater cost-effectiveness, and its introduction has exacerbated problems of equity (see pp. 44–45).

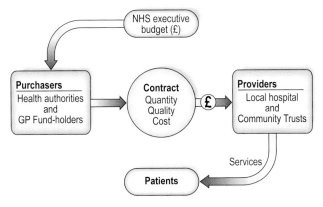

Fig. 1 **Simplified model of 'internal market'.**

Organising and funding health care

- The organisation of a nation's health care system is closely related to the way it is funded.
- Public and private health care and health funding systems both have specific advantages and disadvantages.
- It seems as if the different health care systems are converging.

ASSESSING NEEDS

The health services are constantly in a state of flux due to alterations at the supply side of care, for example the appearance of new drugs, the introduction of new medical technology, and managers' attempts to make services more efficient and effective. Health services are also changing through alterations in demand, for example the changing composition of the population (more people live longer), the appearance of new diseases (HIV/AIDS for instance) and changing preferences among consumers of health care for certain kinds of treatment. Somewhere in this pool of potentially conflicting interests we have to establish the needs of individuals, communities and populations whilst ensuring that each receives maximum benefit within the limits of available resources, such as staff, buildings and funding.

DIFFERENT KINDS OF NEED

The first distinction to make is the difference between (1) the need for health and (2) the need for health care. The former refers to the WHO definition of health: 'all aspects of physical and mental well-being'. The latter refers to the ability to benefit from health care or prevention services. It is therefore more specific and, as such, will depend on the health care and preventive services (potentially) available.

THE NEED FOR 'NEEDS' ASSESSMENT

Why does a service provider, a doctor or a hospital manager set about identifying the needs of people? Providers of health care need to know (a) what users need in the way of health care and (b) what is needed in a particular area, in order to achieve an improvement in the health of the population. These two objectives are not the same. What potential or actual service users feel they need (Fig. 1) might only partially overlap with what policy-makers consider to be the best possible range of services in an area that can improve the health of the people there ('normative needs'). Both types of needs have to be distinguished from 'expressed needs', the actual use or demand for a service, and 'comparative needs', which compares services across similar communities or client groups, for example comparing service available to people with HIV and those with cancer, or comparing services available in the West End of London with those in the East End. Thus need is not a unified concept.

NEEDS ASSESSMENT EXERCISES

It is difficult to assess all needs at the same time, since needs assessment exercises require funding and can be time-consuming like any other piece of research. Consequently, needs assessments usually focus on a specific illness and a limited area of care, thus assessing the needs of a particular group of (potential) patients in order to determine how their need might be met. When we consider the needs of the population in a given area we also have to ask questions such as: 'Whose needs do we take into consideration?' and 'Are we looking at the present needs of people currently ill or the potential future needs of the total population?'. The assessment of the needs of the local population also requires to be performed on a regular basis, since a population might change over time, and their actual or perceived needs might change. Planning health care provision takes time, whether it be training of doctors and nurses or building hospitals. Changing funding from one type of health service to another, such as the transformation from hospital care to community-based services, is also time-consuming.

Thus one of the main issues here is 'How do we firstly define, and secondly measure, *need*?'. The next main questions are: 'Who should perform a needs assessment?' and 'Whose definition of 'needs' is it to be based on: (a) lay people; (b) professionals; (c) researchers; (d) politicians; (e) managers; or (f) a combination of these groups?'.

STOP THINK | Can ordinary people assess their own health care needs, or does this process always require professional input?

One main issue in needs assessment exercises is the way one goes about researching health needs. We can focus on all people (healthy or unhealthy), or only on those with the specific disease or illness. The former is the most equal way of assessing the overall need in a population, whilst the latter ensures that those who know what it is to have a particular illness help to establish an overview of the needs of its sufferers. Both approaches also have drawbacks. Asking a sample of *all* people to identify needs will result in highlighting the need for provisions related to more common illnesses and related health services, and will underrepresent specific needs for people with 'rarer' or less 'acceptable' conditions (Hopton and Dlugolecka 1995). Conducting a needs assessment among

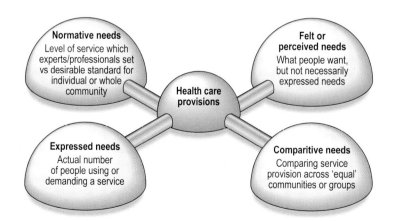

Fig. 1 **Types of needs in health care provision.** (Source: Bradshaw 1972)

Normative needs
Level of service which experts/professionals set vs desirable standard for individual or whole community

Felt or perceived needs
What people want, but not necessarily expressed needs

Health care provisions

Expressed needs
Actual number of people using or demanding a service

Comparitive needs
Comparing service provision across 'equal' communities or groups

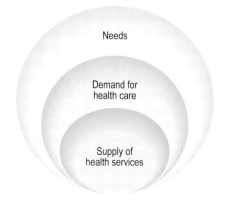

Fig. 2 **The relationship between needs, demand and supply.**

Needs

Demand for health care

Supply of health services

people with specific conditions will highlight needs which might be specific to them only, but not to the general population or to people with other conditions. Thus although previous users are likely to have a bias towards existing services, non-users are likely to lack experience and knowledge of the topic and will generally opt for provision for more common conditions.

The way a needs assessment is conducted can have an influence on its outcome. An uncritical social marketing approach may lead to more service for the general population, at the expense of specific services for those most in distress. Researchers can use the survey method in an attempt to reach a large sample of the total population of people whose needs we are assessing, or they can conduct focus groups with users to get to the depth of the issue.

 Would it be possible to combine the two research methods and investigate both the range and the depth of the perceived need? What problem might such an approach encounter?

The case study shows that the needs as assessed by different people all have a role to play in the provision of health services.

Case study
The organisation of maternity care

Epidemiologists and policy makers can establish the likely number of healthy babies that will be born in a city, region or any other area. This estimate will be based on (1) the number of women of childbearing age in the area and (2) the birth rate for that area, subtracting the likely number of mothers and babies needing specialist obstetric care before, during or after the delivery.

This information in itself will not be sufficient to predict the need for maternity services in the area. We need to ask women and their partners how and where they want the maternity services to provide health care. Do women want a predominantly midwife-led care, or do they want General Practitioner maternity care, or do they want shared care between doctors and midwives, or shared care between obstetricians and GPs? A further set of questions is: Where should these maternity services be delivered — at home, in a GP maternity unit, in a midwifery unit, or in a specialist obstetric hospital?

 Considering the Case study on the organisation of maternity care, what would you think will be the main needs identified by the following groups?

- General practitioners in the community
- Obstetricians in the regional hospital
- Regional health administrators
- Local politicians
- Community midwives
- Pregnant women
- Women of childbearing age but not currently pregnant

Remember to have another look at pages 2–3.

It is important to remember that a prediction of more pregnancies in a certain area does not automatically mean that more hospital beds and doctors are needed to cope with the increase in deliveries. Different illnesses require different approaches to service provision, and the needs assessment itself might vary according to the illness in question. It is likely that service users have less input in a needs assessment of hospital-based orthopaedic surgery than in one of community-based mental health care.

UNMET AND UNLIMITED NEEDS

There is a potential problem of unmet needs, as well as unlimited needs. The former issue refers to missing out people in assessing needs, whilst the latter refers to whether we will be able to fulfil the needs we identify in a needs assessment exercise. Asking people about their health problems in order to identify unmet needs might raise expectation about the service they expect to receive, but which we cannot provide. This has been exemplified in some areas of England in relation to needs assessment for community care services.

In Figure 2 three circles represent needs, demand and supply. Demand in this figure can be seen as the 'expressed needs' mentioned above. Figure 1 indicates that there might be needs (in the left hand corner) which are not as such recognised by those who have them. This implies that people other than the users have conducted the needs assessment.

The realisation that health needs are far more than demands from patients presented to the medical profession gave rise to the idea of a *clinical iceberg* or *iceberg of disease*. From a social science perspective the concept of an iceberg of disease is an indication that different perceived needs in different groups of people can lead to different reactions; some will result in seeking medical help while others will lead to self-medication or are simply ignored (see pp. 84–85).

WEAKNESSES OF NEEDS ASSESSMENT LED BY USERS

Needs assessment cannot be left completely to users: for example recreational drug users might not feel that they have a drugs problem, so a needs assessment exercise conducted among this group would indicate that there is no need for a problem drug service. However, we know that a small proportion of these recreational drug users will develop problems in the near future, leading to a need for specific drug services. Furthermore, needs assessment has to be linked to the provision of services. If needs assessments are conducted in different health and social services areas, we (society as a whole, i.e. our politicians) have to decide which of those needs have priority over others.

Assessing needs

- There is a difference between the need for health and the need for health services.
- There are four ways of defining need: normative need, felt need, expressed need and comparative need.
- Needs assessment should include the views of users, as well as lay public, professionals, managers, politicians and researchers.
- Different research methods will result in the identification of different needs.
- Needs assessment runs the risk of raising people's expectations and of not having the resources to meet them.

SETTING PRIORITIES AND RATIONING

The medical profession often has to prioritise treatment and ration services at a patient level. Any doctor who has been practising for some time can tell a personal story of having to choose between patients because resources are limited — whether staff, money, theatres or organ donors.

Rationing of health care has always taken place, however wealthy the country, but until recently it was done implicitly, was often invisible and often inequitable (see pp. 140–141). As spending on health services has increased in most countries, discussion about priorities and rationing has become more explicit. Thus, the question is not 'Will we have rationing?', but 'How will we organise rationing?'.

SECRET SUMMIT PLANS RATIONING FOR NHS: TOP DOCTORS TOLD PRIORITY-SETTING IS INEVITABLE

This headline in the British newspaper The Guardian (27-11-1995) indicates that rationing is regarded by some as (a) unavoidable and (b) neither popular nor desirable, hence the secrecy.

SETTING PRIORITIES

Setting priorities implies choosing a limited number of options from a wider range and ranking these in order of importance. Following on from priority setting is a process of rationing. Rationing is often defined as allocating scarce resources by some criteria other than the price mechanism. This does not mean that the price is not an important consideration, but that the price (or cost, which may not be the same as price) of a service, say a hip replacement, is not the only factor in the decision whether or not a patient who is in need of such surgery will receive treatment. Priority setting is a dynamic process, and in every budget cycle new technologies and information on health outcomes are taken into consideration in setting new priorities.

FORMS OF RATIONING

Rationing is a trade-off between providing all services to a limited number of people, or providing a limited number of services to all people. Rationing often involves a limitation of both the range and volume of service provision (example below from BMJ). Decisions regarding rationing also have to be made at different levels: at an individual, local/regional and national level.

'Neonatal care may become too expensive: Doctors at Sheffield's main maternity unit have been told that if demand for neonatal services continues to rise an "arbitrary ban" may have to be introduced, according to Panorama, a British documentary programme. This could mean that babies born more than 15 weeks prematurely could be refused treatment.'

This cutting from the British Medical Journal (1994: 309, p. 282) highlights the issue of limited availability of resources and the ever growing demand for medical services.

A variety of rationing mechanisms have been identified (Klein et al, 1996):

- **Denial:** for example, refusing to treat people over seventy for certain conditions.

- **Deterrence:** putting up social, economic or psychological barriers.
- **Dilution:** prescribing cheaper non-brand name drugs, or reducing length of stay in hospital.
- **Delay:** hospital waiting lists.
- **Deflection:** having GPs as gatekeepers; or referring an elderly person for local authority services rather than keeping him/her in hospital.

Free market provision of care is often not regarded as a form of rationing. Everybody who has enough money can buy any treatment, e.g. expensive operations, privately. However, many people will not have the money either to buy the service directly or to take out comprehensive private insurance. Hence, practically, the effect is similar to rationing.

UNDERLYING PRINCIPLES OF RATIONING

Having itemised some of the ways that services are rationed, we now consider some of the principles that underpin rationing. The key principle is generally considered to be 'equity' but a number of other principles are also important (see: Harrison and Hunter, 1994):

- **Equity:** ideally everyone should have a fair opportunity to attain their full health potential and, more pragmatically, no one should be disadvantaged from achieving their potential if it can be avoided. Equity could refer to access to health care, but also to healthy living conditions or equity of autonomy.
- **Needs:** the British NHS was introduced on the principle that people should receive health services on the basis of their health and medical need rather than their 'ability to pay', but 'need' is not a simple, clear concept (see pp. 142–143).
- **Equality:** all individuals have an equal access to health care. Should a 70-year-old smoker and heavy drinker have the same chance of getting the next available donor kidney as a 21-year-old non-smoker and non-drinker?
- **Effectiveness:** the ability of an intervention to achieve its intended effect in those to whom it is offered (i.e. does it work?).
- **Cost-effectiveness (efficiency):** the effectiveness of an intervention in relation to the resources used (e.g. time, labour, equipment and materials).
- **Quality adjusted life years (QALY's):** a technique for estimating the extra years of life gained from particular interventions, adjusted for the quality of the extra years. They are often combined with costs to give a 'cost per additional QALY', but there are many assumptions built into their calculation (see also pp. 40–41).

 STOP THINK What principles do you think should guide a decision to spend more money on either (a) clinical psychology services for people with depression, or (b) hip replacement surgery, both of which have six-month waiting lists? What information would you need to help you make a decision between them?

What effect would using different principles have on the decision?

DECISION-MAKING

In a democracy, we have to establish who should set priorities and ration services. Should it be doctors, administrators, politicians, service users, courts or some sort of consensus group?

Case study

During the second world war penicillin was scarce on the battlefields. Doctors had to make decisions on which soldiers would be treated and which not. The recovery rate of getting the soldiers back to the front was considerably higher among with those with a STD (sexually transmitted disease) rather than those with serious shot and shrapnel wounds. However, medical considerations (i.e. the highest recovery rate) were overruled by political (what people at home might think) and ethical considerations, such as 'soldiers with a STD are less deserving than those with bullet wounds'.

Case study
The Oregon experiment

The American state of Oregon pioneered a system for prioritising health care in an attempt to address the widespread problem in the US of the growing number of people who are without private health insurance and who are not eligible for federal assistance programmes. Most controversial of the reforms is the use by the legislature of a priority list of health services to determine benefit levels for the insurance programmes. In addition Oregon aimed to bring cover for the rationed services to everyone in the population. Priorities were set by a Health Services Commission initially on the basis of a technical methodology similar to 'cost per QALY', and subsequently on broad-based consensus through public consultation. The Health Services Commission came up with the following list of high priorities:

- acute, fatal conditions where treatment prevents death and leads to full recovery
- maternity care
- acute, fatal conditions where treatment prevents death, but does not lead to full recovery
- preventive care for children
- chronic, fatal conditions where treatment prolongs life and improves quality of care
- comfort or palliative care.

The next step was for the politicians to determine how much could be funded from existing and additional sources. This clearly brought the provision of health care to the centre of the political arena, since an increase in the health budget meant an increase in taxation or a decrease in the provision of other state provisions, for example in education. Thus the Oregon experiment introduced a rational plan for expanding services to the entire population of the state, while acknowledging the limitations of funding resources.

(Based on Kitzhaber, 1993)

Commissioning is one of the growing fields in health care where decisions have to be made by the purchasers of health care regarding the range, the quantity and the quality of health services bought for a specific population at a specific time. Setting priorities in Britain is now confused with purchasing and providing at a local level. The local NHS health care trusts in the 1990s are setting priorities and effectively taking decisions on the rationing of services. This is a case where decision-making about priority setting and rationing lies predominantly with the health care managers, and to a lesser extent the medical profession, but certainly not the services users.

One explicit reason for introducing GP fund-holding (and the subsequent GP purchasing/commissioning) was that GPs were said to be the health care professionals who were most in touch with the needs and wishes of patients and local communities.

Consultation of users

The appeal of the Oregon experiment (see Case study) lies, partly, in its explicit approach to rationing, partly, in community participation in priority setting. It is interesting to note that prevention comes high on the population's priority list.

Figure 1 shows the main possible results of the different forms of rationing, whereby medical and economic considerations are taken in to account. The bottom left-hand corner is the situation often found in the UK, the top right-hand corner is a serious possibility in any country with private medicine working for profit.

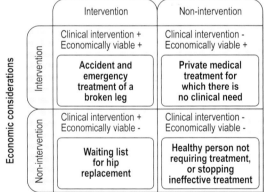

Fig. 1 Overview of medical and economic considerations in decision making.

Setting priorities and rationing

- All health care systems have some in-built form of rationing.
- Rationing takes different forms: denial, deterrence, dilution, delay and deflection.
- The key principles of rationing care are equity, equality, effectiveness and cost-effectiveness. Needs and value are also important but difficult to operationalise.
- Much rationing and setting of priorities takes place implicitly. Explicit rationing forces people to make difficult choices. Who makes these choices and decisions is another key issue.

COMMUNITY CARE

Community care is currently being proposed as the way forward in the development of health services, and in the future many doctors who previously spent their lives in hospitals will now be based in community settings. Community care is a concept embraced by people of all professions and political persuasions, even if they have not quite worked out what they mean by it.

'Community care means providing the right level of intervention and support to enable people to achieve maximum independence and control over their own lives.'

Secretaries of State 1989

At its broadest, community care involves service delivery, economic policy, political rhetoric and philosophical ideology. It can be seen as a treatment used, a way of enhancing quality of life or a way of reducing spending by an out-of-control welfare state. It has come from the New Right in both Britain and the USA and from a Marxist background in Italy. The development of community care throughout developed countries has come about through a variety of clinical, social and political influences (see Fig. 1).

The most numerous group within community care is the elderly, but it also covers people with mental health problems and people with learning, physical or sensory disabilities. Some of the problems in discussing community care come from translating what is a generic policy to services appropriate for different patient and client groups. Guiding users through a variety of different agencies and organisations, all of which should cooperate and interrelate (Fig. 2), adds to the problem.

INFLUENCES ON COMMUNITY CARE

'The community'

There are two powerful beliefs at work here. The first is that there is a community which cares and which will accept its old, its ill and its disabled people and treat them as equal and valued members of that community. The second is that living in the community is, by definition, better than living in an institution. For those who receive good care and support, have appropriate housing and a good social network, living in the community is the empowerment to make choices over their lives, freed from the restrictions of institutions. For those who are ignored by

their neighbours, with a very low income from benefits and little support from services, living in the community can be a nightmare existence of loneliness and poverty.

Anti-institutions

Institutions are visibly expensive and can be dehumanising and lead to new problems (see pp. 102–103). As the population of long-stay psychiatric patients, mainly people with schizophrenia, diminished, their place was taken by the growing number of elderly people with dementia. The true meaning of asylum as sanctuary has been forgotten and, as the number of beds are cut, it can be difficult to admit patients in acute crisis.

Consumerism

The political right supports the view that market forces should dictate services which are thus needs-led not service-led. Consumers (formerly patients) are to be consulted about service delivery. The left supports consumerism more from a position of advocacy and empowerment.

Welfare pluralism

There is a move from the welfare state (in Britain, for example) towards a mixed economy of care in which services are provided by statutory agencies, voluntary organisations and the private sector. This can incorporate means testing for certain kinds of care.

Cost-cutting

The growing elderly population means that the cost of residential care is escalating for welfare state countries. Community care is a way of capping this cost by restricting residential care and moving costs to families. This has also involved trying to make the divide between health care and social care more distinct. In continuing care of elderly people the distinctions are made between medical care, which requires hospitalisation, and nursing care, which can take place in nursing homes and thus is not part of free health care.

Family values

A return to traditional family values has been a major political theme for conservative governments in both Britain and North America for the last decade. The family is promoted as the front

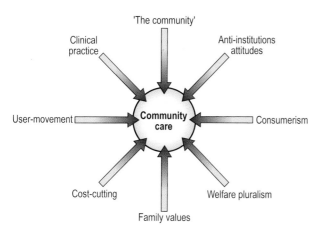

Fig. 1 **Influences on community care.**

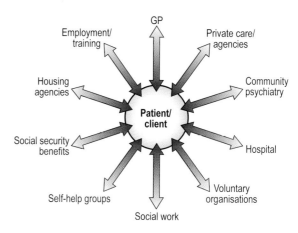

Fig. 2 **Agencies with whom the patient/client may be involved**

line of care and services are directed at helping families care rather than replacing that care with state or private facilities (see pp. 134–135).

User-movement
Although this can be linked to consumerism it has more to do with advocacy, the promotion of patients' rights and often an anti-medical, anti-psychiatry model of mental health problems (see pp. 136–137).

Clinical practice
From the 1950s onwards new advances in treatment, including the introduction of phenothiazines, behaviour therapy, rehabilitation and psycho-social therapies, meant that custodial care for groups such as those with mental health problems became less relevant.

STOP THINK
- Is the community willing and able to accept everyone with a problem?
- Is there a role for institutions/asylums?

UNDERLYING PROBLEMS

Coherence of vision
Community care requires multidisciplinary cooperation at all levels; staff and policy in housing, social work, benefits, medicine, nursing, occupational and physiotherapy, psychology and employment are all involved. Different professional views and priorities can cause practical problems. In mental illness, for example, the bio-medical versus the social-environmental view requires radically different approaches to clients and services. A bio-psychosocial approach brings these together and is advocated by many. The reality of service delivery, however, can be difficult as many agencies which have to cooperate have different views and priorities.

The role of women
By and large women relatives and friends are expected to fill the gaps left by the shortage of public service resources and provide informal care at home (see pp. 134–135). Community services tend to be staffed by low-paid, predominantly female workers with poor conditions and terms of employment.

'Them' and 'Us'
The well-known NIMBY syndrome (Not in My Back Yard) means that the community is often not willing to accept people with problems. Plans to develop hostels or sheltered housing frequently meet with local opposition.

TREATMENT MODEL OF COMMUNITY CARE

As well as seeing the community as a more appropriate place for people to live than hospitals, research has looked at how well people do who are discharged from long-term care. One long-term study by TAPS (Team Assessment of Psychiatric Services) has followed the closure of Friern and Claybury hospitals in London demonstrating the success of the project (Leff et al 1996). Not all studies are completely positive and although people live in the community they may not show improvements in daily living or social skills (Donnelly et al 1996). MIND, however, conducted a survey of users' views which was overwhelmingly positive, with users feeling generally more-independent and active, and having greater control over their lives with more choices open to them (Rogers et al 1993).

COMMUNITY CARE IN THE UK
Community care in Britain has been both defined and limited by the NHS and Community Care Act 1990 which came into operation on April 1st 1993.

Whereas previously patients were fitted into established services, now patients are to be assessed as to their 'needs' and services designed around, and provided, to meet such needs (see pp. 142–143). This ties in with who provides services. Health Boards and Social Work Departments now buy-in services from the mixed economy rather than provide them themselves. Many residential establishments for the elderly, or sheltered housing for those with mental health problems, are expected to be provided by private companies or voluntary organisations rather than social work departments.

The impact of this for patients is that there is no longer free-at-point-of-delivery care by the NHS but means-tested care through social work (LA). Services are targeted to 'concentrate on those with greatest needs'; they should 'allow for a range of options', 'respond flexibly and sensitively to the needs of individuals and carers' and, above all, 'intervene no more than is necessary to foster independence'.

Key objectives for service delivery:

- to promote the development of domiciliary, day and respite services to enable people to live in their own homes wherever feasible and sensible
- to ensure that service providers make practical support for carers a high priority
- to make proper assessment of need and good case management the cornerstone of high quality care
- to promote the development of a flourishing independent sector alongside good quality public services
- to clarify the responsibilities of agencies and so make it easier to hold them to account for their performance
- to secure better value for tax-payers' money by introducing a new funding structure for social care.

Case study
Tom was born with cerebral palsy and had, until he was 21, been cared for by his mother. When she became too old and frail to look after him, he was taken into a large psychiatric hospital (although he was not intellectually impaired) where he was put in a wheel-chair and became dependent for help from staff who had many others to tend to and who worked to fairly fixed timetables. There were few opportunities for privacy and when (25 years later) he met a woman (with learning disabilities) he wanted to marry, they would have had to sleep apart.

He and his wife chose to leave hospital and live in a flat in a newly built block of 50 flats which included two other flats for disabled people. Support was provided by a care worker who also lived in the block, and agency staff who covered the care worker when she was off. Over the subsequent 10 years, Tom has experienced some problems with his health and has had to spend time in hospital, but he is still adamant that living in the community has given him control over his own life and a far higher quality of life than he had experienced in hospital.

Community care
- Is a generic policy.
- Is a needs-led service.
- Places care outside institutions.
- Is both inter- and multidisciplinary.
- Relies on care by families.

MEDICAL STUDENTS' EXPERIENCE

Wherever you train to be a doctor, there are some experiences common to all medical students. These set you apart from the rest of the undergraduate population. Thinking about how you solve problems during this time should enable you to see how you might tackle challenges in the future. It will also facilitate an understanding of how other people (including patients) deal with their own difficulties.

WHAT IS DIFFERENT ABOUT MEDICINE?

The pressures on pre-clinical medical students are not qualitatively different from those on other students: they worry about coursework, exams, money, relationships, but the workload is heavier. Curricula are moving slowly towards greater choice and better integration. The new developments of problem-based, self-directed learning are viewed positively by students, although they require some adjustment and the time spent in preparation is not substantially less than the time spent rote-learning.

Family background may add to the pressure, since parents may have high expectations of medical student offspring. There is evidence that where this is the case, it adds to the stress experienced throughout the medical career (see pp. 52–53). This may operate by setting up specific personal beliefs about the need for high achievement. These then influence both feelings and behaviour.

Personality influences a student's reactions to the medical course. One factor is the student's ability to tolerate ambiguity and uncertainty. Medical students are all excellent at science, but people, including patients, are often irrational and unpredictable. The realisation of this fact can cause distress in students, and there is evidence that this influences career choice. Those most intolerant of ambiguity tend to choose specialities such as pathology, anaesthesiology, radiology, and surgery: those with greater tolerance go into general practice and psychiatry, where they have closer contact with people.

Adjustment takes time. The first term seems to be stressful. Miller (1994) surveyed a complete class cohort of medical students in the UK, at the beginning and end of their first year. He found that in the first term, nearly half the class scored above the threshold on a screening device (the General Health Questionnaire) for psychological distress. By the summer term, only a third showed these levels of distress (see Fig. 1).

THE CLINICAL YEARS

The sources of stress change with clinical experience. Firth-Cozens (1986) found the item most commonly reported as 'particularly stressful' in fourth-year students in the UK was 'relationships with consultants' (Table 1). A common complaint is that some senior staff teach by humiliation rather than encouragement (Allen 1994): some students can become so anxious that they fail to attend ward rounds. Any objective assessment of teaching would recognise this as not only grossly inappropriate and unfair, but a very poor teaching method. Reporting such incidents through a formal feedback mechanism, anonymously if necessary, would help to stop it. Discussing them with others could reduce distress.

COPING STRATEGIES

There are some well-known maladaptive responses. One is avoidance, for example by putting off work that is difficult. Another is alcohol abuse. Firth-Cozens (1986) found that emotionally distressed students were drinking most alcohol. This may be on the increase. Ashton and Kamali (1995) found that

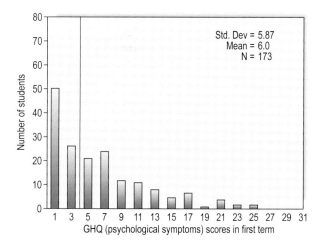

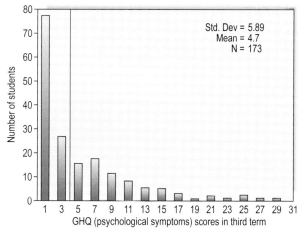

Fig. 1 **Proportion of students above the GHQ threshold in first and third term.** Dotted vertical line indicates threshold for significant psychological symptoms. (Data reproduced by permission of P McC Miller.)

Table 1 **Numbers (%) of fourth year medical students reporting categories of experience as 'particularly stressful'.** (Source: Firth-Cozens, 1986 BMJ 292: 533–536)

Stressful experience	Men	Women	Overall
Relations with academic staff	22 (13)	17 (15)	39 (13)
Relations with consultants	57 (33)	41 (35)	101 (34)
Relations with ward staff	17 (10)	15 (13)	32 (11)
Physical examinations of patients	21 (12)	11 (9)	32 (11)
Talking with terminally ill patients	38 (22)	29 (25)	69 (24)
Too little responsibility	46 (27)	33 (28)	81 (28)
Too much responsibility	35 (21)	34 (29)	73 (25)
Effects on personal life	49 (29)	40 (34)	92 (31)
Total no. who responded	171	117	294*

*Six responders did not give their sex.

alcohol and illicit drug use had risen over the last 10 years in a British university: 25% of medical students were drinking over the recommended low-risk levels. Qualified doctors have a higher than average risk of developing alcohol problems: these student studies suggest that the habit may be established early in the medical career.

Tackling stress can be done on all levels. Try to deal with the source of the stress:

- *Manage the workload.* Prioritise what you are doing, then delegate, delay, or drop things that are not urgent.
- *Seek support.* Talk to others. If you are worried, listen to someone else's point of view.
- *Look at your thinking style.* If you think that you may set unrealistic standards for yourself, try to challenge this (see pp. 128–129). Ask yourself what you would say to a friend in a similar situation, then take your own advice.
- *Relax.* Trying to work all the time leads to tiredness and inefficiency. Set aside time to switch off by doing something else: sport, yoga, music, seeing friends.

In the competitive environment of a medical school, students can sometimes feel inadequate. Classmates may enjoy demonstrating their knowledge and skills. Remember that the requirements for being a good doctor are diverse and not necessarily based on being the first to display textbook knowledge. For example, giving an immediate diagnosis on the basis of the initial information given by a patient can be faulty. Research on students has shown that many of them start off with a wide-ranging interview style (being unsure of possible diagnoses). They explore all possibilities. Over the course of medical school,

however, they gradually use increased medical knowledge to home in early on a diagnosis. They may fail to investigate the other possibilities. In this situation, a more open-minded approach would be more appropriate.

In the early experience of clinical work, remember that you are still a student. Set realistic standards for yourself.

If you have persistent thoughts about leaving medicine, it is important to talk this over with someone. You may feel great pressure from your family or a medical member of staff. It may be helpful to talk to an outsider. Most universities have counsellors or those who can offer careers guidance. It is important that the decision is yours and not dominated by feelings of duty or consideration of how much you have invested already. Remember that there are many branches of medicine that you may not have considered: the choice is not limited to general practice versus hospital medicine.

There is evidence that levels of anxiety and depression in students are to some extent predetermined by personality, but it has also been shown that teaching stress management to medical students enables them to control the symptoms of stress. Another view is that some experience of anxiety and depression may not be a bad thing anyway, since doctors who score more highly on these symptoms are more empathetic and approachable.

Given these various findings, and that lack of support from senior staff is a common complaint, should more be done for students — stress management courses, regular meetings with members of staff, or support groups across years? Or is it the case that 'If you can't stand the stress, you should get out of the medical school?'

SATISFACTION

Despite the demanding conditions of medical training, there are many rewards in the practice of medicine. Students and young doctors can have experience of different specialities and are likely to settle eventually in one that suits their personality and abilities. Those who derive most interest from the science can move towards laboratory research and those who enjoy the 'art' of medicine will go into specialities that include closer contact with patients. Although very different, both types of career can bring enormous personal satisfaction.

Case study

Ian, a third-year medical student, appeared before a Faculty committee appealing to stay on, despite having twice failed an exam in Paediatrics. He said that he had fallen behind in studying, but assured the committee that he would not do so again.

When asked whether there were any relevant circumstances, he described a catalogue of misfortune. During his third year, he had been off for several weeks with abdominal pain that eventually proved to be appendicitis and resulted in an appendectomy. Just before Christmas, his parents separated, and he kept going home at weekends to help his depressed mother. In the spring, his landlord evicted him because a drunken flatmate had smashed furniture. By the summer term, he was camping out in friends' flats, trying to study and missing many days on clinical attachments. He was extremely anxious and unable to sleep or concentrate. Having failed the exam, he attempted to revise over the summer, but had to earn money by working in a bar and made little progress.

The committee took a sympathetic view of his circumstances, but criticised him for not discussing his difficulties with a tutor and arranging to have time off officially, especially when he was ill. He was permitted to repeat his third year, but strongly advised to make contact with the Accommodation Service, the Counselling Service, and with his tutor. He did this and scraped through his repeated year. In subsequent years, he maintained reasonable passes and graduated successfully.

Medical students' experience

- Medical students' experience of stress is different from other students: at first in terms of the amount of work, then later in terms of clinical contact.
- Adaptation to medical school is influenced by family background and personality: these factors also influence career choice.
- Relationships with senior medical staff are stressful in the clinical years.
- Students' use of alcohol to relieve stress may establish a habit that puts them at risk of becoming doctors with alcohol problems.
- If you have doubts about medicine as a career, talk it over with someone, and make your own decision.

BEING A JUNIOR DOCTOR

After graduating from a university course in medicine comes the reality of working with the patient population. In most countries, this period of training is tough. The hours are long and the knowledge to be gained is substantial. At the same time, the pressure of carving out a career path impinges on daily work. New doctors often feel that clinical supervision and support is inadequate and the responsibility for patients can seem overwhelming. Yet this is also a time when new graduates can realise how useful and effective they can be in dealing with health problems and this experience is satisfying.

SOURCES OF STRESS FOR YOUNG DOCTORS

Hours

Young doctors are affected by the long hours that they work. Cognitive performance on medical tasks and standard psychological tests is worse after a night on call: mood is also affected (Lingenfelser et al 1994). In the past, junior doctors have been known to work very long hours. Figure 1 shows the number of hours worked in a week by a sample of junior doctors in a UK survey conducted in 1993, before new guidelines were introduced. For these doctors, long hours over a working week were associated with increased psychosomatic symptoms (e.g. feeling ill, feeling run down, pains in the head) and poorer social functioning (e.g. taking longer over things, inability to make decisions).

Feeling overwhelmed

Despite the relationship between hours worked and somatic symptoms and social dysfunction, long hours were not associated with a feeling of being overwhelmed or of making minor mistakes. Feeling overwhelmed was however, associated with the number of emergency admissions, and the number of deaths in the past week and fetching equipment. Feeling overwhelmed was strongly related to anxiety, depression, somatic symptoms, social dysfunction and physical illness.

Other sources of stress

Other sources of stress for young doctors have been studied systematically. In the UK, Firth-Cozens (1987) has followed medical students from their clinical

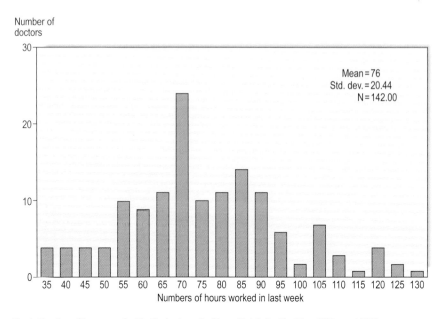

Fig. 1 **Number of hours worked in the last week.** (From Baldwin, Dodd and Wrate, 1997)

undergraduate years through to their final choice of career. The most stressful aspects of the first postgraduate year were 'overwork', 'talking to distressed relatives', 'effects of work on your personal life', and 'serious treatment failures'. Women doctors reported more depression, but otherwise, no more psychological distress.

Similarly, in the USA, long hours, pressure of work, fatigue and lack of time for personal interests were the major sources of stress. Young doctors in the USA complete other degrees before they start medical education and are therefore older: for them marriage appeared to buffer the effects of these stressors (Butterfield 1988).

STOP THINK

How do you think you will react to your first job? Can you predict what will give you satisfaction, and what you will find most difficult?

Although medical students may be aware that the first postgraduate year is tough, many of them seem surprised by the high demands of the early years. When asked 'What is different about medicine from what you thought when applying to university?', a class cohort of British junior doctors in 1994 wrote comments that were grouped into the following factors:

- The hours are even longer than expected   40%
- The work is more demanding/stressful   25%
- There is little respect from patients, or care from other staff   21%
- Inadequate training for the job   13%
- Lack of support/supervision by senior medical staff   13%
- Frequent mundane, routine, non-clinical work   10%

(Baldwin, Wrate and Dodd 1997)

At the same time, a survey of attitudes to work amongst these same doctors showed that despite these conditions, 88% believed that they were useful most of the time; 87% thought that they were developing new skills, and most were satisfied with their choice of medicine as a career.

MISTAKES

In medicine, it is inevitable that doctors will sometimes make mistakes, whatever their grade. The majority of serious mistakes made by young doctors are made through ignorance or inexperience; less common are mistakes through lack of information or poor communication, and tiredness. The most common types of mistake are misdiagnosis (including underestimating the severity of a condition) and procedural errors. The fear of making mistakes is an important source of stress for young doctors and this is exacerbated by the fear of litigation, which is becoming increasingly common (see pp. 124–125).

Where there is doubt about clinical management, it is always wise to get another opinion. In general, senior staff would prefer this to the increased risk of mistakes, no matter how irritable or unapproachable they may appear. Apart from any legal worries associated with making mistakes, there are always emotional effects. Junior doctors, in particular, experience feelings of remorse and guilt, even when they were not responsible for a mistake. In good teams, the incident will be discussed so that feelings of remorse can be shared, put into perspective and lessons learned. Often junior doctors have a distorted perception of the incident, believing themselves to be wholly to blame when in fact they were only partly, or not at all, responsible.

HOW CAN YOU PREPARE TO COPE IN THE EARLY YEARS?

You can approach this stressful situation in the same way as other difficulties (see pp. 124–125). Looking at three different aspects may help you: these are cognitions, feelings and behaviour.

Cognitions

- Put the situation in perspective: this period of training is limited and conditions will improve within a few years.
- Focus on what you have achieved on a day-to-day basis. Junior doctors are highly skilled and learning all the time. The part they play is vital to the clinical team.
- Some mistakes are inevitable: what is important is to learn from them and to assess them objectively.

It will help to discuss them with other people.

- Think about what you want from a career: is it to have a varied job, to be an eminent specialist, to enjoy a balanced work and personal life, or to work part-time? Make choices that fit in with your own needs.

Feelings

- Discuss feelings with others in a similar situation, whether these are feelings of pleasure, fatigue, disillusionment, guilt, incompetence, pride, or anger.
- Discuss feelings with friends, partner or family. They may not know what it is like, but they can still empathise with you and it may help them to understand your situation.

Behaviour

- Look after your health. Try to rest when you can and to eat properly whenever possible. If you are ill, despite the culture of working through illness, take time off and see a doctor if necessary.
- Find good ways to unwind: going away, going out, taking exercise, reading, watching television, socialising. Do whatever works for you.
- Seek support from others: junior medical staff at work, friends and family at home.

Case study

Debbie was in her first job in a teaching hospital, intending to go into Paediatrics. Her boyfriend, Peter, was training in surgery 350 miles away. On one of their rare weekends together, Peter was very bitter and depressed and expressed doubts about medicine as a career.

Debbie returned after the weekend and was herself then very low. She worked a 72-hour week during which she contracted tonsillitis. One night she admitted an elderly man but did not realise the severity of his unstable angina. He was not treated and died in the early hours of the morning. Although a more senior member of staff said that this was likely to have happened even with appropriate treatment, her consultant implied that she was negligent, and said so in front of nursing staff. She was devastated and decided to give up hospital medicine and go into General Practice where she would be away from hospitals and able to be nearer Peter. On telephoning him, she learned that he had decided to leave surgery. Being now less concerned about her consultant's reference, she took time off to recover from tonsillitis. She then went to stay with Peter for the weekend and told him what had happened on the ward. He was sympathetic and helped put the incident in perspective.

A year later, Debbie was in another teaching hospital in Paediatrics, and despite regularly working long hours, was enjoying good clinical supervision and had resumed her original career plans. Peter was in medical publishing and only 60 miles away.

Several factors had helped her to get through her crisis: the temporary relief of knowing that she could leave hospital medicine if she wanted to; taking time off to recover from illness; catching up on sleep; and talking about her misery had been enough help at a critical period. Her next job was one with better senior support and this was enough to sustain her in working towards her career in Paediatrics.

Being a junior doctor

- Long hours have been shown to affect young doctors' cognitive performance, mood, general health and functioning.
- Stressful factors reported by young doctors are long hours, the effects on personal life and concern about making mistakes.
- Mistakes happen most often through ignorance and inexperience. It is important to seek help, however uncomfortable this may be.
- Most junior doctors feel useful and are satisfied with their choice of medicine as a career.
- Stress management techniques can be helpful: focus on cognitions, feelings and behaviour.

THE PROFESSION OF MEDICINE

Being a medical student means learning about the discipline of medicine. However, much more is learnt that is not part of the official medical curriculum. Implicit in medical training is showing students how to behave and act as doctors. Your medical education is a socialisation into medicine. Socialisation refers to a new recruit being exposed to the predominant norms (expected ways of behaving) and values of an occupation, and this recruit gradually absorbing these ideas until they become 'natural'. Students, for example, learn to take decisions, to deal or cope with cutting up bodies in pathology practicals, but also to adhere to a dress code on the wards, or to talk to patients and nursing staff in a certain way. In other words, one learns to become a medical professional, as much as a medical doctor.

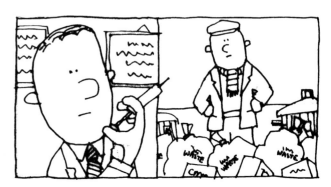
Fig. 1 'Which is more important for public health?'

THE NATURE OF PROFESSIONS

The importance of the profession of medicine does not just lie in the process of becoming a doctor. Professions are also an important element in the organisation of medical care and the structure of our wider society. The former refers to the position that the medical profession has in the health services, the latter refers to the way professions are regarded as special occupations in society (Fig. 1). We could ask ourselves: 'What do professionals such as doctors, clergy, and lawyers have in common?' or 'What is the difference between doctors and rubbish collectors, two occupations we cannot really do without?'

 STOP THINK What makes medicine a 'profession' rather than just an 'occupation'?

There are two main perspectives on the origin and nature of professions. Professions, in the older of the two perspectives, represent the institutionalisation of altruistic values, since the professions are seen as committed to providing services for the common good. Thus stockbrokers and company directors differ from teachers, lawyers and doctors in that the former occupations consist of people working for an immediate personal gain, be it money, prestige, or promotion. The latter occupations consist of people who are not motivated only by personal interest or by financial gains. The Declaration of Geneva states that doctors 'consecrate their lives to the service of humanity'. Those engaged in a profession are often said to have a 'vocation', or a 'calling'. Sociologists who studied professions in the 1950s drew up lists of characteristics of professions as opposed to other occupations. Greenwood

(1957) developed one such list with qualities required by an occupation if it was to be regarded as a profession:

1. systematic theory
2. authority recognised by its clientele
3. broader community sanction
4. code of ethics
5. professional culture sustained by formal professional sanctions.

The medical profession incorporates all the above features. (1) It has a theoretical basis; (2) patients come to doctors for advice/help, and also governments come to the medical profession for advice/help; (3) no one is allowed to practise medicine without a licence; (4) the Hippocratic oath and the Declaration of Geneva are its code of ethics (see pp. 154–155) and (5) it has strong professional organisations that guard the quality of the work done by its members, leaving it relatively free of lay evaluation or legal contracts.

 STOP THINK How altruistic is medicine as a profession?

PROFESSIONS AND COMPETITION

More recent thinking approaches professions from the notion of 'autonomy', which is based on the profession being able to exercise power and control over, for example, other occupations, policy makers, and clients (Turner 1995). Such approaches emphasise competition between different occupations. For example, the crucial feature of the division of labour in health care is the control that doctors exercise over their own work and that of allied occupations. The original function of nursing, for example, was to serve the doctor: '…what the nurse did for the patient was a function of what the doctor felt was required for the care of the patient… All nursing work flowed from the doctor's orders' (Freidson 1975: 61). Today nursing has developed to a more autonomous profession with its own education (with professors of nursing in many universities), field of knowledge, its control over its members and some power to exclude other occupations from its area of expertise. The maintenance of the medical profession requires the continuing exercise of dominance over allied and competing occupations. As a result

---

The World Medical Association Declaration of Geneva: Physician's Oath

At the time of being admitted as a member of the medical profession:

I solemnly pledge to consecrate my life to the service of humanity;

I will give to my teachers the respect and gratitude which they are due;

I will practise my profession with conscience and dignity; the health of my patients will be my first consideration.

I will maintain by all means of power the honour and the noble traditions of the medical profession; my colleagues will be my brothers;

I will not permit considerations of religion, nationality, race, party politics or social standing to intervene between my duty and my patient;

I will maintain the utmost respect of human life from the time of conception, even under threat; I will not use my medical knowledge contrary to the laws of humanity;

I make these promises solemnly, freely and upon my honour.

the medical profession can be seen to possess an officially approved monopoly of the right to define health and illness and to treat illness. For example, in Britain death certificates must be signed by two doctors and in many countries it is illegal to practise medicine without a licence.

Depending on which approach one takes, a profession is either defined as an altruistic occupation serving the common good or a particularly successful competitor in the occupational arena. Perhaps we can see elements of both approaches at different times or in different types of doctors.

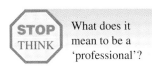 What does it mean to be a 'professional'?

In many countries doctors tend to belong to the best paid categories of professionals. One way of being able to guarantee jobs for medical graduates is to limit the intake of medical students. Matching the supply of and demand for doctors maintains a sense of exclusiveness and enables the medical profession to claim a high renumeration. It is interesting that in Italy, the European Union (EU) country where it is easiest to enter medical school, more medical students graduate than in other EU countries. Consequently, the average income of general practitioners is considerably lower than in countries such as the UK, Denmark, the USA, Germany and the Netherlands, where entry to medical school is more restricted.

Professions can be seen as occupations that somehow reduce risk and uncertainty in our lives. The priest, the lawyer and the doctor look after our soul, our well-being, and/or our body. Some have argued that this gives these occupations a higher status in society.

THE ORGANISATION OF THE MEDICAL PROFESSION

Doctors in nearly every country in the world have a strong professional organisation, which acts both as an advisory body to governments and the public and as a trade union. The medical view is often aired in prestigious medical journals, which are in themselves part of the organisation of the profession. More significantly, such medical journals are regarded as important by the general population and government officials, which makes them highly influential. After all, the importance and influence of professions is not so much based on their claims, as on society's reaction to these claims. Aromatherapists, clinical psychologists, kinesiologists and faith healers make claims which are often not dissimilar to those made by doctors, but most people in industrialised societies put their faith most of the time in the medical profession and not in the other healers.

CHALLENGES TO MEDICAL AUTONOMY

The medical profession is self-regulating in many countries, and in Britain it is regulated by the General Medical Council. Doctors often dismiss claims from outsiders ('lay people') arguing that the only person who can evaluate the work of a doctor is a fellow doctor. However, medical autonomy has been increasingly challenged and eroded in recent years:

- The state has varying degrees of control over professionals, such as regulating their income, their training or the right to practice.
- Hospital administrators/managers and health insurance companies have a certain amount of control over doctors. Managers can direct funding from one medical speciality to another, or from hospital-based medicine to community-based practitioners, while insurance companies can influence the kind and amount of medical interventions conducted by doctors.
- Challenges have also come from the increasing professionalisation of the other 'paramedical' occupations, particularly nursing.
- Within the profession of medicine itself, there have been attempts to change the hierarchical structure of the profession and to embrace 'complementary' therapies like homeopathy and acupuncture.
- Over the past three decades we have seen an increase in consumer power in many industrialised countries. Consumers (and patients) have begun to question the kind of services they receive from companies and state services. In Britain the recent introduction of the Patient Charter has changed the balance towards the lay public.
- The effectiveness of medical treatments and procedures has been challenged and the number of complaints against doctors has increased over the years, and the number of court cases against doctors, especially in the United States, has made indemnity insurance very costly. The consequence of all these societal factors is that doctors have increasingly limited autonomy over medical issues.

Case study
The development of the medical profession in Britain

It was only as the nineteenth century progressed that doctors became the dominant group in treating illness. The British Medical Association was founded in 1832, and one role of the BMA was to transform the status of medicine into a profession ranking with other learned professions.

After 15 unsuccessful attempts to convince Parliament that doctors could be trusted with monopoly powers, the 1858 Medical Act unified the profession, combining surgeons, physicians and apothecaries and created the General Medical Council which was empowered to keep a register of suitably qualified practitioners. As a result, employment positions were increasingly open only to registered doctors, particularly those posts controlled by the state's Poor Law hospitals and by the mutual Friendly Societies which provided insurance protection and medical care to working class patients, often through trade unions. In 1911, again after successful political lobbying, the National Insurance Act brought the control of these Friendly Societies under local health committees with strong medical representation, thereby reducing the degree of external and lay control over these doctors' activities.

The profession of medicine

- Professionals are said to work towards professional standards, which are regarded as being higher than the standards to which other occupations work.
- Professional standards combine an element of altruism with a well-developed system of quality control.
- Students are socialised into the profession.
- The state is the most limiting factor on professional freedom.
- The rise in importance of managers, other health practitioners and patients has eroded the professional power of doctors.

ETHICAL ISSUES

Ethics is about what ought or ought not to be done, what is morally right or wrong, good or bad. The words 'ethical' or 'moral' refer to questions about human conduct to which there are often no agreed or 'right' answers. This does not mean that ethics is just a matter of personal opinion. One reason for studying ethics is to learn how to distinguish good (or better) moral arguments from bad (or worse) ones. Patients whose future will be crucially affected by what is done are entitled to share in the relevant decision-making, and a doctor's ability to think clearly and communicate sensitively about such issues is essential for this.

ETHICAL ISSUES AND MORAL JUDGEMENT

On some issues there are broadly agreed conclusions — for example: professional 'medical ethics', the standards of competence and conduct agreed by the medical profession and expected of all doctors, as set out in General Medical Council (UK) (Table 1). While maintaining agreed ethical standards, doctors also need to consider carefully ethical questions on which opinion is divided or uncertain — for example: abortion, prenatal screening, organ donation and transplantation, resuscitation and the scope and limits of appropriate investigation and treatment.

To think clearly about ethical issues involves recognising the different ways of arguing which we use in coming to moral judgements. Some ways (for example attacking the character rather than the arguments of people who disagree with us, or making hasty generalisations from our own personal experiences) are prejudiced or illogical, but quite common. In contrast, mild scepticism about our own and others' argumentative motives can be morally healthy. It is also worth trying to distinguish ethical from legal or religious arguments. Doctors must respect the law, their own consciences and the religious or other basic values of their patients. But what is legally required may not be all that is morally required. And in a multicultural society, the practical implications of patients' beliefs and values about their care and treatment may need to be explored sensitively.

STOP THINK Are you thinking? See Figure 1

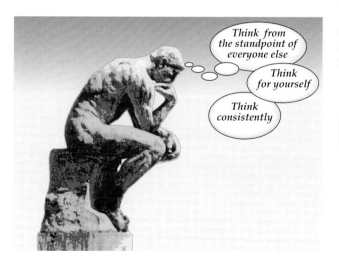

Think from the standpoint of everyone else

Think for yourself

Think consistently

Fig. 1 **Kant's three rules for clear thinking.**

Table 1 **The duties of a doctor**

- Make the care of your patient your first concern.
- Treat every patient with courtesy and consideration.
- Respect patients' dignity and privacy.
- Listen to patients and respect their views.
- Give patients information in a way they can understand.
- Respect the rights of patients to be fully involved in decisions about their care.
- Keep your professional knowledge and skills up to date.
- Recognise the limits of your professional competence.
- Be honest and worthy of trust.
- Respect and protect confidential information.
- Make sure that your personal beliefs do not prejudice your patient's care.
- Act quickly to protect patients from risk if you have good reason to believe that you or a colleague may be unfit to practise.
- Avoid abuse of your position as a doctor.
- Work with colleagues in the ways that best serve patients' interests.

General Medical Council (UK) 1995

TWO TYPES OF ETHICAL ARGUMENT

Ethical arguments can be seen as either Deontological or Consequentialist. Deontological arguments are about duties (deontological means the logic of duties) and rights (which usually means that someone has a duty to respect them). They often take the form of a command. The Golden Rule 'Do unto others as you would have them do to you' is the oldest and most universal example. A philosophical version of it is Kant's Categorical Imperative: 'Act only on that maxim through which you can at the same time will that it can become a universal law', and 'Act in such a way that you always treat humanity, whether in your own person or the person of any other, never simply as a means, but always at the same time as an end'.

Consequential arguments are less concerned with duty than with happiness and less with actions than their outcomes. The most familiar is Bentham's Utilitarian principle that we should act, or live by, rules which will produce the greatest happiness or utility for the greatest number. This can raise problems: for example of quantifying and calculating happiness or utility, and of foreseeing the unpredictable. But so can deontological arguments. Even when we agree on specific duties or rights, there are situations when one may conflict with another: for example when telling someone the truth may cause them hurt or even harm. In practice, most ethical questions need to be examined in the light of both approaches.

STOP THINK You are the registrar in a busy Accident and Emergency department. An unconscious victim of a serious motorway pile-up is brought in. He is unaccompanied and the ambulanceman thinks he is not local. He has lost a lot of blood and urgently requires a transfusion. A card drops out of his pocket; you pick it up without anyone noticing. It states that he is a Jehovah's Witness and should not be given blood under any circumstances. The rest of the staff are busy with the other victims. What ought you do?

FOUR PRINCIPLES OF BIOETHICS

A widely-agreed framework for examining ethical issues in medicine is that of the 'four principles': beneficence (doing good), non-maleficence (avoiding harm), respect for autonomy, and justice (Gillon 1994). These can be stated as:

- Act in the patient's best interest.
- Avoid harm.
- Respect the patient's judgement.
- Be fair to everyone, including yourself.

If we were able to act according to all four principles simultaneously, it is quite likely that we would be doing the morally right or best thing. But often this is not possible. A patient may disagree with what the doctor judges are his/her best interests (for example a Jehovah's Witness refusing a life-saving blood transfusion); or neither the best interests nor the wishes of the patient may be clear (for example a severely disabled neonate, or someone in a persistent vegetative state or with advanced dementia); or again the interests of different patients or groups of patients may be in conflict, and the doctor may have conflicting responsibilities as a patient's own doctor but also as a manager of resources.

In such cases, the four principles are a useful checklist to ensure that all the ethical angles of a particular case have been covered. When a case raises moral dilemmas or conflicts, it can also be helpful (having first made sure that we know all the knowable clinical facts and views of patient, family and carers) to analyse it by asking the following questions:

- What is a good example of a case with similar clinical and moral features but where we all agree what should be done?
- What details of that case would have to be changed to persuade us that something radically different should be done? Consider the range of options.
- Where does our case fit into this spectrum?
- What does that tell us about which of the four (or other) moral principles carries most weight in our case?

STOP THINK

You are a country doctor. One of your patients is a bus driver who has had a heart attack. You have advised him that his stressful occupation may make it more likely that he will have another. Later he tells you that he has been transferred to lighter but much more poorly paid duties in the bus station office, which is in a city 10 miles away. He travels there as a bus passenger daily. Visiting the city you catch sight of him driving a long-distance coach. You know that he has a sick wife and three small children to support. What should you do?

This procedure can be helpful but is not foolproof. Moral judgement, like clinical judgement, is not an exact science but a 'science of individuals', from which a degree of uncertainty can never be excluded. It is also an art, acquired over time by attention to detail in undramatic cases which present no great moral dilemmas, and by attention to patients as persons as well as cases. It means becoming comfortably 'bilingual' not just in the technical jargon of medicine (including medical ethics), but also in the unique emotional dialect of individual patients. It also means having enough self-confidence to sift justified from unjustified criticism (from others or from our own conscience) and to learn from mistakes. For 'In order to get anything right, we are obliged first to get a great many things wrong' (Lewis Thomas).

Case study
Confidentiality

After a few years in a country practice, Dr Brown and his wife decided to add a conservatory to their house. They employed Mr Black, a prosperous local builder. The final bill was far greater than they expected, but in the end they decided that it was less trouble to pay it than to take Mr Black to court. The conservatory subsequently lets in rain, and Dr Brown had to employ another builder to repair it. A year or two later, Mr Black's wife (a patient of Dr Brown's partner, who was on holiday) came to Dr Brown's surgery. A sexually transmitted disease was diagnosed. At dinner that evening Mrs Brown asked her husband if anything interesting had happened today.

Points to think about:

- Hippocratic Oath: 'All that may come to my knowledge in the exercise of my profession or outside of my profession or in daily commerce with men, which ought not to be spread abroad, I will keep secret and never reveal.'
- Deontological argument: doctors have always been assumed to have promised to keep patients' secrets. Promises ought to be kept.
- Consequentialist argument: patients may not seek medical help if they feel their secrets will not be kept.
- Action rules:
  a) A doctor's only justification for disclosing confidential information (even with the patient's consent) to a third party is that the third party has 'a need to know'.
  b) Keeping secrets can be difficult. 'Know yourself' and develop trusting relationships with colleagues.

Ethical issues

- Thinking clearly about ethical issues involves recognising that we use different ways of arguing in making our particular moral judgements.
- There are two main types of ethical argument: deontological and consequentialist.
- There are four basic principles of bioethics: beneficence, non-maleficence, respect for autonomy, and justice.

REFERENCES

Abraham-Van der Mark E (ed.) 1993 Successful home birth and midwifery: the Dutch model. Bergin & Garvey, Westport, CT, USA

Ajzen I, Madden T J 1986 Prediction of goal-directed behaviour: attitudes, intentions and perceived behavioural control. Journal of Experimental Social Psychology 22: 453–474

Allbutt H, Amos A, Cunningham-Burley S 1995 The Social Image of Smoking among Young People in Scotland. Health Education Research 10: 443–454

Allen I 1994 Doctors and their careers: a new generation. Policy Studies Institute, London

Alonzo A A, Reynolds N R 1995 Stigma, HIV, and AIDS: an exploration and elaboration of a stigma trajectory. Social Science and Medicine 41: 303–15

Amos A, Cunningham-Burley S, Kerr E A 1998 The social and cultural impact of the new genetics. ESRC Risk and human behaviour programme, Grant No. L21125003

Anderson E A 1987 Preoperative preparation for cardiac surgery facilitates recovery, reduces psychological distress and reduces the incidence of acute postoperative hypertension. Journal of Consulting and Clinical Psychology 55: 513–520

Anionwu E N 1993 Sickle cell and thalassaemia: community experiences and official response. In: Ahmad W (ed.) 'Race' and health in contemporary Britain. Open University Press, Buckingham

Armstrong D 1994 An outline of sociology as applied to medicine. Butterworth/Heinemann, London

Ashton C H, Kamali F 1995 Personality, lifestyles, alcohol and drug consumption in a sample of British medical students. Medical Education 29: 187–192

Baldwin P J, Dodd M, Wrate R M 1997 Young doctors' health: attitudes health and behaviour. Social Science and Medicine 45: 35–40

Baldwin P J, Wrate R M, Dodd M 1997 Unpublished data

Bancroft J 1989 Human sexuality and its problems. Churchill Livingstone, Edinburgh

Beale N, Nethercott S 1985 The health of industrial employees four years after compulsory redundancy. Journal of the Royal College of General Practitioners 37: 390–394

Becker H M, Heafner D P, Kasl S V, Kirscht J P, Maiman L A, Rosenstock I M 1977 Selected psychosocial models and correlates of individual health-related behaviours. Medical Care 15 (suppl.): 27–46

Berkman L F, Breslow L 1983 Health and ways of living: the Alameda County Study. Oxford University Press, Oxford

Bibace R, Walsh M E 1980 Development of children's concepts of illness. Pediatrics 66: 912–917

Birkhead J S on behalf of the Joint Audit Committee of the British Cardiac Society and a Cardiology Committee of the Royal College of Physicians of London 1992 Time delays in provision of thrombolytic treatment in six district hospitals. British Medical Journal 305: 445–448

Blackburn I M, Bishop S, Glen I M, Whalley L J, Christie J E 1981 The efficacy of cognitive therapy in depression: a treatment trial using cognitive therapy and pharmacotherapy, each alone and in combination. British Journal of Psychiatry 139: 181–189

Blaxter M 1990 Health and lifestyles. Tavistock Routledge, London

Blaxter M, Paterson E 1982 Mothers and daughters: a three-generational study of health attitudes and behaviour. Heinemann, London

Blaxter M 1987 Self reported health. In: Cox, B D (ed) The Health and Life style Survey. Health promotion trust, London

Bloor M, McKeganey N P, Finlay A, Barnard M A 1992 The inappropriateness of psycho-social models of risk behaviour for understanding HIV-related risk practices among Glasgow male prostitutes. Aids Care 4: 131–137

Blytheway B 1995 Ageism. Open University Press, Buckingham

Boakes R A, Popplewell D A, Burton M 1987 Eating habits. John Wiley, Chichester

Bond J, Coleman P 1990 Ageing in Society: An introduction to social gerontology. Sage, London

Bower T G R 1977 A Primer of Infant Development. W. H. Freeman, San Francisco

Bowling A 1995 Measuring Disease: A review of disease-specific quality of life measurement scales. Open University Press, Buckingham

Bowling A 1997 Measuring Health: A review of quality of life measurement scales. Open University Press, Buckingham

Bradshaw J 1972 A taxonomy of social need. In McLachlan G (ed) Problems and Progress in Medical Care, 7th series. Oxford University Press, Oxford

Bramley G, Doogan K, Leather P et al (eds) 1987 Homelessness and the London housing market. School for Advanced Urban Studies, Bristol

Brenner M H, Mooney A 1983 Unemployment and health: the context of economic change. Social Science and Medicine 17: 1125–1138

BMA 1995 Alcohol: guidelines on sensible drinking. British Medical Association, London

Bromley D B 1990 Behavioural Gerontology: Central Issues in the Psychology of Ageing. London, Wiley

Brown G W 1978 Depression. In: Tuckett D, Kaufert J M (eds) Basic readings in medical sociology. Tavistock, London

Brown G W, Moran P 1994 Clinical and psychological origins of chronic depression episodes I: a community survey. British Journal of Psychiatry 165: 447–456

Brown G, Brolchain M, Harris T 1975 Social class and psychiatric disturbance among women in an urban population. Sociology 9: 225–254

Brown G, Davison S 1978 Social class, psychiatric disorder of mother and accidents to children. Lancet, 1, 368–380.

Bruner J S 1983 Child's talk. Norton, New York

Buckman R 1994 How to break bad news. Pan Macmillan, London

Bunton R, Burrows R 1995 Consumption and health in the 'epidemiological' clinic of late modern medicine. In: Bunton R, Nettleton S, Burrows R (eds) The sociology of health promotion. Routledge, London

Butterfield P S 1988 The stress of residency Archives of Internal Medicine 148: 1428–1435

Cairns E, Wilson R 1984 The impact of political violence on mild psychiatric morbidity in Northern Ireland. British Journal of Psychiatry 145: 631–635

Campbell J, Elton R A 1994 Consultation, waiting, prescribing and referral patterns: some methodological considerations. Family Practice 11: 182–186

Cartwright A 1982 The role of the general practitioner in helping the elderly widowed. Journal of the Royal College of General Practitioners 32: 215–227

Cattell R B 1971 Abilities: their structure, growth and action. Houghton Mifflin, Boston

Chipuer, Rovine, Plomin 1990 LISREL modelling: Genetic and environmental influences on IQ revisited. Intelligence 14: 11–29

Clarke A 1995 Population screening for genetic susceptibility to disease. BMJ 311: 35–38

Committee on Health Promotion 1996 Women and coronary heart disease (Guidelines for Health Promotion No. 45). Faculty of Public Health Medicine, London

Common Services Agency 1994 Scottish health statistics 1994. HMSO, Edinburgh

Conger J J 1991 Adolescence and youth. Psychological development in a changing world, 4th edn. Harper Collins, New York

Cornwell J 1984 Hard-earned lives: accounts of health and illness from East London. Tavistock, London

Cox J 1986 Postnatal depression. A guide for health professionals. Churchill Livingstone, Edinburgh

Cox T 1995 Coping and physical health. In: Broome A, Llewelyn S (eds) Health psychology: processes and applications. Chapman & Hall, London

Cromarty I 1996 What do patients think about during their consultations? A qualitative study. British Journal of General Practice 46: 525–528

Cunningham-Burley S, Irvine D A, Maclean U 1983–85 The cultural context of children's illnesses. SHHD

Cunningham-Burley S, Irvine S 1987 'And have you done anything so far?' An examination of lay treatment of children's symptoms. British Medical Journal 295: 700–702

Cunningham-Burley S, Maclean U 1991 Dealing with children's illness: mothers' dilemmas. In: Wyke S, Hewison J (eds) Child Health Matters. Open University Press, Milton Keynes

Cunningham-Burley S, Milburn K 1995 Health, health promotion and middle age. SOHHD Grant No. K/OPR/212/D64

Davey Smith G, Shipley M, Rose G 1990 The magnitude and causes of socioeconomic differentials in mortality: further evidence from the Whitehall Study. Journal of Epidemiology and Community Health 285: 265–270

Davis M S 1968 Physiologic, psychological and demographic factors in patient compliance with doctor's orders. Medical Care 5: 115–122

Davison C, Davey Smith G, Frankel S 1991 Lay epidemiology and the prevention paradox: the implications of coronary candidacy for health education. Sociology of Health and Illness, 13: 1–19

de Beauvoir S 1960 The second sex. Four Square Books Ltd., London

Dennehy A, Smith L, Harker P 1997 Not to be ignored: young people, poverty and health. Child Poverty Action Group, London

Department of Health 1991 Drug misuse and dependence: guidelines on clinical management. HMSO, London

Doll R, Peto R 1981 The causes of cancer. Oxford Medical Publications, Oxford University Press, Oxford

Donaldson M 1978 Children's minds. Fontana, London

Donaldson M L, Elliot A J 1990 Children's explanations. In Grieve R, Hughes M (eds) Understanding children. Blackwell, Oxford

Donnelly M, McGilloway S, Mays N, Knapp M, Kavanagh S, Beecham J, Fenyo A 1996 Leaving hospital: one and two-year outcomes of long-stay psychiatric patients discharged to the community. Journal of Mental Health 5: 245–255

Doyle D, Hanks G W C et al 1993 Oxford textbook of palliative medicine. Oxford University Press, Oxford

Drever F, Whitehead M, Roden M 1996 Current patterns and trends in male mortality by social class (based on occupation). Population Trends No. 86, HMSO, London

Drewett R F, Young B, Wright P. 'From Feeds to Meals: the development of hunger and food intake in infants and young children. In: Niven C A & Walker A. The Psychology of Reproduction Vol. 3 Butterworth Heinmann (in press)

Egan G 1990 The skilled helper: a systematic approach to effective helping, 4th edn. Brooks/Cole, California

Egbert L D, Battit G E, Welch C E, Bartlett M K 1964 Reduction of post-operative pain by encouragement and instruction of patients. New England Journal of Medicine 270: 825–827

Egeland J A, Hotstetter A M 1983 Amish study, 1: affective disorders among the Amish, 1976–1980 American Journal of Psychiatry 140: 56–61

Eiser C, Havermans T, Casas R 1993 Healthy children's understanding of their blood: implications for explaining leukaemia to children. British Journal of Educational Psychology 63: 528–537

Emerson E, Hatton C 1994 Moving out: relocation from hospital to community. HMSO, London

Erikson E H 1968 Identity: youth and crisis. Norton, New York

Erikson K T 1976 Loss of communality at Buffalo Creek. American Journal of Psychiatry 133: 302–305

European Bureau for Action on Smoking Prevention 1993 The labelling of tobacco products in the European Union. European Bureau for Action on Smoking Prevention, Brussels

Eyer J 1977 Prosperity as a cause of death. International Journal of Health Services 7: 1

Eysenck H J 1992 Psychosocial factors, cancer, and ischaemic heart disease. British Medical Journal 305: 457–459

Eysenck M 1996 Simply psychology. Psychology Press, Hove, pp. 115–131

Fagin L, Little M 1984 The forsaken families. Penguin, Harmondsworth

Faulkner A 1995 Working with bereaved people. Churchill Livingstone, Edinburgh

Faulkner A et al 1994 Breaking bad news — a flow diagram. Palliative Medicine 8: 145–151

Festinger L 1957 A theory of cognitive dissonance. Row Peterson, Evanston, Illinois

Fhanér G, Hane M 1979 Seat-belts: opinion effects of law-induced use. Journal of Applied Psychology 64: 205–212

Field T M, Woodson R, Greenberg R, Cohen D 1982 Discrimination and imitation of facial expression by neonates. Science 218: 179–181

Firth S 1993 Cultural issues in terminal care. In: Clark D (ed.) The future for palliative care. Issues of policy and practice. Open University Press, Buckingham, pp. 98–110

Firth-Cozens J 1986 Levels and sources of stress in medical students. British Medical Journal 292: 533–536

Firth-Cozens J 1987 Emotional distress in junior house officers. British Medical Journal 295: 533–536

Firth-Cozens J 1996 Stress in doctors: a longitudinal study, unpublished report for the Department of Health, Research and Development Division

Fisher S 1986 Stress and strategy. Lawrence Erlbaum, London

Fitzpatrick R 1994 Health needs assessment, chronic illness and the social. In: Popay J, Williams G (eds) Researching the People's Health. Routledge, London

Foxwell M, Alder E 1993 More information equals less anxiety. Anxiety and screening: an intervention by nurses. Professional Nurse 9: 322–336

Frasure-Smith N, Lesperance F, Talajic M 1995 Coronary heart disease/myocardial infarction: depression and 18-month prognosis after myocardial infarction. Circulation 91: 999–1005

Freidson E, 1975 Profession of medicine — a study of the sociology of applied knowledge. University of Chicago Press, London

Friedman M, Thoresen C E, Gill J J et al 1986 Alteration of type A behavior and its effect on cardiac recurrences in post myocardial infarction patients: summary results of the Recurrent Coronary Prevention Project. American Heart Journal 112: 653–665

Fulder S J, Munro R 1982 The status of complementary medicine in the United Kingdom. Threshold Foundation, London

General Medical Council (UK) 1995 Duties of a doctor. GMC, London

Gillon R 1994 Principles of health care ethics. Wiley, Chichester

Goffman E 1968 Asylums. Penguin, Harmondsworth

Goffman E 1968 Stigma. Penguin, London

Goldberg E M, Morrison S L 1963 Schizophrenia and social class. British Journal of Psychiatry 109: 785

Gordon R A 1990 Anorexia and bulimia. Blackwell, Oxford

Gossart-Maticek R , Schmidt P, Vetter H, Arndt S 1984 Psychotherapy research in oncology. In: Steptoe A, Mathews A (eds) Health care and Human Behaviour. Academic Press, London

Graham H 1984 Women, health and the family. Harvester Wheatsheaf, Hemel Hempstead

Graham H 1989 Women and smoking in the United Kingdom: the implications for health promotion. Health Promotion Vol 3 (No 4): 371–382

Green H 1988 Informal carers: agenda for action. A Report to the Secretary of State for Social Services. HMSO, London

Greenwood 1957 Attributes of a profession. Social Work 2: 45–55

Greer S, Morris T E, Pettingale K W 1979 Psychological responses to breast cancer: effect on outcome. Lancet ii: 785–787

Griffiths R 1989 Community care: agenda for action. HMSO, London (The Griffiths Report)

Hajek P 1997 Group therapy. In: Baum A, Newman S, Weinman J, West R, McManus C (eds) Cambridge handbook of psychology, health and medicine. Cambridge University Press, Cambridge

Hannay D 1979 The symptom iceberg — a study of community health. Routledge and Kegan Paul, London

Harrison S, Hunter D J 1994 Rationing Health Care. Institute for Public Policy Research, London.

Harvey S 1988 Just an occupational hazard. Kings Fund, London

Haster F 1991 The international year of disabled people. Disability Now, January

Hawton K, Salkovskis P M, Kirk J, Clark D M 1989 Cognitive behaviour therapy for psychiatric problems: a practical guide. Oxford Medical Publications, Oxford

Health Committee 1992 Maternity Services Second Report. Vol 1 (Winterton Report), HMSO, London

Hill M J, Harrison R H, Talbot V 1973 Men out of work. Cambridge University Press, Cambridge

Hilts P J 1995 Memory's ghost. Simon & Schuster, New York

Holland M, Youngs C 1990 Mental handicap. In: Primary Care for People with a Mental Handicap. Occasional Paper 47. Royal College of General Practitioners, London

Holmes T, Rahe R 1967 The social readjustment rating scale. Journal of Psychosomatic Research 11: 213–218

Hopton J L, Dlugolecka M 1995 Patients' perceptions of need for primary health care services: useful for priority setting? British Medical Journal 310: 1237–1240.

Howe M J A 1997 IQ in question: the truth about intelligence. Sage, London

Howells G 1991 Mental handicap – care in the community. British Journal of General Practitioners 41: 2–4

Howie J G R, Hopton J L, Heaney D J, Porter A M D 1992 Attitudes to medical care, the organisation of work, and stress among general practitioners. British Journal of General Practice 42: 181–185

Howie J G R, Porter A M D, Heaney D J, Hopton J L 1991 Long to short consultation ratio: a proxy measure of quality of care for general practice. British Journal of General Practice 41: 48–54

Hunt S 1997 Housing-related disorders. In: Charlton J & Murphy M (eds) The Health of Adult Britain 1841–1994. Vol 1. Office for National Statistics. Decennial Supplement No 12, The Stationery Office, London. Chapter 10, pp 156–170.

Hunter M 1993 Counselling in obstetrics and gynaecology. BPS Books, Leicester

Ineichen B 1987 Measureing the rising tide: how many dementia cases will there be by 2001? British Journal of Psychiatry. 150: 193–200

Information and Statistics Division 1996 Scottish Health Statistics 1995. Common Services Agency, Edinburgh

Information and Statistics Division 1996, Scottish Health Statistics 1995. Common Services Agency, Edinburgh

Janis LL 1958 Psychological stress. Wiley, New York

Janz N K, Becker H M 1984 The health belief model: a decade later. Health Education Quarterly 11: 1–47

Johnston M 1980 Anxiety in surgical patients. Psychological Medicine 10: 145–152

Johnston M 1987 Emotions and cognitive aspects of anxiety in surgical patients. British Journal of Clinical Psychology 21: 255–261

Johnston M 1988 Impending surgery. In: Fisher S, Reason J (eds) Handbook of life stress, cognition and health. Wiley, London: pp. 79–100

Johnston M, Vogele C 1993 Benefits of psychological preparation for surgery: a meta-analysis. Annals of Behavioral Medicine 15: 245–256

Jones P K, Jones S L, Katz J 1987 Improving compliance in asthmatic patients visiting the emergency department using a health belief model intervention. Journal of Asthma 24: 199–206

Judge K, Mays N, 1994 Allocating resources for health and social care in England. British Medical Journal 308: 1363–1366

Katz A H, Bender E I (eds) 1976 The strength in us: self-help groups in the modern world. Franklin Watts, New York

Kelleher D 1994 Self-help groups and their relationship to medicine. In: Gabe J, Kelleher D, Williams G 1994 Challenging medicine. Routledge, London: pp.104–117

Kelly M 1991 Coping with an ileostomy. Social Science and Medicine 33: 115–125

Kelly M 1992 Colitis. Routledge, London

Kelly M P, Sullivan F 1992 The productive use of threat in primary care: behavioural responses to health promotion. Family Practice 9: 476–80

King J B 1982 The impact of patients' perceptions of high blood pressure on attendance at screening. An extension of the health belief model. Social Science and Medicine 16: 1079–1091

Kister M C, Patterson C J 1980 Children's conceptions of the causes of illness: understanding of contagion and use of immanent justice. Child Development 51: 839–46

Kitzhaber J A 1993 'Prioritising health services in an era of limits: the Oregon experience' British Medical Journal 307: 373–7

Klein R, Day P, Redmayne S 1996 Managing Scarcity. Open University Press, Buckingham.

Kleinman A 1985 Indigenous systems of healing: questions for professional, popular and folk care. In: Salmon J (ed.) Alternative medicines: popular and policy perspectives. Tavistock, London

Korsch B M, Gozzi E K, Francis V 1968 Gaps in doctor–patient communication: 1. Doctor-patient interaction and patient satisfaction. Pediatrics 42: 855–871

Kubler-Ross E 1970 On death and dying. Tavistock Publications, London

Lam D H 1991 Psychosocial family intervention in schizophrenia: a review of empirical studies. Psychological Medicine 21: 423–441

Langrish M 1981 Assertiveness training. In: Cooper C L (ed) Improving interpersonal relations. Gower Press, Epping

Lazarus R 1980 Stress and coping paradigm. In: Bond L, Rosen J (eds) Competence and coping during adulthood. University Press of New England, Hanover, NH

Lazarus R S 1991 Cognition and motivation in emotion. American Psychologist 46: 352–367

Leeson J, Gray L 1978 Women and health. Tavistock, London

Leff J, Trieman N, Gooch C 1996 The TAPS Project 33: Prospective follow-up of long stay patients discharged from two psychiatric hospitals. American Journal of Psychiatry 153: 1318–24

Lemert E 1951 Social pathology. McGraw Hill, New York

Levine J D, Gordon N C, Fields H L 1978 The mechanisms of placebo analgesia. The Lancet: 654–57

Levine M 1988 An analysis of medical assistance. American Journal of Community Psychology 16: 167–188

Levinson D J, Darrow D N, Klein E B, Levinson M H, McKee B 1978 The seasons of a man's Life. Knopf, New York

Levy L H, Derby J F 1992 Bereavement support groups: who joins; who does not; and why? American Journal of Community Psychology 20: 649–662

Ley P 1997 Communicating with patients; improving communication, satisfaction and compliance. Stanley Thornes Publishers, Cheltenham

Ley P, Llewelyn S 1995 Improving patients' understanding, recall, satisfaction, and compliance. In: Broome A K (ed.) Health psychology: processes and applications. Chapman and Hall, London

Ley P, Whitworth M A, Woodward R, Pinsent R J F H, Pike L A, Clarkson M E, Clark P B 1976 Improving doctor–patient communication in general practice. Journal of the Royal College of General Practitioners 26: 720–724

Lingenfelser T, Kaschel R, Weber A, Zaiser-Kapel H, Jakober B, Kuper J 1994 Young hospital doctors after night duty: their task specific cognitive status and emotional condition. Medical Education 28: 566–572

Lock P et al 1985 Action on smoking at work. ASH, London

Lydeard S, Jones R 1989 Factors affecting the decision to consult with dyspepsia: comparison of consulters and non-consulters. Journal of the Royal College of General Practitioners 39: 495–498

MacDonald M L, Butler A K 1974 Reversal of helplessness: producing walking behavior in nursing home wheelchair residents using behavior modification procedures. Journal of Gerontology 29: 97–101

MacLeod S 1981 The art of starvation. Virago, London

Maguire P, Fairbairn S, Fletcher C 1986 Consultation skills of young doctors. British Medical Journal 292: 1573–1578

Manuck S B, Kaplan J R, Clarkson T B 1983 Social instability and coronary artery atherosclerosis in cynomolgus monkeys. Neuroscience and Behavioural Reviews 7: 485–491

Marks I M 1986 Genetics of fear and anxiety disorders. British Journal of Psychiatry 149: 406–418

Marteau T M 1989 Psychological costs of screening. British Medical Journal 299: 527

Marteau T M 1993 Health related screening: psychological predictors of uptake and impact. In: Maes S, Leventhal H, Johnston M (eds) International review of health psychology. Wiley, Chichester

Marteau T, Anionwu E 1996 Evaluating carrier testing: objectives and outcomes. In: Marteau T, Richards M (eds) The Troubled Helix. Cambridge University Press, Cambridge

Martin M, Block J E, Sanchez S D, Arnaud C D, Beyene Y 1993 Menopause without symptoms: the endocrinology of menopause among rural Mayan Indians. American Journal of Obstetrics and Gynecology 168: 1839–1845

Masters W H, Johnson V E 1970 Human sexual inadequacy. Churchill, London

Mathews A, Ridgeway V 1984 Psychological preparation for surgery. In: Steptoe A, Mathews A (eds) Health Care and Human Behaviour. Academic Press, London

McDonald I G et al 1996 Opening Pandora's box: the unpredictability of reassurance by a normal test result. British Medical Journal 313: 329–332

McKeown T 1979 The role of medicine: dream, mirage or nemesis? Blackwell, Oxford

McLauchlan C A J 1990 Handling distressed relatives and breaking bad news. British Medical Journal 301: 1145–1149

McNally R J, Steketee G S 1985 The etiology and maintenance of severe animal phobia. Behavior Research and Therapy 23: 431–436

Melzack R 1987 The short form McGill pain questionnaire. Pain 20: 191–7

Miles A 1991 Women, health and medicine. Open University Press, Buckingham

Milgram S 1974 Obedience to authority. Tavistock, London

Miller P McC 1994 The first year at medical school: some findings and student perceptions. Medical Education 28: 5–7

Mischel W 1968 Personality assessment. Wiley, New York

Morgan A, Whent H, Sayers M 1991 Smoking. Health Education Authority, London

Morris J K, Cook D G, Shaper A G 1994 Loss of employment and mortality. British Medical Journal 308: 1135–1139

Moser K A, Fox A J, Jones D R 1984 Unemployment and mortality in the OPCS longitudinal study. Lancet ii: 1324–9

Mullen K 1993 A healthy balance: Glaswegian men talking about health, tobacco and alcohol. Avebury, Aldershot

Mullen P D 1997 Compliance becomes concordance. British Medical Journal 314: 691–692

Myers F 1982 Nonbehavioural testing of the newborn infant. Clinics in perinatology 9: 191–214

National Center for Health Statistics 1995 Health, United States 1994. Public Health Service, Hyattsville MD: Table 77

Navarro V, 1989 Why some countries have national health insurance, others have national health services, and the U.S. has neither. Social Science and Medicine 28: 887–898

Naysmith A, O'Neill W 1989 Hospice. In: Sherr L (ed.) Death, dying and bereavement. Blackwell Scientific Publications, Oxford: 1–16

Neisser U et al 1996 Intelligence: knowns and unknowns. American Psychologist 51: 77–101

Nerenz D R, Leventhal H, Love R R 1982 Factors contributing to emotional distress during chemotherapy. Cancer 50: 1020–1027

Nichols T 1975 The sociology of accidents and the social production of industrial injury. In: People and work. Open University, Buckingham

North F, Syme S L, Feerey A, Head J, Shipley M J, Marmot M G 1993 Explaining socioeconomic differences in sickness absence: the Whitehall II study. British Medical Journal 306: 361–366

Nuffield Council 1993 Genetic Screening. Ethical Issues. Nuffield Council on Bioethics, London

Office for National Statistics 1997 Living in Britain 1995, HMSO, London

Ostrowski J 1989 Thinking about drug legalization. Cato Institute Paper No. 121. Cato Institute, Washington DC

Palmore E 1997 Facts on Aging: A Short Quiz. The Gerontologist Magazine.

Parkes C M 1975 Bereavement. Studies of grief in adult life. Penguin Books, Harmondsworth

Parkes C M 1980 Bereavement counselling: does it work? British Medical Journal 281: 3–6

Parsons L, Macfarlane A, Golding J 1993 Pregnancy, birth and maternity care. In: Ahmad W (ed.) 'Race' and health in contemporary Britain. Open University Press, Buckingham

Pearce S, Erskine A 1989 Chronic pain. In: Pearce S, Wardle J 1989 The practice of behavioural medicine. BPS/Oxford University Press, Oxford

Pearce S, Wardle J 1989 The practice of behavioural medicine. Oxford Scientific Publications/BPS, Oxford

Pelosi A J, Appelby L 1992 Psychological influences on cancer and ischaemic heart disease. British Medical Journal 304: 1295–1298

Petty R E, Cacioppo J T 1986 The elaboration likelihood model of persuasion. In: Berowitz L (ed.) Advances in experimental social psychology. Academic Press, New York, pp. 123–205

Plant M, Peck D, Samuels E 1985 Alcohol, drugs and school leavers. Tavistock, London

Platt S 1985 Measuring burden of psychiatric illness on the family. An evaluation of some rating scales. Psychological Medicine 15: 383–393

Platt S, Martin, C J, Hunt, S M, Lewis C W 1989 Damp housing, mould growth and symptomatic health state. British Medical Journal 298: 1673–1678

Porter A M D, Howie J G R, Forbes J F 1989 Stress in general medical practitioners of the UK. In: McGuigan F J, Sime W E, Macdonald Wallace J 1989 Stress and tension control, 3rd edn. Plenum Press, London

Prior L 1995 Chance and modernity: accidents as a public health problem. In: Bunton R, Nettleton S, Burrows R (eds) The sociology of health promotion. Routledge, London.

Prochaska J O, Diclemente C C 1983 Stages and processes of self-change of smoking: toward an integrative model of change. Journal of Consulting and Clinical Psychology 51: 390–395

Puri B, Laking P J, Treasaden I H 1996 Textbook of psychiatry. Churchill Livingstone, Edinburgh

Raw M, White P, McNeill A 1990 Clearing the air. A guide for action on tobacco. WHO/BMA, London

Registrar General's Mortality Statistics 1994. HMSO, London

Richards M 1993 The new genetics: some issues for social scientists. Sociology of Health and Illness 15: 567–586

Richards T 1990 Chasms in communication. British Medical Journal 301: 1407–1408

Rintala M, Mustajoki P, 1992 Do mannequins menstruate? British Medical Journal 305: 1575–6

Roberts H, Smith S, Bryce C 1993 'Prevention is better ...' Sociology of Health & Illness 15: 447–463

Rogers A, Pilgrim D, Lacey R 1993 Experiencing Psychiatry: Users' views of services. Macmillan in Mind Publications

Rudd P, Price M G, Graham L E, Beilstein B A, Tarbell S J, Bacchetti P, Fortmann S P 1986 Consequences of worksite hypertension screening: differential changes in psychosocial function. American Journal of Medicine 80: 853–861

Sacks O 1986 The Man Who Mistook His Wife for a Hat. Picador, London

Saile H, Burgemeir R, Schmidt L R 1988 A meta-analysis of studies on psychological preparation of children facing medical procedures. Psychology and Health 2: 107–132

Saunders C, Sykes N 1993 The management of terminal malignant disease, 3rd edn. Edward Arnold, London

Saunders, Pearce and Amato 1983 The Original Australian Test of Intelligence.

Savage R, Armstrong D 1990 Effects of a general practitioner's consulting style on patients' satisfaction: a controlled study. British Medical Journal 301: 968–970

Scambler G, Hopkins A 1986 Being epileptic: coming to terms with stigma. Sociology of Health and Illness 8: 26–43

Scambler G 1997 Sociology as applied to medicine. Saunders, London

Schachter S, Singer J E 1962 Cognitive, social, and physiological determinants of emotional state. Psychological Review 69: 379–399

Schaffer H R 1990 Making decisions about children: psychological questions and answers. Blackwell, Oxford

Schaie K W 1990 The optimization of cognitive functioning in old age: prediction based on cohort-sequential and longitudinal data. In: Baltes P B, Baltes M M (eds) Successful aging: perspectives from the behavioural sciences. Cambridge University Press, New York

Schaie K W 1996 Intellectual development in adulthood. In J E Birren and K W Schaie (eds) Handbook of the Psychology of Aging. Academic Press, London

Schwarzer R (ed.) 1992 Self-efficacy: thought control of action. Hemisphere Publishing Corporation

SCIEH 1997 Answer (AIDS News Supplement to the Weekly Report) Issue 7 (AM-37)

Seyle H 1956 The stress of life. McGraw-Hill, New York, NY

Shapira K, McClelland H A, Griffiths N R, Newell D J 1970 Study of the effects of tablet colour in the treatment of anxiety states. British Medical Journal 2: 446–449

Shapiro D A, Shapiro D 1983 Meta-analysis of comparative therapy outcome studies: a replication and refinement. Psychological Bulletin 92: 581–604

Shapiro R S, Simpson D E, Lawrence S L, Talsky A M, Sobocinski K A, Schiedermayer D L 1989 A survey of sued and nonsued physicians and suing patients. Archives of Internal Medicine 149: 2190–2196

Sharma U 1990 Using alternative therapies: marginal medicine and central concerns. In Abbot P, Payne G (eds) New Directions in the Sociology of Health, Falmer Press, Basingstoke

Sidell M 1995 Health in Old Age: Myth, Mystery and Management. Open University Press, Buckingham

Slade P 1984 Premenstrual changes in normal women: fact or fiction. Journal of Psychosomatic Research 28: 1–7

Smaje C 1995 Health, 'race' and ethnicity. Making sense of the evidence. King's Fund Institute, London

Smith R 1987 Unemployment and Health. Oxford University Press, Oxford

Snodden R 1992 The good, the bad and the unacceptable. Faber and Faber, London

Social trends 26 1996 HMSO, London

Social trends 27 1997 HMSO, London

Spearman C 1923 The nature of intelligence and the principles of cognition. Macmillan, London

Spiegel D, Bloom J R, Kraemer H C, Gottheil E 1989 Effect of psychosocial treatment on survival of patients with metastatic breast cancer. Lancet 334: 888–891

Stevenson B S, Coles P M 1993 A breast cancer support-group: activities and value to mastectomy patients. Journal of Cancer Education 8: 239–242

Stewart M A, McWhinney I R, Buck C W 1979 The doctor–patient relationship and its effect upon outcome. Journal of the Royal College of General Practitioners 29: 77–82

Stroebe W, Stroebe M S 1987 Bereavement and health: the psychological and physical consequences of partner loss. Cambridge University Press, Cambridge

Stuart-Hamilton I 1994 The Psychology of Ageing. Jessica Kingsley, London

Stubbs P 1993 'Ethnically sensitive' or 'anti-racist'? Models for health research and service delivery. In: Ahmad W (ed.) 'Race' and health in contemporary Britain. Open University Press, Buckingham

Sudnow D 1967 Passing on: the social organization of dying. Prentice Hall, New York

Swanston M, Abraham S C S, Macrae W A, Walker A, Rushmer R, Methven H 1993 Pain assessment with interactive computer animation. Pain 53: 347–351

Taylor K M 1988 Telling bad news: physicians and the disclosure of undesirable information. Sociology of Health and Illness 10 (2):

Taylor S 1986 Health psychology. Random House, New York

Tew M 1990 Safer childbirth? A critical history of maternity care. Chapman & Hall, London

Thomas L 1995 The youngest science. Penguin, New York

Tizard B, Hughes M 1984 Young children learning. Fontana, London

Tones K, Tilford S 1994 Health Education: effectiveness, efficiency and equity. Chapman & Hall, London

Townsend P, Davidson N, Whitehead M (eds) 1992 Inequalities in health: The Black Report and The Health Divide. Penguin, Harmondsworth

Tuckett D, Boulton M, Olsen C, Williams A 1985 Meetings between experts: an approach to sharing ideas in medical consultations. Tavistock, London

Tudor Hart J 1971 The inverse care law. The Lancet 27: 405–12

Turner B 1995 Medical power and social knowledge, 2nd edn. Sage, London

Turner J A 1982 Comparison of group progressive-relaxation training and cognitive-behavioural group therapy for chronic low back pain. Journal

of Consulting and Clinical Psychology 50: 757–765

Twigg J, Atkin K 1991 Evaluating support to informal carers. Social Policy Research Unit, York

Twycross R 1994 Pain relief in advanced cancer. Churchill Livingstone, Edinburgh

Usherwood T P 1991 Development and randomised controlled trial of a booklet of advice for parents. British Journal of General Practice 41: 58–62

Walker A 1993 Poverty in old age. In J Bond, P Coleman, S Peace (eds) Ageing in Society: An introduction to social gerontology. Sage, London

Warr P B 1978 Work, unemployment and mental health. Oxford University Press, Oxford

Watson J B and Raynor R 1920 Conditioned emotional responses. Journal of Experimental Psychology 3: 1–14

Wellings K 1988 Perceptions of risk — media treatment of AIDS. In: Aggleton P, Homans H (eds) Social Aspects of AIDS. Falmer Press, London pp 83–85

Wellings K, Wadsworth J, Johnson A M et al 1995 Provision of sex education and early sexual experience: the relation examined. British Medical Journal 311: 417–420

Wells C G 1983 Talking with children: the complementary roles of parents and teachers. In: Donaldson M (ed.) Early childhood development and education. Blackwell, Oxford

West P, Sweeting H 1992 Distribution of basic information from 1990. Follow-up of the Twenty-07 Study Youth Cohort. MRC Medical Sociology Unit, Working Paper No. 32 MRC, Glasgow

White A, Freeth S, O'Brien M 1992 Infant Feeding 1990. OPCS, Social Survey Division. HMSO, London

Whitehead M 1988 The health divide. Health Education Council, London

Whitehead M 1995 Tackling inequalities: a review of policy initiatives. In: Benzeval H, Judge K, Whitehead M (eds) Tackling inequalities in health: an agenda for action. King's Fund, London

White Paper, Secretaries of State 1989 Caring for people. Community care in the next decade and beyond. HSMO, London

WHO 1990 Cancer relief and palliative care: report of a WHO expert committee. World Health Organization Technical Report Series 804 World Health Organization, Geneva

Wilkinson R G 1992 Income distribution and life expectancy. British Medical Journal 304: 165–168

Wilkinson R G 1996 Unhealthy societies: the afflictions of inequality. Routledge, London

Winokur G, Pitts F N 1965 Affective disorder VI: a family history study of prevalences, sex differences and possible genetic factors Journal of Psychiatric Research 3: 113–123

Winterton Report 1992 Maternity Services Second Report Vol 1 (Health Committee) HMSO, London

Wong D, Whaley L 1986 Clinical handbook of pediatric nursing, 2nd edn. Mosby, St Louis

Woodroffe C, Glickman M, Barker M, Power C 1993 Children, teenagers and health: the key data. Open University Press, Buckingham

Worden J W 1991 Grief counselling and grief therapy. A handbook for the mental health practitioner. Routledge, London

World Health Organisation 1946 Constitution. World Health Organisation, Geneva

World Health Organization 1980 International classification of impairments, disabilities and handicaps. WHO, Geneva

Zigler E, Valentine J 1979 Project Head Start: a legacy of the war on poverty. Free Press, New York

INDEX